Respiratory
Pharmacology and
Pharmacotherapy

Cystic Fibrosis Pulmonary Infections: Lessons from Around the World

Edited by
A. Bauernfeind
M. I. Marks
B. Strandvik

Birkhäuser Verlag
Basel · Boston · Berlin

Editors:

Professor Dr. Adolf Bauernfeind
Max von Pettenkofer-Institut
Pettenkoferstrasse 9a
D-80336 Munich
Germany

Melvin I. Marks, MD
Professor and Vice Chair of Pediatrics
University of California at Irvine
Medical Director/Administrator
Memorial Miller Children's Hospital
Long Beach Memorial Medical Center
2801 Atlantic Avenue
Long Beach, California 90801
USA

Birgitta Strandvik, MD, PhD
Professor of Pediatrics
Department of Pediatrics
Faculty of Medicine
Göteborg University
S-416 85 Göteborg
Sweden

Library of Congress Cataloging-in-Publication Data

Cystic fibrosis pulmonary infections : lessons from around the world /
edited by A. Bauernfeind, M I. Marks, B. Strandvik
    (Respiratory pharmacology and pharmacctherapy)
Includes bibliographical references and index.
  ISBN 978-3-0348-7361-1   ISBN 978-3-0348-7359-8 (eBook)
  DOI 10.1007/978-3-0348-7359-8
    1. Respiratory organs – Infections –Treatment. 2. Cystic fibrosis – Complications –
Treatment. I. Bauernfeind, A. (Adolf) II. Marks,
Melvin I.   III. Strandvik, B. (Birgitta) IV. Series.
    [DNLM: 1. Cystic Fibrosis – complications 2. Cystic Fibrosis –
therapy. 3. Lung Diseases – complications. 4. Lung Diseases –
therapy. WI 820 C9997 1996]
RC740. C96 1996
616.2' 4 – dc20
DNLM/DLC
for Library of Congress

Deutsche Bibliothek - Cataloging-in-Publishing Data

**Cystic fibrosis pulmonary infections: lessons from around the
world** / ed. by A. Bauernfeind... – Basel ; Boston ; Berlin :
Birkhäuser, 1996
    (Respiratory pharmacology and pharmacotherapy)
    ISBN 978-3-0348-7361-1

NE: Bauernfeind, Adolf [Hrsg.]

© 1996 Birkhäuser Verlag, P.O. Box 133, CH-4010 Basel, Switzerland
Softcover reprint of the hardcover 1st edition 1996

Printed on acid-free paper produced from chlorine-free pulp. TCF ∞

ISBN 978-3-0348-7361-1

9 8 7 6 5 4 3 2 1

Contents

Contributors

G. S. Adam, Cystic Fibrosis Centre, "Aghia Sophia" Children's
Hospital, 11527 Athens, Greece

S. Alvarez de Garcia Tuñon, Department of Pediatrics, University
School of Medicine, Central University of Venezuela, Venezuela

Ö. Ăng, Department of Microbiology, Istanbul Faculty of Medicine,
University of Istanbul, 34390 Çapa, Istanbul, Turkey

F. Baquero, Cystic Fibrosis Unit of the Ramón y Cajal Hospital,
28034 Madrid, Spain

A. Bauernfeind, Max von Pettenkofer-Institut, Ludwig-Maximilians-
Universität, München, Germany

T. Baykal, Division of Nutrition and Metabolism, Department of
Pediatrics, Istanbul Faculty of Medicine, University of Istanbul,
34390 Çapa, Istanbul, Turkey

J. Biolek, Department of Pediatrics, Most Hospital, 434 64 Most,
Czech Republic

S. M. Cabeza, Scientific Medical Advisory Committee, Association of
Cystic Fibrosis in Uruguay, Costa Rica 2061, Montevideo,
Uruguay

E. G. Cafferata, Instituto Nacional de Genetica Medica, Las Heras
2670, 1425 Buenos Aires, Argentina

S. Carrasco, Cystic Fibrosis Unit, La Paz Children's Hospital, 28046
Madrid, Spain

J. M. Collée, Department of Human Genetics, Free University, 1081
HV Amsterdam, The Netherlands

M. Corey, Canadian Cystic Fibrosis Foundation, Toronto, Ontario,
Canada M4S 2B4

J. Dankert, Department of Medical Microbiology, University of
Amsterdam, Academic Medical Centre, 1105 AZ Amsterdam, The
Netherlands

J. E. Dankert-Roelse, Department of Pediatrics and Pediatric
Pulmonology, Free University, 1081 HV Amsterdam, The
Netherlands

M. Demirkol, Division of Nutrition and Metabolism, Department of
Pediatrics, Istanbul Faculty of Medicine, University of Istanbul,
34390 Çapa, Istanbul, Turkey

J. Dodge, Department of Child Health, Royal Victoria Hospital,
Belfast, UK

S. Elborn, Adult Cystic Fibrosis Unit, Belfast City Hospital, Belfast BT9 7AB, UK

Z. Erturan, Department of Microbiology, Istanbul Faculty of Medicine, University of Istanbul, 34390 Çapa, Istanbul, Turkey

H. C. Farrar, Department of Pediatrics, University of Arkansas for Medical Sciences, Little Rock, Arkansas, and Divisions of Pediatrics, Clinical Pharmacology, and Emergency Medicine, Arkansas Children's Hospital, Little Rock, Arkansas 72202, USA

A. Gentile, Hospital de Ninos "Ricardo Gutierrez", 1425 Buenos Aires, Argentina

A. Giunta, Centre for the Diagnosis, Prevention and Therapy of Cystic Fibrosis, "De Marchi" Pediatric Clinic, University of Milan, 20122 Milan, Italy

T. E. Guembitskaia, Cystic Fibrosis Centre, State Research Centre for Pulmonology, St. Petersburg, Russia

K. Gyurkovits, Hospital for Chest Diseases, County Somogy, 7257 Mosdós, Hungary

L. Hjelte, Department of Pediatrics, Karolinska Institutet, Huddinge Hospital, S-14186 Stockholm, Sweden

M. E. Hodson, Department of Cystic Fibrosis, Royal Brompton National Heart and Lung Hospital, London SW3 6NP, UK

M. Hofmann, IBMP – Institute for Biomedical and Pharmaceutical Research, D-90562 Nürnberg-Heroldsberg, Germany

N. Høiby, The Cystic Fibrosis Center, Rigshospitalet, DK-2100 Copenhagen, Denmark

A. Holčiková, University Children's Hospital, 662 63 Brno, Czech Republic

H. Honomichlová, Department of Pediatrics, University Hospital Plzen, 305 99 Plzen, Czech Republic

G. Hüner, Division of Nutrition and Metabolism, Department of Pediatrics, Istanbul Faculty of Medicine, University of Istanbul, 34390 Çapa, Istanbul, Turkey

N. J. Kapranov, Cystic Fibrosis Centre, State Research Centre for Pulmonology, St. Petersburg Institute for Medical Genetics, Moscow 197089, Russia

G. L. Kearns, Department of Pediatrics and Pharmaceutics, University of Arkansas for Medical Sciences, Little Rock, Arkansas, and Divisions of Pediatrics and Clinical Pharmacology, Arkansas Children's Hospital, Little Rock, Arkansas 72202, USA

E. Kerem, Cystic Fibrosis Center, Shaare Zedek Medical Center, Jerusalem 91031, Israel

M. Kinzig, IBMP – Institute for Biomedical and Pharamceutical Research, D-90562 Nürnberg-Heroldsberg, Germany

C. Koch, The Cystic Fibrosis Center, Rigshospitalet, DK-2100 Copenhagen, Denmark

A. Kolek, Department of Pediatrics, University Hospital Olomouc, 775 20 Olomouc, Czech Republic

H. Krásničanová, 2nd Medical Faculty, Charles University Prague, University Hospital Prague-Motol, 150 18 Prague, Czech Republic

G. Kurdoğlu, Division of Nutrition and Metabolism, Department of Pediatrics, Istanbul Faculty of Medicine, University of Istanbul, 34390 Çapa, Istanbul, Turkey

C. Labisch, Department of Radiology, University of Essen, D-45122 Essen, Germany

J. L. Lezana-Fernandez, Mexican Cystic Fibrosis Association, Altavista 21, CP 01000, Mexico D.F.

J. Littlewood, Regional Cystic Fibrosis Unit, St. James' University Hospital, Leeds LS9 7TF, UK

O. Lochmann, 2nd Medical Faculty, Charles University Prague, University Hospital Prague-Motol, 150 18 Prague, Czech Republic

M. C. Luna, Instituto Nacional de Genetica Medica, Las Heras 2670, 1425 Buenos Aires, Argentina

N. MacDonald, Canadian Cystic Fibrosis Foundation, Toronto, Ontario, Canada M4S 2B4

M. Macek, 2nd Medical Faculty, Charles University Prague, University Hospital Prague-Motol, 150 18 Prague, Czech Republic

M. Macek Jr., Johns Hopkins University, Baltimore, USA

C. N. Macri, Hospital de Ninos "Ricardo Gutierrez", 1425 Buenos Aires, Argentina

B. P. Madden, Department of Cardiological Sciences, St. George's Hospital, Tooting, London SW17 0QT, UK

E. Mahenthiralingam, Division of Infectious and Immunological Diseases, Department of Paediatrics and the Canadian Disease Network, University of British Columbia, Vancouver, Canada V5Z 4H4

A-S. Malmborg, Department of Clinical Microbiology, Karolinska Institutet, Huddinge Hospital, S-14186 Stockholm, Sweden

D. Maza Gonzales, Mexican Cystic Fibrosis Association, Altavista 21, CP 01000, Mexico D.F.

L. V. Möller, Department of Medical Microbiology, University of Amsterdam, Academic Medical Centre, 1105 AZ Amsterdam, The Netherlands

R. Morrison, Policy Development and Medical/Scientific Program, Canadian Cystic Fibrosis Foundation, Toronto, Ontario, Canada M4S 2B4

J. Musil, 2nd Medical Faculty, Charles University Prague, University Hospital Prague-Motol, 150 18 Prague, Czech Republic

S. Nagata, Department of Pediatrics, Juntendo University School of
Medicine, Tokyo, Japan 113

S. Oguchi, Department of Pediatrics, Juntendo University School of
Medicine, Tokyo, Japan 113

Y. Ohtsuka, Department of Pediatrics, Juntendo University School of
Medicine, Tokyo, Japan 113

R. Padoan, Centre for the Diagnosis, Prevention and Therapy of
Cystic Fibrosis, "De Marchi" Pediatric Clinic, University of Milan,
20122 Milan, Italy

K-D. Paul, Department of Bronchopneumology, Children's Hospital,
Technical University of Dresden, D-01307 Dresden, Germany

S. S. Pedersen, The Cystic Fibrosis Center, Rigshospitalet, DK-2100
Copenhagen, Denmark

P. D. Phelan, Department of Pediatrics, University of Melbourne,
Parkville 3052, Victoria, Australia

A. Pianaroli, Centre for the Diagnosis, Prevention and Therapy of
Cystic Fibrosis, "De Marchi" Pediatric Clinic, University of Milan,
20122 Milan, Italy

O. H. Pivetta, Instituto Nacional de Genetica Medica, Las Heras
2670, 1425 Buenos Aires, Argentina

H-G. Posselt, Zentrum der Kinderheilkunde, Abteilung für
Allgemeine Pädiatrie I, Pädiatrische Gastroenterologie und
Mukoviszidose, Klinikum der Johann Wolfgang
Goethe-Universität, D-60590 Frankfurt am Main, Germany

A. Prince, College of Physicians and Surgeons, Columbia University,
New York NY 10032, USA

B. Przyklenk, University Children's Hospital, Ludwig-Maximilians-
Universität, D-80337 München, Germany

H. Reyes, Department of Pediatrics, University School of Medicine,
Central University of Venezuela, Venezuela

J. Rivlin, Cystic Fibrosis Center, Carmel Medical Center, Haifa
34362, Israel

L. Saiman, College of Physicians and Surgeons, Columbia University,
New York NY 10032, USA

I. Sekyrová, Department of Pediatrics IPVZ, 370 87 České
Budějovice, Czech Republic

I. Shalit, Infectious Disease Unit, Tel-Aviv Medical Center, Tel-Aviv
64239, Israel

T. Shimizu, Department of Pediatrics, Juntendo University School of
Medicine, Tokyo, Japan 113

T. Shioya, Department of Pediatrics, Juntendo University School of
Medicine, Tokyo, Japan 113

F. Sörgel, IBMP – Institute for Biomedical and Pharmaceutical
Research, D-90562 Nürnberg-Heroldsberg, Germany

D. P. Speert, Department of Microbiology and Immunology,
University of British Columbia, Vancouver, Canada V5Z 4H4

U. Stephan, Department of Pediatrics, University of Essen, D-45122
Essen, Germany

B. Strandvik, Department of Pediatrics, Faculty of Medicine,
University of Göteborg, S-41685 Göteborg, Sweden

H. R. Stutman, Pediatric Infectious Disease, Memorial Miller
Children's Hospital, Long Beach, California 90801, USA

M. Šuláková, 1st Department of Pediatrics, University Hospital Brno,
656 91 Brno, Czech Republic

A. Szeinberg, Cystic Fibrosis Center, Sheba Medical Center, Tel
Hashomer 52621, Israel

A. Tal, Cystic Fibrosis Center, Soroka Medical Center, Ben-Gurion
University, Beer Sheva 84101, Israel

L. Ťouкláková, Department of Pediatrics, Batta's Hospital, 760 01
Zlín, Czech Republic

L. van Alphen, Department of Medical Microbiology, University of
Amsterdam, Academic Medical Centre, 1105 AZ Amsterdam, The
Netherlands

H. Vaníček, Department of Pediatrics, Hradec Kralové University
Hospital, 500 36 Hradec Králové, Czech Republic

V. Vávrová, 2nd Medical Faculty, Charles University Prague,
University Hospital Prague-Motol, 150 18 Prague, Czech Republic

L. A. Vishnyakova, Cystic Fibrosis Centre, State Research Centre for
Pulmonology, St. Petersburg, Russia

B. Wiedemann, Institute of Medical Informatics and Biometry, Carl
Gustav Carus Faculty of Medicine, Technical University of
Dresden, D-01307 Dresden, Germany

P. Wunderlich, Department of Bronchopneumology, Children's
Hospital, Technical University of Dresden, D-01307 Dresden,
Germany

Y. Yahav, Cystic Fibrosis Center, Sheba Medical Center, Tel
Hashomer 52621, Israel

Y. Yamashiro, Department of Pediatrics, Juntendo University School
of Medicine, Tokyo, Japan 113

A. Zapletal, 2nd Medical Faculty, Charles University Prague,
University Hospital Prague-Motol, 150 18 Prague, Czech Republic

D. Zemková, 2nd Medical Faculty, Charles University Prague,
University Hospital Prague-Motol, 150 18 Prague, Czech Republic

L. A. Zhelenina, Cystic Fibrosis Centre, State Research Centre for
Pulmonology, St. Petersburg, Russia

Introduction

Infection of the lower respiratory tract is a major determinant of the course of cystic fibrosis. Although numerous efforts have been made to elucidate the specific mechanisms predisposing the respiratory mucosa of cystic fibrosis patients to infection, so far no clinically relevant procedures for completely effective prevention or control of infection have resulted. Hence, in dealing with infections in cystic fibrosis, we continue to rely mainly on antimicrobials. Antiinfective measures are inseparably correlated with microbiology, and the quality of antiinfective therapy directly reflects the quality of microbial monitoring. Validated guidelines for microbiologic testing and antiinfective use need to be developed and made available to all health providers and their cystic fibrosis patients.

Several years ago, the editors cochaired a symposium at the International Congress of Chemotherapy on the Global Perspectives of Microbiological and Clinical Infectious Diseases in Patients with Cystic Fibrosis. During this half-day symposium, the editors heard reports from several countries around the world with an alarming range of survival for patients with cystic fibrosis. This sent a dramatic message to us that the understanding of this disease, its diagnosis, management and prevention was different in various countries and that patients may be inconsistently served. That is how our journey began.

We set out with a major objective of improving the understanding of infections in cystic fibrosis around the world. We chose, in fact, a sharing of experience from CF leaders in many countries. We concentrated on pulmonary infections in cystic fibrosis because it is the major cause of morbibity and mortality in cystic fibrosis and understanding the pathogenesis, diagnosis and management of infections in these patients can dramatically improve the quality and duration of life for these patients and their families. The editors also share an interest in microbiology and clinical infectious diseases, an expertise valuable in accomplishing our tasks.

One of the goals of our project was to underline the necessity to optimize the application of antimicrobials according to the actual state of cystic fibrosis disease of the individual patient. Another objective was to draw attention to the microbiological dynamics of pulmonary infection in cystic fibrosis patients and to emphasize the value of sensitivity testing and other measures to guide antimicrobial therapy. We reached out to colleagues around the world with the simple message that we want to share information based on their clinical experience and to publish this for others to read and understand. The response was overwhelming and gratifying.

We are impressed with the outstanding efforts our authors have made to organize, communicate and interpret data from their specific regions. The editors gratefully acknowledge the work of this international group of authors as well as the excellent editorial assistance of the publisher and Joyce Bagan. The regional diversities in many aspects of cystic fibrosis (including local health care systems) have to be considered thoroughly to establish the optimal treatment of patients in various areas around the world. The editors do not presume to judge any experiences or methods as superior but rather to facilitate learning and teaching through sharing of experience and information among the contributors and readers.

Interest in this book has escalated since word of its impending publication has begun to spread. We have had inquiries from physicians, patients, health care organizations and support foundations, the pharmaceutical industry and others. Cystic fibrosis patients suffer from an important genetic disease that can be controlled, and through that control, the patients can lead high quality lives with survival that is considerable compared to former years. For example, at the time of diagnosis in 1940, a patient had a life expectancy of approximately one year, whereas nowadays more than half of the patients survive into their third decade. This information and the methods whereby this success is achieved need to be delivered to patients and their caretakers around the world. That is our message, the purpose of this book and the collective mission of the authors, editors and publisher.

Adolf Bauernfeind
Melvin I. Marks
Birgitta Strandvik

Cystic Fibrosis Pulmonary Infections:
Lessons from Around the World
ec. by A. Bauernfeind, M. I. Marks and B. Strandvik
© 1996 Birkhäuser Verlag Basel/Switzerland

CHAPTER 1
Viral, Fungal and Atypical Bacterial Infections in Cystic Fibrosis

Barbara Przyklenk[1] and Adolf Bauernfeind[2]

[1]University Children's Hospital, Ludwig-Maximilians-Universität, 80337 München, Germany
[2]Max von Pettenkofer-Institut, Ludwig-Maximilians-Universität, 80336 Munchen, Germany

Summary. The role of respiratory viral and fungal agents in cystic fibrosis (CF) was investigated. Among the serologically proven viral infections, adenovirus was the most frequent (53%), followed by parainfluenza (24%) and RSV (20%); 54% of the episodes lead to hospital admission. A significant change in microbial flora of respiratory secretions was seen in 88% of the episodes, mainly with *P. aeruginosa*, and 65% of cases with initial colonization with *P. aeruginosa* are associated with a viral respiratory tract infection. It is hypothesised that viral respiratory infections to a predamaged lung in CF predispose to colonization with *P. aeruginosa*. Many of the CF-patients show elevated serum IgG to *C. albicans*, and therefore, *C. albicans* should not be considered a harmless colonizing mold. The prevalence of *A. fumigatus* increases with age. Of the CF-patients with *A. fumigatus*, 73% showed elevated specific serum IgG to this fungus. No correlation was found between culture, specified IgG to *A. fumigatus* and either specific Aspergillus IgE or total serum IgE. Maintaining good pulmonary condition and reduction of exposure to *A. fumigatus* may prevent colonization and infection with this mold.

Introduction

The clinical course of patients with cystic fibrosis (CF) is characterized by progressive pulmonary dysfunction, resulting in respiratory failure and death. However, the time of onset and the course of the lung disease in the individual patient are highly variable. Typically, acute exacerbations of the pulmonary disease which contribute to further lung damage are seen in these patients. Each of these exacerbations may be associated with the isolation of high concentrations of *S. aureus* and/or *H. influenzae* in the respiratory tree in the youngest CF-patients, and of *P. aeruginosa* in older CF-populations. One third of these exacerbations are thought to be induced by viral respiratory tract pathogens [1]. As well as the main bacterial pathogens *P. aeruginosa* and *S. aureus*, various bacterial and fungal species may occasionally be recovered from respiratory secretions of CF-patients. In this study the role of non-bacterial respiratory tract infections in CF-patients is evaluated, especially

Correspondence address: Dr B. Przyklenk, Dr von Haunersches Kinderspital der Universität München, Lindwurmstr. 4, 80337 München, Germany.

those induced by viral and fungal pathogens. Further, the role of occasionally isolated microorganisms will be estimated.

Methods

Viral Respiratory Tract Infections

1289 serum samples from 276 patients with laboratory and clinical signs of cystic fibrosis (139 male, 137 female; age 0.3–34 years, mean age 15.6 ± 7.2 years) were collected during the study period (from November 1984 until November 1991). 902 serum samples were taken from 258 CF-patients, outpatients at the Dr. von Haunersches Kinderspital München.

Of the 276 CF-patients, 161 (58.3%) had been chronically (> 6 months continuously) and 19 (6.9%) intermittently colonized with *P. aeruginosa* at their entry into this study. Of the 276 CF-patients, 96 (34.8%) had not been colonized with *P. aeruginosa* before. Of 387 serum samples collected during a hospital stay, 332 were from 110 CF-patients who had been admitted to the hospital because of pulmonary exacerbations (overall, 243 admissions). Of the 110 patients, 70 were chronically colonized, 6 intermittently and 34 not colonized with *P. aeruginosa* at the start of the study. Pulmonary exacerbations were defined as an acute change in health associated with increasing cough, sputum production, dyspnea, hemoptysis or fever. Antibodies to influenza A, influenza B, influenza C, parainfluenza types 1 to 3, and respiratory syncytial virus (RSV) were detected by complement fixation. Antibodies to adenovirus were measured by an IgG-ELISA using purified hexon antigen [2]. Some serum samples were tested in purified IgM-fractions for antibodies to adenovirus, parainfluenza viruses and RSV by indirect immunofluorescence technique. 20% of the serum samples had been tested for antibodies to mycoplasma and *C. burnetti*, as described previously [3]. A fourfold or greater increase of antibody titer between paired serum samples in the complement fixation, or a threefold or greater increase of U/1 in the adeno IgG-ELISA were considered to indicate a recent infection, as well as titers $\geq 1:32$ for influenza A, B and RSV, $\geq 1:16$ for parainfluenza and influenza C [4], a positive IgM-immunofluorescence test and ≥ 80 U/ 1 in the adeno-IgG-ELISA in single serum samples.

Standardized quantitative microbiological analyses of sputum or throat swabs [5] were performed at the same time as serology.

Fungal and Atypical Bacterial Infections in Patients with Cystic Fibrosis

For consideration of the role of fungal and atypical bacterial infections in patients with cystic fibrosis, the data of 3500 microbiological samples (sputum samples and throat swabs) of 386 CF-patients (199 female, 187 male) were analyzed over a period of 8 years (November 1984 to November 1992). The mean age of the patients was 10.6 ± 7.8 years (range 0.2–33.5 years). The microbiological analyses were performed by standardized procedures [5]. Cultures for mycoplasma, chlamydiae, typical and atypical mycobacteria were not performed.

Serum IgG-antibodies to *Candida albicans* and *Aspergillus fumigatus* were determined as described previously (6).

Results

Viral Respiratory Tract Infections

In 116 of 276 CF-patients 168 viral respiratory infectious episodes (mean 1.4 infections per patient, range 1–5) were detected, by serological methods. 29 of the 168 (17%) episodes were simultaneous infections with more than one viral agent (Table 1). Infections caused by adenoviruses were the most frequent (89/168; 53%), followed by RSV (34/168; 20%), influenza A (25/168; 15%), parainfluenza type 2 (20/168; 12%), parainfluenza type 3 (14/168; 8%), influenza B (11/168; 7%) and parainfluenza type 1 (7/168; 4%). Deterioration of the pulmonary condition occurred in 144/168 (86%) episodes leading in 78/144 (54%) cases to hospital admission. Infections with RSV, adenovirus and parainfluenza type 2 tended to be more severe than episodes caused by other agents, leading more frequently to hospital admission (Table 2). Ten episodes (adenovirus 4, influenza B 3, RSV once, influenza A once, adenovirus + influenza B + RSV once) were probably nosocomial.

The serum samples tested for antibodies against respiratory viral pathogens were collected regularly during the four seasons of the year

Table 1. Simultaneous infections with more than one viral agent (n = 29) in patients with cystic fibrosis

Serological diagnosis	No. of patients
Adenovirus + RSV	6
Adenovirus + influenza A	5
Adenovirus + parainfluenza type 2	3
RSV + parainfluenza type 3	3
Adenovirus + parainfluenza type 1	2
RES + influenza A	2
RSV + parainfluenza type 2	2
RSV + parainfluenza type 1	1
Adenovirus + influenza B	1
Influenza A + influenza B	1
Adenovirus + RSV + influenza B	1
Adenovirus + RSV + parainfluenza type 1	1
Adenovirus + influenza A + parainfluenza type 1	1

Table 2. Clinical features of viral respiratory tract infections in patients with cystic fibrosis

Virus	Leading to hospital admission	Nosocomial infection	Occurrence and treatment at home	No. of infections
Adenovirus	41	5	43	89
RSV	19	2[1]	14	34
Influenza A	11	1[1]	14	25
Parainfluenza type 2	11		9	20
Parainfluenza type 3	7	7		14
Influenza B	2	4[2]	6	11
Parainfluenza type 1	2		5	7

[1]One patient with RSV infection and one patient with influenza A. treated at home after discharge from the ward.
[2]One patient with influenza B. readmitted to the hospital.

(Table 3). Infections with adenovirus, RSV, and parainfluenza occurred throughout the year whereas influenza A and B were more frequent in winter and spring time (Table 3). Taking into account the combined viral infections, the incidence of respiratory infectious episodes was highest in winter (44 episodes/304 serum samples being tested; 14.4%), followed by spring (50/372; 13.4%), fall (37/304; 12.2%) and summer (37/309; 11.9%).

Infections in preschool CF-patients were most frequently caused by adenovirus (39%), followed by RSV (33%) and parainfluenza types 1 to 3 (27%). The prevalence of influenza A and B is higher in the second and third decade of life, whereas infections by RSV and parainfluenza become less frequent (Table 4).

63% (15/24) of the infectious episodes without clinical deterioration and 78% (113/144) of the infections with acute pulmonary exacerbation

Table 3. Seasonal variation of viral respiratory tract infections in patients with cystic fibrosis

	Winter months 12/1/2	Spring months 3/4/5	Summer months 6/7/8	Fall months 9/10/11
Serum samples tested	304	372	309	304
Serological diagnosis				
Adenovirus	20	28	20	21
RSV	9	9	7	9
Influenza A	9	11	3	2
Parainfluenza type 2	5	3	6	6
Parainfluenza type 3	4	1	4	5
Influenza B	5	4	1	1
Parainfluenza type 1	4		1	2
Total number of infections	56	56	42	46
% of serum samples tested	18.4	15.1	13.6	15.1

Table 4. Viral etiology of respiratory tract infections in different age groups of patients with cystic fibrosis

| | Age (years) | | | | | |
	< 1	1–2	3–5	6–9	10–19	≥ 20
Serum samples tested	14	41	88	186	588	372
Serological diagnosis						
Adenovirus	1	2	10	23	32	21
RSV	1	2	8	3	16	4
Influenza A				3	15	7
Parainfluenza type 2	1	1	3	4	6	5
Parainfluenza type 3			2	3	8	1
Influenza B				1	10	
Parainfluenza type 1			2	2	2	1
Total number of infections	3	5	25	39	89	39
% of serum samples tested	21.4	12.2	28.4	21.10	15.0	10.5

were evaluable, as microbiological cultures had been performed at the same time as the serology and the infection did not occur at the beginning of the study. An increase of a bacterial or fungal pathogens in the sputum of CF-patients was considered to be significant if the ratio of the number of colony-forming units (CFUs) per millilitre in the sputum before and after the viral infection was greater than 1:3. A significant change in the microbial flora was found in 88% (99/113) of the infections with pulmonary exacerbation compared with 73% (11/15) of the infections without pulmonary deterioration (Table 5). These changes were mainly caused by *P. aeruginosa* (74/128; 58%), followed by *C. albicans* (38/128; 30%), *S. aureus* (21/128; 16%), *A. fumigatus*

Table 5. Sputum or nasopharyngeal flora and clinical condition of CF-patients with viral respiratory tract infections (n = 168 episodes; 128 microbiologically evaluable)

	Pulmonary exacerbation no. of episodes	No pulmonary exacerbation no. of episodes
No significant change of the microbial flora	14	4
Significant increase of		
P. aeruginosa	67	7
S. aureus	19	2
X. maltophilia	12	
Enterobacteriaceae	6	3
H. influenzae and *parainfluenzae*	5	1
coagulase-negative staphylococci	5	
Others (*S. pneumoniae* twice; *E. faecalis*, *A. denitrificans*, *P. fluorescens*, *P. vesiculare* each once)	5	1
C. albicans	37	1
A. fumigatus	14	

(14/128; 11%) and *X. maltophilia* (12/128; 9%). The proportion of proven viral respiratory tract infections with significant changes of the microbial flora did not differ for the viral agents investigated.

17 of 74 episodes with a significant increase of *P. aeruginosa* were due to the first isolation of *P. aeruginosa* associated with a viral respiratory tract infection (adenovirus 6, parainfluenza 4, RSV 2, RSV + parainfluenza type-3 2, adenovirus + RSV once, adenovirus + parainfluenza type-1 once, adenovirus + RSV + parainfluenza type-1 once). These patients were 12.1 ± 7.9 years (range 0.6–25.1 years) old at the onset of initial colonization with *P. aeruginosa*, which was also the onset of chronic colonization in 6/17 (35%) patients.

Nine CF-patients, who had not been colonized with *P. aeruginosa* at the beginning of the study but became initially colonized during the observation period, did not show elevated antibody titers against the viruses investigated. Thus, 65.4% (17/26) of cases with initial colonization with *P. aeruginosa* in cystic fibrosis seem to be associated with viral respiratory tract infections.

56/60 (93%) CF-patients, who became initially colonized with *P. aeruginosa* between 1984 and 1992 (independently of whether they were tested for antiviral antibodies or not) had the onset of their initial colonization in winter, spring or fall and only 4/60 (7%) during the summer. The onset of chronic colonization shows the same seasonal variation (Figure 1).

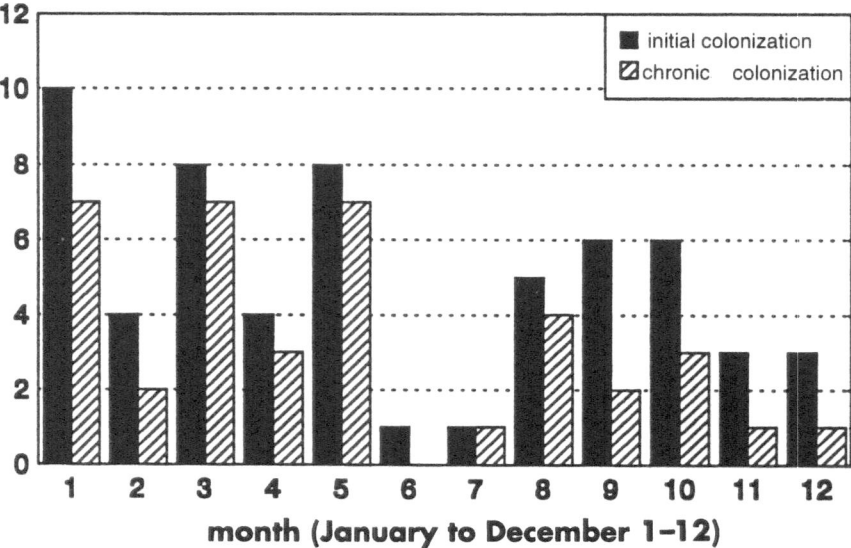

Figure 1. Month of onset of initial/chronic colonization with *P. aeruginosa* in patients with cystic fibrosis from 1984 to 1992.

Fungal and Atypical Bacterial Infections in Patients with Cystic Fibrosis

Overall, 72 different bacterial and fungal species were identified in the 3500 samples of 386 CF-patients investigated. The dominating species with a prevalence higher than 5% of patients or an overall mean isolation rate of more than 1% were *P. aeruginosa* (72.8% of the patients; 69.9% of the samples), *C. albicans* (77.9%; 46.8%), *S. aureus* (49.5%; 18.3%), *Aspergillus* spp. (33.4%; 14.1%), *X. maltophilia* (24.4%; 11.8%), *E. coli* (16.8%; 4.4%), *H. influenzae* (14.8%; 2.3%), *E. cloacae* (9.1%; 1.7%), *K. oxytoca* (6.7%; 1.2%), *S. pneumoniae* (6.5%; 0.8%), *S. marcescens* (4.9%; 1.1%), and *B. cepacia* (3.4; 1.8%).

The role of various species in the respiratory secretions of CF-patients may be determined by considering the persistence of these species or the immune response of the patients to these microbial pathogens. The persistence of a species was defined as the ratio of the number of isolates which were recovered in consecutive samples and of the number of all isolates of that species minus the number of isolates recovered only from the last sample examined of the patients. The persistence was most extended for *P. aeruginosa* (95.1%), followed by *C. albicans* (93.8%), *X. maltophilia* (87.5%), *B. cepacia* (86.9%), *A. fumigatus* (77.1%), *S. aureus* (75.6%), *Acinetobacter* spp. (65.6%), *M. catarrhalis* (60%) and enteric bacilli (54.9%). Other species including *Haemophilus* spp., *S. pneumoniae* and other glucose non-fermenting bacilli were intermittently isolated. The serologic response to *C. albicans* in CF-patients has been reported previously [6]. 28/36 (78%) of CF-patients (mean age 16.9 ± 4.3 years) from whom *C. albicans* was recovered in respiratory secretions and each of six CF-patients (mean age 14.8 ± 6.4 years) with repeatedly negative cultures for *C. albicans* showed significantly increased serum IgG to *C. albicans*. In 17 of 22 (77%) patients with more than one serum sample tested significant rises of the specific IgG could be observed concurrently to the isolation of *C. albicans*.

The prevalence of *A. fumigatus* in sputum of CF-patients increases with age from 13% in the first decade to 22% in the second, 25% in the third, and 45% in the fourth decade of life. CF-patients colonized with *P. aeruginosa* in the respiratory secretions are not more frequently colonized by *A. fumigatus* than patients without *P. aeruginosa*. 73% (40/55) of the CF-patients with cultures positive for *A. fumigatus* (mean age 16.3 ± 6.7 years, range 5–33 years) who were tested for specific serum IgG to *A. fumigatus* showed elevated IgG to *A. fumigatus*, whereas only 40% (14/35) of CF-patients without *A. fumigatus* (mean age 16.1 ± 5.9 years, range 4–28 years) and 30% (3/10) of healthy young adults were seropositive. There was no correlation between specific Aspergillus IgG and either specific Aspergillus IgE or total serum IgE level. This was true in all CF-patients investigated and of those CF-patients from whom *A. fumigatus* could be isolated. In addition, no correlation was found between the presence or absence of *A. fumigatus* and Aspergillus-specific IgE.

Discussion

Determination of antibodies to different viral respiratory tract pathogens revealed 168 infectious episodes mainly caused by adenoviruses (53%), parainfluenza viruses types 1 to 3 (24%) and RSV (20%) in the CF-patients investigated. Viral cultures and antigen detection procedures from respiratory secretions were omitted, together with assays for antibodies to rhinoviruses, coronavirus, echovirus and *Legionella* species. Furthermore, serum samples were not collected during each acute episode of upper respiratory tract disease. The real incidence of viral respiratory tract infections therefore, in CF-patients, is not reflected by these data. However, the effect of a proven viral respiratory tract infection for the further clinical and microbiological course of the patients can be evaluated. The consequences of viral infections are more severe in CF-patients than in healthy individuals: deterioration of pulmonary condition occurred in 86% of the episodes. A respiratory virus was serologically identified in association with 32% (78/243) of the admissions to hospital brought about by major respiratory exacerbations. These data are comparable with those previously published [7, 8]. Some of the admissions associated with viral disease of the upper respiratory tract were the first required by CF-patients. The detection of ten probable nosocomial infections reveals the importance of rapid diagnosis of viral respiratory disease and of measures to reduce cross-infections. In contrast to other studies [9, 10], the rate of proven viral infections in association with an admission to hospital due to pulmonary deterioration was not significantly different in CF-patients whether not colonized (41%; 19/46); intermittently colonized (38%; 6/16) or chronically colonized with *P. aeruginosa* (29%; 53/181).

A viral–bacterial synergism may be responsible for the onset of colonization with *P. aeruginosa*. Nearly two thirds of patients who became colonized with *P. aeruginosa* had a serologically proven single or mixed viral respiratory tract infection associated with the first isolation of *P. aeruginosa*. These illnesses were caused by adenoviruses (53%; 9/17), parainfluenza types 1 to 3 (47%; 8/17) and RSV (35%; 6/17). The point-prevalence for *P. aeruginosa* increases with age in the first two decades of life in our CF-population: 21% (0–2 years), 58% (3–5 years), 49% (6–9 years), 68% (10–15 years), and 89% (16–19 years). These data show that many patients become colonized with *P. aerugi-nosa* after the age of 10 years, corresponding to the mean age of CF-patients becoming initially colonized with *P. aeruginosa* in association with a proven viral infection. The high frequency of respiratory tract infections as documented in young non-CF infants and preschool-children and the still increasing prevalence of *P. aeruginosa* at school age in CF leads to the hypothesis that the extent of lung damage prior to the viral infection predisposes to initial colonization with *P. aeruginosa*. The seasonal variation of the onset of initial and chronic colonization is pronounced, confirming the data from Denmark [11].

CF-patients already intermittently or chronically infected with *P. aeruginosa* at the time of the proven viral infection developed a significant rise of *P. aeruginosa* CFUs per millilitre of sputum in 52% of illnesses (57/109 episodes microbiologically evaluable). Considering all significant rises in CFUs/ml of *P. aeruginosa* in patients chronically or intermittently colonized, 46% (57/123) of episodes were associated with a serologically proven respiratory infection. Therefore, even in patients intermittently or chronically infected with *P. aeruginosa*, a viral–bacterial synergism may be assumed.

Evaluating the role of other bacterial species recovered from respiratory secretions during viral illnesses, *S. aureus* plays a dominant role in CF-patients still not colonized by *P. aeruginosa* (26%; 9/35 episodes microbiologically evaluable) in contrast to CF-patients already colonized with this species (11%; 12/109 episodes microbiologically evaluable; $\chi^2 = 4.599$; $p = 0.05$). This may be explained by a bacterial antagonism between *P. aeruginosa* and *S. aureus*.

The high isolation rate and persistence of *C. albicans* in patients with cystic fibrosis as well as the pronounced seroprevalence and the frequency of significant rises of specific IgG concurrently to the isolation of this fungus reflects the clinical role of *C. albicans* in cystic fibrosis, underestimated in the past.

The inhalation of *A. fumigatus*, can lead to bronchial asthma, allergic bronchopulmonary aspergillosis (ABPA), invasive aspergillosis and aspergilloma, alone or in combination with ABPA. CF-patients with *A. fumigatus* in their respiratory tree showed significantly higher specific IgG to *A. fumigatus* than CF-patients of comparable age without this fungus. 86% (24/28) CF-patients with repeatedly positive cultures (≥ 3 isolations in consecutive samples) were seropositive in contrast to 59% (16/27) with less frequent isolations ($\chi^2 = 4.850$, $p < 0.05$). The highest specific IgG to *A. fumigatus* was seen in a female patient with ABPA and aspergilloma. *A. fumigatus* is an ubiquitous fungus to which all lungs are constantly exposed. The increase of prevalence with age may be explained by progressive pulmonary damage leading to impaired mucosal defence and ineffective removal of the spores from the airways. The consequence in CF-patients is a pronounced immune response to *A. fumigatus* which may lead to further lung damage eg. by antibody-dependent cellular cytotoxicity. In agreement with previous studies [12], no correlation was found between specific Aspergillus IgG and either specific Aspergillus IgE or total serum IgE level. By multiple step regression analysis we found a negative effect of the level of specific IgE to *A. fumigatus* on FVC, FEV_1, MEF_{50}, MEF_{25}, and sGAW, and an additional effect of the specific IgG to *A. fumigatus* on MEF_{50} and MEF_{25}. In contrast to the effect of specific IgE, the consequences of specific IgG on lung function have been confirmed [12]. An additional fungal species *Exophiala/Wangiella dermatidis* can be isolated from 9% of German CF-patients, using long-term culture [13]; with repeated isolation this leads to elevated specific serum antibodies in 89%, indicating an invasive process rather than superficial colonization.

Only limited data are available on atypical bacteria in cystic fibrosis. Thomassen *et al.* [14] found that two of ten CF-patients had anaerobes in sputum as well as in thoracotomy specimens. However, the level of *P. aeruginosa* was comparable with that of the anaerobes suggesting that the anaerobes played only a minor role in these patients.

The culture of mycobacteria from respiratory secretions of CF-patients may be challenged by frequent contamination with *P. aeruginosa*. A decontamination technique of 0.25% N-acetyl-L-cysteine and 1% sodium hydroxide (NALC–NaOH) followed by 5% oxalic acid treatment reduces the overgrowth with *P. aeruginosa* from 74% to only 5% [15]. 1.3 to 1.8% of CF-patients seem to be infected with atypical mycobacteria and 0.3 to 1.4% with typical mycobacteria [16]. Recently a prevalence of about 20% of atypical mycobacteria in respiratory secretions from adult CF-patients has been reported [17].

Our study proves the clinical and mircobial relevance of respiratory viral infections in young CF-patients not colonized with *P. aeruginosa* as well as in older CF-patients already colonized with this species. Therefore vaccination against influenza A and B should be strictly recommended to CF-patients, and all efforts made for rapid diagnosis of viral illness as well as the development of effective vaccines against adenoviruses, parainfluenza and RSV. In addition the roles of *C. albicans* and of *A. fumigatus*, which become more and more prevalent with increasing age, were estimated.

Acknowledgements

We thank Prof. Dr. K. Harms and Dr R. M. Bertele from the cystic fibrosis outpatient department at the University Children's Hospital for their collaboration. In addition, we thank colleagues from the viral laboratory of the University Children's Hospital, supported by the Friedrich-Baur-Stiftung for providing us with the results of the IgM-immunofluorescence tests.

References

1. Wright PF, Khaw KT, Oxman MN, Shwachman H. Evaluation of the safety of amantadine HCl and the role of respiratory viral infections in children with cystic fibrosis. J Infect Dis 1976; 134: 144–149.

2. Roggendorf M, Wigand R, Deinhardt F, Frösner G. Enzyme-linked immunosorbent assay for acute adenovirus infection. J Virol Methods 1982; 4: 27–35.
3. Przyklenk B, Bauernfeind A, Bertele RM, Deinhardt D, Harms K. Viral infections of the respiratory tract in patients with cystic fibrosis. Serodiagn Immunother Infect Dis 1988; 2: 217–225.
4. Enders G. Virusinfektionen. In: Thomas L, editor. Labor und Diagnose. 3rd edition. Marburg: Medizinische Verlagsgesellschaft, 1988: 1285–1330.
5. Bauernfeind A, Bertele RM, Harms K, Hörl G, Jungwirth R, Petermüller C, Przyklenk B, Weisslein-Pfister C. Qualitative and quantitative microbiological analysis of sputa of 102 patients with cystic fibrosis. Infection 1987; 15: 270–277.
6. Przyklenk B, Bauernfeind A, Hörl G, Emminger G. Serologic response to *Candida albicans* and *Aspergillus fumigatus* in cystic fibrosis. Infection 1987; 15: 308–310.
7. Wang EEL, Prober CG, Manson B, Corey M, Levison H. Association of respiratory viral infections with pulmonary deterioration in patients with cystic fibrosis. N Engl J Med 1984; 311: 1653–1658.
8. Pribble CG, Black PG, Bosso JA, Turner RB. Clinical manifestations of exacerbations of cystic fibrosis associated with non-bacterial infections. J Pediatr 1990; 117: 200–204.
9. Ramsey BW, Gore EJ, Smith AL, Cooney MK, Redding GJ, Foy H. The effect of respiratory viral infections on patients with cystic fibrosis. Am J Dis Child 1989; 143: 662–668.
10. Stroobant J. Viral infections in cystic fibrosis. J R Soc Med 1986; 79(12): 19–22.
11. Johansen HK, Hoiby N. Seasonal onset of initial and chronic infection with *Pseudomonas aeruginosa* in patients with cystic fibrosis in Denmark. Thorax 1992; 47:109–111.
12. Forsyth KD, Hohmann AW, Martin AJ, Bradley J. IgG antibodies to *Aspergillus fumigatus* in cystic fibrosis: a laboratory correlate of disease activity. Arch Dis Child 1988; 63: 953–957.
13. Haase G, Skopnik H, Groten T, Kusenbach G, Posselt H-G. Long-term cultures from sputum of patients with cystic fibrosis. Mycoses 1991; 34: 373–376.
14. Thomassen J, Klinger JD, Badger SJ, van Heckeren DW. Cultures of thoracotomy specimens confirm usefulness of sputum cultures in cystic fibrosis. J Pediatr 1984; 104: 352–356.
15. Whittier S, Hopfer RL, Knowles MR, Gilligan PH. Improved recovery of mycobacteria from respiratroy secretions of patients with cystic fibrosis. J Clin Microbiol 1993; 31: 861–864.
16. Gilligan PH. Microbiology of airway disease in patients with cystic fibrosis. Clin Microbiol Rev 1991; 4: 35–51.
17. Kilby JM, Gilligan PH, Yankaskas JR, Highsmith WE, Edwards LJ, Knowles MR. Nontuberculous myobacteria in adult patients with cystic fibrosis. Chest 1992; 102: 70–75.

Cystic Fibrosis Pulmonary Infections:
Lessons from Around the World
ed. by A. Bauernfeind, M. I. Marks and B. Strandvik

CHAPTER 2
Pharmacokinetics of Antibacterials in Cystic Fibrosis

Fritz Sörgel[1,2], Martina Kinzig[1], Christoph Labisch[2],
Martina Hofmann[1] and Ulrich Stephan[3]

[1]IBMP – Institute for Biomedical and Pharmaceutical Research, D-90562
Nürnberg-Heroldsberg, Germany
[2]Department of Radiology, University of Essen, D-45122 Essen, Germany
[3]Department of Pediatrics, University of Essen, D-45122 Essen, Germany

This chapter is dedicated to Christiane Herzog, who founded the German National Cystic Fibrosis Foundation ("Mukoviszidose Hilfe e.V.") in 1986 and has served this organization with great enthusiasm and untiring energy since then. She is the wife of the President of the Federal Republic of Germany, Professor Dr. Roman Herzog, who was elected in 1994.

Summary. There has been a controversy about the pharmacokinetics of drugs in cystic fibrosis. This article reviews the different concepts and reports available. Our findings show that neither the kidney nor the liver are "hyperorgans" in CF nor does the distribution of antibiotics follow different characteristics in this disease. There is also no evidence of impaired absorption of antibiotics in CF. Since the pharmacodynamic effect of antibiotics has recently been related to their plasma concentrations to MIC-relationships, our findings should lead to a complete reevaluation of antibiotic therapy in cystic fibrosis on rational data analysis.

Introduction

Present Situation

Cystic fibrosis (CF) is a complex disease with many manifestations. Although the exact location of the gene has now been found [1, 2], the condition is not well understood. The interpretation of results obtained in pharmacokinetic studies with these patients adds to the complexity. Reports that CF affects the function of organs such as the kidney and liver (relevant for the pharmacokinetics of drugs and antibiotics in particular) are addressed.

The confusion around the pharmacokinetics of antibiotics in CF patients started when Jusko *et al.* [3] published in 1975 the findings of a "hyperkidney" in patients with cystic fibrosis which seemed to eliminate dicloxacillin far more quickly than a kidney in a non-affected individual. In 1985 an editorial in *Lancet* stated that ". . . high doses of antibiotics

Correspondence address: Fritz Sörgel, IBMP – Institute for Biomedical and Pharmaceutical Research, Schleifweg 3, D-90562 Nürnberg-Heroldsberg, Germany.

in CF are rational in the context of their pharmacokinetics in these patients" [4]. A representative example of how this great confusion about altered pharmacokinetics was created is shown in Table 1. As was common practice at that time, the authors used data from different sources to compare pharmacokinetics between CF patients and non-affected individuals. Depending on which data from healthy volunteers or patients were compared, a significant increase, decrease, or no change in clearance values were obtained for comparison between CF patients and healthy controls. The arbitrary opinion of the investigator, reviewer, or editor therefore, affected the pharmacokinetic result.

Two years after the *Lancet* editorial we critically analyzed [10] the severe problems arising from such arbitrary comparisons. In Table 1 evidence for a hyperkidney, normal kidney, and impaired kidney function could be obtained. In 1987 [10] we gave recommendations on how pharmacokinetic studies trying to compare CF vs. non-CF pharmacokinetics should be performed. The use of an appropriate control group with similar age, weight, and body surfaces studied at the same time by the same laboratory was to our mind mandatory to any pharmacokinetic comparison between CF patients and non-affected individuals. Also, most investigations before 1985 were performed using a microbiological assay for the determination of antibiotics in plasma and urine. These methods may have been inadequate for pharmacokinetic studies especially in CF with "unknown" plasma constituents. We showed evidence that the "hyperfunction" of excretory organs and alterations in volume of distribution are clearly caused by the weight correction of pharmacokinetic parameters which becomes necessary when the weight differences between normals and CF patients were too large. Until most recently these important considerations would seem to have been ignored by some review authors in the Anglo-American literature [11–13] and work which was not of North American origin may have been

Table 1. Pharmacokinetics of cefsulodin in healthy volunteers (C) and CF patients

Comparison	Population	Comparison	Total clearance (ml/min)	Renal clearance (ml/min)	Authors
	C		128–148	52–60	Grannemann *et al.* [5]
	C		99	77	Ahrens *et al.* [6]
	C		181	141	Arvidsson *et al.* [7]
	CF		117	90	Reed *et al.* [8]
	CF		178	140	Arvidsson *et al.* [7]
	CF		89	—	Michalsen *et al.* [9]

Comparison of total clearance with the result:
———— = no difference between C and CF.
– – – – = CF-clearance < C-clearance.
.... = CF-clearance > C-clearance.

overlooked. Only in 1992 our criticism (expressed as early as 1987) was accepted by a "letter to the editor" of an American Journal [14]. We will discuss the rational physiological basis for antibiotic treatment or drug treatment in general for patients with cystic fibrosis.

Physiologic Functions Affecting Pharmacokinetics

As in a normal individual, it is the function of the kidney, the liver, and the gastrointestinal tract which affect the pharmacokinetics most significantly. Most antibiotics are primary eliminated by the kidney. Alteration in their pharmacokinetics would therefore have to be expected when kidney function is altered in CF. As Table 2 shows the available literature does not allow a clear conclusion on whether kidney function is normal or enhanced in CF patients. In all studies published until now no abnormal pathology was found in cystic fibrosis kidneys to explain the enhanced renal clearance of antibiotics.

The findings from autopsy liver samples in CF patients report liver pathology abnormalities in the majority of patients. These would make one expect a decrease in drug metabolizing capacity. Yet, what many authors seem to have shown was an enhancement of drug elimination in

Table 2. Kidney function in cystic fibrosis and controls

	Inulin-clearance (ml/min/1.73 m^2)		Creatinine-clearance (ml/min/1.73 m^2)		Renal blood flow (ml/min/1.73 m^2)
Jusko et al. [3]	—		CF	196	—
			C	127	
Levy et al. [15]	CF	147.5 ± 29.2*	C	133.8 ± 24.6	—
	C	142.9 ± 33.3*	C	145.8 ± 23.4	
Yaffe et al. [16]	—		CF	163 ± 38	—
	—		C	171 ± 52	—
Arvidsson et al. [7]	CF	142 ± 38	—		—
	C	102 ± 15	—		—
Marra et al. [17]	CF	142 ± 40	—		—
	C	137 ± 28	—		—
MacDonald et al. [18]	CF	111 ± 26	—		770 ± 140
Aladjem et al. [19]	—		CF	83.8 ± 17.4	—
	—		C	93.3 ± 19.3	—
Rosbon et al. [20]	CF	120	—		—
Spino et al. [21]	CF	95.8 ± 20.0**	—		499.8 ± 60.2***
	C	98.9 ± 12.9**	—		496.9 ± 102.3***
Berg et al. [22]	CF	127 ± 18	—		616 ± 78 +
	C	112 ± 10	—		601 ± 67 +
Reed et al. [8]	—		CF	112.4 ± 24.5	—

* Iothalamate-clearance.
** ^{99m}Tc-DTPA (diethylentriamine-penta-acetic acid)-clearance.
*** ^{125}I-OIH (orthoiodohippurate)-clearance.
$^-$ = PAH-clearance.
C = Controls.
CF = Cystic fibrosis.

their patients. Most recently O'Sullivan *et al.* [23] showed in an excellent study using duplex ultrasound scanning that there is no change in either hepatic vein or portal vein blood flow.

The gastrointestinal tract plays an important role in the absorption of drugs. Soon after CF had been defined as a disease it became apparent that normal development of children with the disease may not take place because of gastrointestinal abnormalities. It was then speculated that pancreatic insufficiency reduces nutrient absorption. It has now been established that gastric hypersecretion, decreased pancreatic sodium bicarbonate secretion, pancreatic insufficiency and altered bile acid metabolism are characteristics of the pathology of the gastrointestinal tract in CF. Vitamin absorption has been shown to be affected by pancreatic function [12].

Pharmacokinetic Studies of Antibiotics in Cystic Fibrosis

As mentioned above, the pharmacokinetic differences one observes between normals and CF patients may be artificial and simply originate from weight correction [10]. The biasing effect on these comparisons is particularly prominent when the CF patient group is very different in body weight from the healthy volunteer group. In the following the data available to us will be reviewed with this caution in mind.

The absorption of a drug can be characterized by the extent and rate of absorption. The extent of absorption represents the amount of drug which is taken up from the gastrointestinal tract. The rate of absorption is the amount of drug absorbed per unit time. It is characterized by k_a, and when this is not available C_{max} and t_{max} may give an idea of rate of absorption for agents with short half-lives.

Extent of Absorption of Antibiotics in Cystic Fibrosis (Table 3)

It has been shown with elegant in vivo perfusion techniques that absorption of phenylalanine and glycine is impaired in CF [12]. The rate of absorption of exogenous sugars did not lead to unequivocally accepted results. These conflicting data on amino acids and sugars are not surprising as when different drugs are studied contradictory results may be obtained.

The extent of absorption can only be reliably studied when the drug is once administered orally and once intravenously. By dividing the AUC (area under the plasma concentration time curve) of the oral form by the AUC of the intravenous form, the fraction (F) of drug absorbed may be determined. Very few studies have been published determining F appropriately. The group of Spino investigated cloxacillin and theo-

Table 3. Absorption of antibiotics in patients with cystic fibrosis (from [24])

	AUC (μg · h/ml)	
	Control group	CF patients
Cefaclor (1 g)	30.0 ± 8.6	39.0
Cefadroxil (1 g)	103.5 ± 11.3	105.5 ± 10.2
Ciprofloxacin (750 mg)	10.2 ± 3.47	14.0 ± 5.9
Pefloxacin (400 mg)	47.7 ± 15.3	61.8 ± 18.0
	F	F
Pefloxacin (400 mg)	1.04 ± 0.21	1.02 ± 0.30

F = absolute bioavailability.

phylline and found the coefficient of variation to be higher in CF than in controls (C) with coefficient of variation for cloxacillin being as high as 53% [12]. When we used pefloxacin, a quinolone antibacterial, we found that the variability (C = 20.2%, CF = 29.4%) in general was much smaller than for cloxacillin (C = 43.5%, CF = 52.7%) in both normals and CF patients [10]. Whether significant differences like these originate from analytical problems or are affected primarily by the different physicochemical nature of the compounds may not be easily differentiated. Our studies have all implemented Good Laboratory Practices (GLP)-conditions with appropriate assay validation and quality controls. Exclusively metabolite and degradation product(s)-specific HPLC-assays were used. Other factors which can influence the results have been extensively discussed [10].

If the higher variability of extent of absorption in CF vs. C have to be explained on physiological/physicochemical grounds one could speculate that when a drug has the characteristics of complete absorption (like pefloxacin in our study) the CF-specific pathological changes of the gastrointestinal tract (GI-tract) may affect the fraction absorbed less than when absorption in controls is already clearly below 100%. Oral penicillins like cloxacillin, studied by Spino [12], do not have complete absorption from the GI-tract and hence the variability of the absorption process is considerable.

In p.o. studies with cefadroxil, a completely absorbed oral cephalosporin, we found similar AUC and renally excreted amounts of the compound. In situations like this, where i.v. administration may not be as critical because of complete availability, the similarity of renal excretion may be sufficient to show identical absorption between groups. The data from our laboratory therefore favor the hypothesis of a high F-value being important for differences between controls and CF patients to be expected. The slightly higher variance of F in CF is not surprising in a disease where the gastrointestinal effects are so variable between individual patients. Studies with cefaclor, which is not

Table 4. Rate of absorption of antibiotics (from [10])

	C_{max} ($\mu g/ml$)		t_{max} (h)		$k_a{}'$ (h^{-1})	
	C	CF	C	CF	C	CF
Cefaclor (1 g)	20.4 ± 4.2	21.7 ± 2.7	0.83 ± 0.26	1.31 ± 0.37*	n.c.	n.c.
Cefadroxil (1 g)	27.2 ± 2.89	30.4 ± 4.8	1.67 ± 0.41	2.00 ± 0.71	n.c.	n.c.
Ciprofloxacin (750 mg)	2.34 ± 0.42	3.46 ± 1.26*	1.12 ± 0.44	1.25 ± 0.38	1.71 ± 1.96	1.34 ± 0.79
Ciprofloxacin (500 mg)	3.51 ± 1.33	3.78 ± 0.97	1.04 ± 0.42	1.72 ± 0.44**	2.301 ± 0.824	0.862 ± 0.662***
Pefloxacin (400 mg)	4.13 ± 0.87	4.94 ± 1.74	1.6 ± 1.0	1.28 ± 0.81	n.c.	n.c.

+ = using two compartment-model.
n.c. = not calculated.
* = $p < 0.05$.
** = $p < 0.01$.
*** = $p < 0.001$.
C = control group.
CF = CF patients.

completely absorbed, also suggest identical extent of absorption in C vs. CF.

Rate of Absorption of Antibiotics in Cystic Fibrosis (Table 4)

Where there is relatively much accordance between authors is in the impaired rate of absorption of antibiotics in CF. The majority of data suggest that absorption of antibiotics is delayed in CF – this may be a result of prolonged small intestinal transit time. Data from our group and LeBel are summarized in Table 4. They show delayed absorption as expressed by a later t_{max} of cefaclor, cefadroxil, and ciprofloxacin. There was no such effect observed for pefloxacin probably because its long half-life blurs this effect.

In conclusion, the extent of absorption of antibacterials and non-antibacterials as calculated from the AUC of oral and intravenous administration is probably unaltered in most CF patients. Assuming passive absorption processes for these exogenous agents this suggests that the physicochemical permeability of the GI-tract is unaltered in CF. However, the time to reach the maximum concentration is prolonged, probably caused by altered transit times. This prolongation does not require any change in administration of antibiotics between CF patients and normals since in many cases of our studies C_{max} was not even reduced. In oral antibiotic treatment of acute and specific chronic infections t_{max}-changes are irrelevant while C_{max} has been shown in i.v.-studies with quinolones and aminoglycosides to be of importance when significantly altered. Since the effects of food on oral availability have not yet been investigated in CF patients these assumptions are only true for fasting conditions. Food has been shown to reduce C_{max} and to increase t_{max} significantly in individuals with a normal GI-tract and this may be more relevant in CF, where food digestion is altered.

Drug Metabolism in Cystic Fibrosis

Until recently there has been very little work on the metabolism of drugs in CF. This was mostly due to the fact that until the early 80s only betalactams and aminoglycosides were investigated. These agents are little metabolized and/or their metabolites (e.g. those of the betalactams) are very difficult to detect. Furthermore the metabolism of antibiotics (e.g. betalactams) is very often by hydrolysis which is not a metabolic step limited to the liver but also occurs in plasma and tissues. Hence differences between CF and controls may be very difficult to find. For non-antibacterial agents elevations of drug metabolism as well as non-alterations were reported in CF and not too surprisingly the contradictory results are as numerous as for the presumed gastrointestinal or renal effects on antibiotic kinetics.

One of the few results which is in accordance with what has been known for many years in pharmacokinetics is that when liver function is impaired (as in CF) drug metabolism is impaired. We administered pefloxacin, a quinolone metabolized to about 90%, to CF and controls and found the excretion of the metabolites relative to parent compound (metabolic ratio) different in the two groups. The non-weight-corrected non-renal clearance (which in the case of pefloxacin reflects metabolism) was smaller in CF patients. These two data fit well with the expected impairment of drug metabolism in CF due to liver impairment. Most recently O'Sullivan et al. [25], in one of the most elegant studies on drug metabolism in CF, probed the CYP2C9 activity in the liver by administering (S)-warfarin. They found no differences between both groups but this may in part be explained by the large standard deviations which were for some parameters higher than 50% and even 100%. We doubt that the unpaired t-test is an appropriate statistical test in this situation. In spite of non-significance, the authors conclude that the "in vivo activity of cytochrome P_{450} isoforms is selectively affected in subjects with cystic fibrosis" [26].

Renal Elimination of Antibiotics in Cystic Fibrosis

Most betalactams have dominating renal excretion. Some antibiotic agents such as ceftazidime and aminoglycosides have almost exclusive renal elimination. The index case of "increased renal clearance" of antibiotics in CF was cloxacillin [3]. Ever since then this work was used as a proof of enhanced renal elimination. Again, we may refer to our 1987 paper [10] in which we describe the obvious problems of earlier work. Most recent work shows that the vision of some authors is still blurred while others have adopted our approach. From our work we conclude that there are no such dramatic differences in total or renal clearance between CF and controls when these clearance parameters were uncorrected for weight (Tables 5 and 6). As in some of our work,

Table 5. Renal clearance (ml/min) of antibiotics in patients with cystic fibrosis (from [10])

	Control group	CF patients
Cefaclor	481.2	321.1
Cefadroxil	180.2	163.0
Cefotiam	202	232
Piperacillin	109	102
Ceftazidime	83	89
Ciprofloxacin	266	245
Pefloxacin	11.3	14.8

Table 6. Comparison of renal clearance with and without weight correction (statistics were done by Student's impaired t-test) (from [24]). C = Controls, CF = CF-patients

	Renal clearance (ml/min)			Renal clearance/kg (ml/min/kg)			Renal clearance/1.73 m² (ml/min/1.73 m²)		
	C	p-value (t-test)	CF	C	p-value (t-test)	CF	C	p-value (t-test)	CF
Cefaclor	481.0	0.027	321.0	6.67	NS	6.79	461.3	NS	365.9
Cefadroxil	180.1	NS	163.0	2.67	0.065	3.40	173.1	NS	184.2
Cefotiam	201.9	NS	245.9	2.97	0.001	5.23	192.9	0.02	264.8
Ceftazidime	83.2	NS	88.6	1.25	NS	1.92	78.9	NS	100.9
Piperacillin	109.1	NS	101.5	1.56	0.001	2.84	102.3	0.025	124.4
Ciprofloxacin	265.4	NS	245.4	4.32	NS	4.56	267.0	NS	257.6
Pefloxacin	11.5	0.072	14.8	0.16	0.001	0.31	16.9	0.001	10.4

there were slightly higher clearances in CF patients when they were corrected for weight.

In a recent paper by Wang et al. [27] on the pharmacokinetics of ticarcillin "enhanced renal clearance" was again observed. But again that group only used weight-corrected data. Moreover, they administered in mg/kg and did a weight correction which automatically increases the error. This is particularly a pity since their study design was very sophisticated. In Table 6 we have completed the data from our laboratory which are clearly against the theory of changed tubular secretion of betalactams and other agents in CF.

Volume of Distribution

An analysis very similar to the ones on gastrointestinal, hepatic, and renal aspects could be made here. As Table 7 shows again the weight correction leads to the false conclusion of an elevated volume of distribution of antibiotics in CF. Since we believe that nobody assumes that CF patients have abnormalities in their extra- to intracellular ratio of the magnitude "observed" for changes in volume of distribution, we are convinced that an increased volume of distribution of drugs with low or no protein binding such as ceftazidime or aminoglycosides cannot occur.

Sputum Penetration

There is agreement among authors that there is a lack of information of the pharmacodynamics of antibacterials in patients with cystic fibrosis. Modern pharmacodynamics relate plasma levels to MIC. Site concentrations and tissue levels have been determined and also used for pharmacodynamic considerations. We are not aware of many studies with reliable determination of antibiotics in the lung or sputum of patients with cystic fibrosis. A study by Autret et al. [28] showed that for 5 and 7.5 mg/kg amikacin doses plasma levels were above the MIC for 21 and 41%, respectively of the dosing interval. The AUC_{sputum}/ AUC_{plasma} was between 0.028 and 0.61 and it increased during multiple dosing. Only with a dose of 15 mg/kg could sputum levels above the MIC be observed. The authors suggested increasing the dose to 7.5 mg/ kg in cystic fibrosis.

We analyzed sputum concentrations of pefloxacin and found drug levels on average of about 60–80% of the plasma levels, with far smaller variation than seen in the amikacin study [28–30]. Whether this is caused by the higher lipophilicity and hence better penetration is difficult to tell. We suspect that also the stability of amikacin in sputum

Table 7. Comparison of volume of distribution with and without weight correction (statistics were done by Student's impaired t-test) (from [24])

	Volume of distribution (VDss) [l]			Volume of distribution (VDss)/kg [l/kg]		
	C	CF	p-value (t-test)	C	CF	p-value (t-test)
Cefotiam	13.39 ± 2.4	13.94 ± 3.11	NS	0.2 ± 0.03	0.3 ± 0.04	0.000
Ceftazidime	13.8 ± 2.2	9.6 ± 5.2	0.08	0.205 ± 0.026	0.211 ± 0.07	NS
Piperacillin	13.23 ± 3.86	8.4 ± 1.8	0.003	0.19 ± 0.066	0.197 ± 0.026	NS
Pefloxacin	121.1 ± 27.8	101.4 ± 41.3	NS	1.69 ± 0.43	2.14 ± 0.55	0.073

Table 8. Pharmacokinetic measurements and parameters relevant for pharmacodynamics after intravenous administration of antibacterials (from [24])

	C_{max} (μg/ml)		AUC (μg·h/ml)		$t_{1/2}$ (h)	
	C	CF	C	CF	C	CF
Ceftazidime (1 g)	251.5 ± 86.5	474.2 ± 251.5*	317.5 ± 68.6	345.5 ± 133.5 n.s.	1.93 ± 0.4	1.33 ± 0.4*
Piperacillin (4 g)	479.9 ± 127.2	727.0 ± 204.3**	571 ± 124	456.7 ± 98.4*	1.25 ± 1.0	0.818 ± 0.25 n.s.
Pefloxacin (400 mg)	4.76 ± 1.38	7.53 ± 2.53**	47.0 ± 14.6	63.2 ± 18.8*	10.2 ± 2.0	11.6 ± 1.4 n.s.
Cefotiam (1 g)	108.7 ± 19.8	123.3 ± 50.0 n.s.	57.3 ± 6.6	54.8 ± 14.1 n.s	0.88 ± 0.23	0.923 ± 0.08 n.s.

n.s. = not significant.
* = p < 0.07.
** = p < 0.01.

samples and difficulty of sensitive and reliable measurement may cause these variable results.

Pharmacokinetics of Antibiotics in Cystic Fibrosis – an Ongoing Confusion?

As discussed above many authors have not considered other people's work in that important area of treating CF patients with antibiotics. To the present there is no convincing publication which shows any enhanced drug elimination in patients with cystic fibrosis. Thus our 1987 article [10] is still a most valid up-date and no really new evidence of enhanced organ functions in cystic fibrosis has been offered.

Any News for the Clinician?

Based on the original work by Jusko et al. [3] in 1975, clinicians have used high doses of antibiotics in CF. The Lancet supported that view in 1985 [4]. The principles of pharmacodynamics suggest that the plasma levels of an antibiotic predict the outcome of infection [31]. For betalactams the time above MIC was shown to be a crucial factor, while for aminoglycosides the ratio of C_{max} divided by MIC should be higher than eight to obtain a sufficient pharmacological and therapeutic response.

The plasma levels of antibiotics we found in our investigations using similar age and weight groups of CF and non-CF populations (Table 8) do not support the idea of using three to five times higher doses in CF as suggested from Jusko et al.'s data. We cannot exclude the possibility, however, that penetration to the site of infection is greatly impaired in CF when compared with respiratory infections in non-CF patients and which therefore requires higher doses. The viscous sputum has often been considered a barrier but the sputum is not the site of action. Data on sputum penetration are rare and the rationale for measuring sputum concentrations as a surrogate for the pharmacodynamic response has never been proven scientifically.

It is interesting that when the quinolones were introduced no high doses were used although similar data as with betalactams were obtained by some authors with these agents: increased clearance and volume of distribution when weight corrections were made. This was probably so because quinolones were considered to be more toxic than betalactams and even aminoglycosides. The latter fact shows that megadose treatment of CF patients was done because the excellent tolerance to those agents did not pose limits to those physicians and has allowed that irrational treatment of CF patients with antibiotics ongoing for many years.

We feel that our suggestions of 1987 [10] to increase the dose by about 30% is still rational in view of the pharmacodynamics of antibiotics and the available findings on their pharmacokinetics.

References

1. Riordan JR, Rommens JM, Kerem B, et al. Identification of the cystic fibrosis gene: cloning and characterization of complementary DNA. Science 1989; 245: 1066–1072.
2. Anderson MP, Rich DP, Gregory RJ, Smith AE, Welsh MJ. Generation of cAMP-activated chloride currents by expression of CFTR. Science 1991; 251: 679–682.
3. Jusko WJ, Mosovich LL, Gerbracht LM, Mattar ME, Yaffe SJ. Enhanced renal excretion of dicloxacillin in patients with cystic fibrosis. Pediatrics 1975; 56: 1038–1044.
4. Editorial. Antibiotic dosage in cystic fibrosis. Lancet 1985; I: 1020–1021.
5. Grannemann GR, Sennello LT, Sonders RC, Wynne B, Thomas EW. Cefsulodin kinetics in healthy volunteers after intramuscular and intravenous injection. Clin Pharmacol Ther 1982; 31: 95–103.
6. Ahrens T, Fischer W, Imhof P, Füllhaas J, Zak O, Kradvefer F. Human pharmacology of CGP 7174/E (SCE-129) and initial results of clinical trials in Europe. Drugs Exptl Clin Res 1979; 5: 61–70.
7. Arvidsson AG, Alvan G, Strandvik B. Difference in renal handling of cefsulodin between patients with cystic fibrosis and normal subjects. Acta Paediatr Scand 1983; 72: 293–294.
8. Reed MD, Stern RC, Yamashita TS, Ackers I, Myers CM, Blumer JL. Single dose pharmacokinetics of cefsulodin in patients with cystic fibrosis. Antimicrob Agents Chemother 1984; 25: 579–581.
9. Michalsen H, Bergmann T. Pharmacokinetics of netilmicin in children with and without cystic fibrosis. Antimicrob Agents Chemother 1981; 19: 312–318.
10. Sörgel F, Stephan U, Wiesemann HG, Gottschalk B, Stehr C, Rey M, Böwing HB, et al. High dose treatment with antibiotics in cystic fibrosis – a reappraisal with special reference to the pharmacokinetics of betalactams and new fluoroquinolones in adult CF-patients. Infection 1987; 15: 385–396.
11. Lindsay CA, Bosso JA. Optimisation of antibiotic therapy in cystic fibrosis patients – pharmacokinetic considerations. Clin Pharmacokinet 1993; 24: 496–506.
12. Spino M. Pharmacokinetics of drugs in cystic fibrosis. In: Gershwin E, editor. Clinical reviews in allergy, vol 9: Cystic fibrosis. The Humana Press, 1991: 169–210.
13. De Groot R, Smith AL. Antibiotic pharmacokinetics in cystic fibrosis – differences and clinical significance. Clin Pharmacokinet 1987; 13: 228–253.
14. Weinberger MM. Drug clearance in patients with cystic fibrosis (letter to the editor). Clin Pharmacol Ther 1992; 52: 106.
15. Levy J, Smith AL, Koup JR, Williams-Warren J, Ramsey B. Disposition of tobramycin in patients with cystic fibrosis: A prospective controlled study. J Pediatr 1984; 105: 117–124.
16. Yaffe SJ, Gerbracht LM, Mosovich LL, Mattar ME, Danish M, Jusko WJ. Pharmacokinetics of methicillin in patients with cystic fibrosis. J Infect Dis 1977; 135: 828–831.
17. Marra G, Tirelli S, Cavanna G, Amoretti M, Giunta A, Appiani AC, Assael BM. Renal function in cystic fibrosis (CF). Ped Res Meeting 1984; Abstr. 365.
18. MacDonald NE, Anas NG, Peterson RG, Schwartz RH, Brooks JG, Powell KR. Renal clearance of gentamicin in cystic fibrosis. J Pediatr 1983; 103: 985–990.
19. Aladjem M, Lotan D. Boichis H, Orda S, Katznelson D. Renal function in patients with cystic fibrosis. Nephron 1983; 34: 84–86.
20. Robson AM, Tateishi S, Ingelfinger JR, Strominger DB, Klahr S. Renal function in patients with cystic fibrosis. J Pediatr 1971; 79: 42–50.
21. Spino M, Chai RP, Isles AF, Balfe JW, Brown RG, Thiessen JJ, et al. Assessment of glomerular filtration rate and effective renal plasma flow in cystic fibrosis. J Pediatr 1985; 107: 64–70.
22. Berg U, Kusoffsky E, Strandvik B. Renal function in cystic fibrosis with special reference to the renal sodium handling. Acta Paediatr Scand 1982; 71: 833–838.

23. O'Sullivan TA, Bauer LA, Horn JR, Zierler BK, Strandness DE, Williams-Warren J, et al. Disposition of drugs in cystic fibrosis. II. Hepatic blood flow. Clin Pharmacol Ther 1991; 50: 450–455.

24. Sörgel F. Pharmakokinetische Grundlagen der Antibiotikatherapie bei Mukoviszidose. Habilitationsschrift, Universität-Gesamthochschule-Essen, Germany, 1987.

25. O'Sullivan TA, Wang J-P, Unadkat JD, Al-Habet SMH, Trager WF, Smith AL, et al. Disposition of drugs in cystic fibrosis. V. In vivo CYP2C9 activity as probed by (S)-warfarin is not enhanced in cystic fibrosis. Clin Pharmacol Ther 1993; 54: 323–328.

26. Wang J-P, Unadkat JD, McNamara S, O'Sullivan TA, Smith AL, Trager WF, et al. Disposition of drugs in cystic fibrosis. VI. In vivo activity of cytochrome P450 isoforms involved in the metabolism of (R)-warfarin (including P450 3A4) is not enhanced in cystic fibrosis. Clin Pharmacol Ther 1994; 528–533.

27. Wang J-P, Unadkat JD, Al-Habet SMH, O'Sullivan TA, Williams-Warren J, Smith AL. Disposition of drugs in cystic fibrosis. IV. Mechanisms for enhanced renal clearance of ticarcillin. Clin Pharmacol Ther 1993; 54: 293–302.

28. Autret E, Marchand S., Breteau M, Grenier B. Pharmacokinetics of amikacin in cystic fibrosis: A study of bronchial diffusion. Eur J Clin Pharmacol 1986; 31: 79–83.

29. Metz R, Sörgel F, Federspil P, Malter U, Koch HU, Stephan U, Gottschalk B, Manoharan M. Penetration of pefloxacin into saliva, sputum, sweat, tears, and nasal secretions. Rev Infect Dis 1988; 10, Suppl. 1: 97.

30. Sörgel F., Stephan U, Brüning I, Wiesemann G, Dominick HC, Heidböhmer A. The pharmacokinetics of pefloxacin in patients with cystic fibrosis and healthy volunteers. 14th International Congress of Chemotherapy, Kyoto, Japan, June 23–28, 1985; Abstract No. 6141.

31. Craig WA. Summary and future directions. In: Cars O, Craig, WA, editors: Pharmacodynamics of antibiotics – consequences for dosing. Proceedings of a Symposium, June 7–9, 1990, Stockholm, Sweden. Scand J Infect Dis 1991; Suppl 74: 284–286.

Cystic Fibrosis Pulmonary Infections:
Lessons from Around the World
ed. by A. Bauernfeind, M. I. Marks and B. Strandvik
© 1996 Birkhäuser Verlag Basel/Switzerland

CHAPTER 3
Antimicrobial Pharmacotoxicity

Henry C. Farrar[1,3,4] and Gregory L. Kearns[1,2,3]

Departments of Pediatrics[1] and Pharmaceutics[2], University of Arkansas for Medical Sciences, Little Rock, Arkansas and the Divisions of Pediatrics Clinical Pharmacology[3] and Emergency Medicine[4], Arkansas Children's Hospital, Little Rock, Arkansas 72202, USA

Introduction

The management of acute pulmonary exacerbations in patients with cystic fibrosis (CF) may be complicated by the development of adverse drug reactions. In the general population, antimicrobial agents are frequently associated with drug-related toxicity. As reviewed by Anderson [1], antimicrobial agents, particularly the beta-lactam antibiotics, may account for 20–50% of the adverse drug effects reported in hospitalized patients.

Several factors increase the risk of antibiotic-related adverse drug effects in patients with CF. Because drug penetration into the lung parenchyma is often impaired and the bioactivity of specific drugs (eg. aminoglycoside antiobiotics) may be reduced in the liquid milieu of the infected and/or colonized lung, higher serum concentrations of drugs for extended periods of time are frequently required to achieve effective tissue levels of these agents. Accordingly, aggressive dosing strategies for several antimicrobial agents in patients with CF may increase the risk of concentration-related toxicities. The unusual and multiple pathogens causing endobronchial infections in these patients often necessitates the concomitant use of multiple antibiotics, which may increase the risk of toxicity through either additive effects (ie. potential for increased nephrotoxicity in patients receiving aminoglycosides and vancomycin) and/or drug interactions (eg. the potentiation of theophylline toxicity by inhibition of hepatic metabolism by quinolones). Finally, the recurrent nature of pulmonary exacerbations in patients with CF results in the need for repeated courses of antimicrobial therapy, resulting in cumulative doses of many antimicrobial agents which far exceed those routinely adminstered to other patients without the disease. Thus, CF patients are at greater risk of developing adverse drug reactions related to drug accumulation (eg. oto- and nephrotoxicity from aminoglycosides) or the appearance of hypersensitivity reactions (eg. acquired, delayed hypersensitivity reactions to beta lactams).

While it is beyond the scope of this review to recapitulate the complete adverse effect and side effect profile for all antimicrobial agents from both a mechanistic and clinical perspective, it is important to provide summary information concerning the pharmacotoxicity (ie. clinically relevant toxicities which might be expected in the context of therapeutic use) of antimicrobial agents common to the treatment of patients with CF. Accordingly, this review will focus on those antimicrobial agents typically used in the management of acute pulmonary exacerbations in patients with CF. The overall incidence of adverse drug effects will be described as well as specific drug-related toxicities.

Aminoglycosides

For almost two decades, aminoglycoside (AG) antibiotics have been both revered and feared as primary agents in the treatment of pulmonary exacerbations in patients with CF. As discussed elsewhere in this text, AG have maintained their key role in therapy primarily as a consequence of their activity against *Pseudomonas* sp. However, because of their propensity to produce both nephrotoxicity and ototoxicity, these agents have received a high degree of attention, both scientific and clinical, with regard to the importance of pharmacodynamics (ie. concentration vs effect relationships) and pharmacokinetics (eg. alterations of drug disposition characteristic of patients with CF) in the selection of dosing regimen. Indeed, in many hospitals throughout the U.S., Canada, and the European Community, the monitoring of AG serum concentrations comprises a significant proportion of all therapeutic drug monitoring and clinical pharmacokinetic service resources available at the present time.

In view of the ever changing patterns of microbial resistance which frequently characterize patients with CF, the proven utility of the AGs in treating these patients and the prospects for the development of less toxic alternatives, it would appear that these antibiotics will retain an important place in the therapeutic armamentarium. Accordingly, practitioners involved in the selection and monitoring of antibiotic therapy in CF patients should remain familiar with the salient features of AG toxicity. To this regard, the following sections are intended to provide a clinically oriented overview of the major toxicities of the aminoglycosides relevant to their therapeutic use in patients with CF.

Nephrotoxicity

Aminoglycoside-associated nephrotoxicity has been reviewed from a mechanistic and clinical basis relevant to both pediatric [2] and adult

[3–5] patients. While the term "nephrotoxicity" implies a dire, drug-induced event, the clinical observation of AG-induced renal injury is generally one of nonoliguric renal failure that is usually completely reversible and rarely, if ever, requires dialysis [5–7].

Aminoglycosides are predominantly (eg. 90–99%) eliminated by glomerular filtration with a small amount of active tubular secretion [4]. Accumulation of these drugs in proximal tubular cells occurs by active reabsorption of a small percent (eg. 5–10%) of the filtered load from the luminal surface and by a smaller contribution from the basolateral membrane [2, 3, 5, 8]. Walker and Duggin (9) have summarized the following sequence of events leading to AG-induced nephrotoxicity: i) glomerular filtration producing high AG concentrations in tubular urine, ii) binding of the AG to apical cell membrane phosphoinositols, iii) pinocytosis of the AG–endocytotic vacuole complex with the development of high intracellular concentrations, iv) incorporation of the complex into lysozomes with inhibition of phospholipid metabolism (ie. normal lysosomal function) and the release of toxic hydrolases into the cytosol, v) mitochondrial interaction leading to the generation of reactive oxygen intermediates causing disruption of cellular function and structure, vi) impairment of cellular transport processes resulting in an increased distal delivery of sodium and vii) reduction in the glomerular filtration rate as the functional nephron pool is reduced. Histologically, the end result of AG-related nephrotoxicity is a marked reduction in the microvillae of the brush border cells, swelling and disruption of the cellular organelles and frank cellular necrosis. The nephrotoxic debris is then sloughed into the lumen of the proximal tubule which forms casts, leaving a denuded basement membrane upon which regenerative activity begins [10].

The pathophysiologic manifestations of AG-associated nephrotoxicity occur 48 to 72 hours after cellular changes (9). Schentag and coworkers [11], have described the functional alterations occuring in AG-induced nephrotoxicity: i) increased urinary excretion of β-2 microglobulin with a peak at approximatley two to three days, ii) tubular enzymuria (eg. N-acetyl-β-glucosaminidase and alanine aminopeptidase) with a peak at four to five days, iii) an increase in urinary cast count that peaks at approximately six days and iv) a progressive increase in serum creatinine that may begin at five to six days and may not peak until ten days into the course of injury. Because AGs accumulate in renal tubular cells following the administration of appropriate doses, subclinical alterations in renal function may occur in all patients who receive the drug.

Since elevations of serum creatinine are generally late findings in patients with AG-induced nephrotoxicity, early indicators of toxicity have been sought to potentially minimize the progression of symptoms. In contrast to early animal studies of this adverse reaction [12], a reduction of urinary concentrating ability in man does not appear to be uniformly present early in the course of renal injury (5). Because β-2 microglobulin has been shown to be a more reliable indicator of early AG-induced renal injury than tubular enzymuria [13], and the renal handling of this protein is normal in patients with CF [14], monitoring of urinary β-2 microglobulin concentrations may afford the best means of detecting nephrotoxicity for up to a week before significant elevations in serum creatinine are seen. It is important to note that elevations in serum AG concentrations seen in association with nephrotoxicity generally correlate with the later phase of injury (ie. a reduction in glomerular filtration rate) and reflect a reduction in the clearance of the drug. Accordingly, these elevations are the result of renal impairment and not the cause. Correlation of a particular post-dose serum AG concentration with the development of nephrotoxicity is limited by the differences between AG concentrations and pharmacokinetics in the plasma and tissues due to tissue accumulation [2].

The reported incidence of AG-associated nephrotoxicity varies widely over a range of 0.5–63% [5]. Because of variations in the criteria used for evaluating and defining AG-induced renal injury (ie. use of serum creatinine vs plasma concentration monitoring, evaluation of patients who have received >5 days of therapy, etc.), the reported incidence of nephrotoxicity has varied among different investigations of the same AG and between different AGs. In a review of 144 clinical trials representing over 10 000 patients, average frequencies of AG nephrotoxicity were 14% for gentamicin, 12.7% for tobramycin, 9.4% for amikacin and 8.7% for netilmicin [15]. These data were supported by those from a more recent review [3] which ranked the propensity of the AGs to produce nephrotoxicity in an identical fashion. It is important to note that the relative frequencies reported for AG-induced nephrotoxicity are based primarily on data generated in adult patients which have been reviewed and compared [3, 15, 16]. These comparisons of the incidence of AG-associated renal injury are often problematic in that the different studies may not have used standardized methods for the evaluation of nephrotoxicity: comparable treatment regimens, homogeneous patient populations (ie. disease severity, disease state, age and gender distribution, etc.) and prospective methods for the individualization of therapy (ie. therapuetic drug monitoring and/or pharmacokinetic-based dose selection). This is illustrated by the examination of one of the early studies which evaluated 258 adult patients with suspected sepsis and reported that nephrotoxicity with gentamicin (26%) was significantly greater than that seen with tobramycin (12%) [17]. Subsequent examination of these data with those from 11 other clinical trials comparing the nephrotoxic potential of these two agents produced no convincing evidence that differences between tobramycin and gentamicin were of clinical significance [18].

There are no large, controlled investigations of AG-induced nephrotoxicity in pediatric patients which employ strict individualization of dose, application of serum concentration monitoring or the use of sensitive and specific methods to detect renal injury [2]. For these reasons, suggested differences between the respective AGs and their propensity to produce renal injury from adult studies continue to be extrapolated to the pediatric use of these drugs. However, because these drugs may lack clinically significant differences in their ability to produce nephrotoxicity, the selection of a given agent to treat colonization/infection in a patient with CF should be guided primarily by clinical and laboratory data such as culture and sensitivity [19, 20]. Also CF patients do not appear to be predisposed to AG-induced renal injury despite the use of higher doses, shorter dosing intervals and more frequent courses of AG therapy [21–24].

The occurrence of AG-induced nephrotoxicity (and ototoxicity as described below) may be lessened by avoidance of clinical risk factors whenever therapeutically possible and also, by individualization of the AG dosing regimen to accommodate patient and disease specific alterations in the disposition of a given drug. Clinical risk factors have been reviewed by Whelton [3] and are summarized in Table 1 with particular emphasis on patients with CF. It should be noted that these particular risk factors, primarily derived from adult studies, are not uniformly accepted. Moore and colleagues [25] examined data from 214 patients randomized to receive either gentamicin or tobramycin and found that diabetes, dehydration, serum bicarbonate, bacteremia, urinary tract infection, AG use, duration of AG therapy, total AG dose, or the use of clindamycin, furosemide or cephalothin did not correlate with AG-nephrotoxicity and hence, were not regarded as specific risk factors. In a more recent study of 1489 patients who were prospectively monitored with AG therapy guided by pharmacokinetic individualization [26],

Table 1. Clinical risk factors for aminoglycoside nephrotoxicity in patients with cystic fibrosis

---

Factors easily influenced by the prescriber
  – selection of dose and dosing interval based on disease and age-specific alterations in drug disposition characteristics
  – duration of systemic therapy
  – avoidance of dehydration and electrolyte disturbances (eg. hypokalemia)
  – selection of therapeutic combinations with less nephrotoxic potential

Factors not easily influenced by the prescriber
  – requirements for prior and future aminoglycoside therapy
  – gender (women > men incidence of acute interstitial nephritis)
  – underlying renal pathology (eg. glomerulomegaly, microscopic nephrocalcinosis[1]) found in patients with CF
  – preexisting reductions in glomerular filtration rate produced by intrinsic or extrinsic (ie. amphotericin B, cis-platinum, cyclosporine, FK-506) renal disease

---

Adapted from Whelton (3)
[1]Denotes Katz et al. (57)

multiple logistic regression was used to identify that the following were independent risk factors for AG-induced nephrotoxicity: trough serum concentration, concurrent therapy with clindamycin, vancomycin, piperacillin or cephalosporins, ascites, advanced age, female gender, decreased albumin, duration of therapy and leukemia. However, in this particular study, no identifiable risk factor alone or in combination was of sufficient sensitivity to reliably predict AG-associated renal injury.

Since observational and epidemiological trials both suggest a relationship between nephrotoxicity and elevated serum AG concentrations [27, 28], it is clear that individualization of therapy based on determination of patient-specific pharmacokinetic parameters coupled with prudent therapuetic drug monitoring offers the best mechanism to ensure both the safety and efficacy of AG therapy in patients with CF [19, 22–24, 27]. Various therapeutic options for AG therapy in patients with CF may also serve to reduce the risk of drug-induced nephrotoxicity. Two variations are the aggressive use of aerosolized AG and/or colistin [20] and the potential use of once-daily AG therapy. The later is a technique which has either the same or a reduced risk of nephrotoxicity (and ototoxicity) when compared to appropriately administered conventional dosing regimens [29, 30]. Finally, aztreonam is a beta-lactam antibiotic with a similar antimicrobial profile to that of AGs but with a markedly lower risk profile for producing nephrotoxicity [31, 32]. In one study, nephrotoxicity occurred in 15% of those treated with an aminoglycoside compared to 1% of those given aztreonam [33]. Accordingly, substitution of aztreonam for AGs when permitted by culture and sensitivity results may reduce the incidence of all AG-associated adverse effects.

Ototoxicity

Embryologic similarities between the kidney and ear are believed to explain, in part, the propensity of the AGs to produce clinically significant ototoxicity. All AGs have been associated with the development of both auditory and vestibular dysfunction during a course of therapy or up to four to six weeks following discontinuation of therapy [2]. In pediatric patients treated with gentamicin or kanamycin, reports of ototoxicity outnumber those of nephrotoxicity. Early investigations comparing the AGs with respect to their ability to produce ototoxicity reported a 2–10% incidence [34], with an average incidence of cochlear toxicity of 13.9% for amikacin, 8.3% for gentamicin, 6.1% for tobramycin and 2.4% for netilmicin [15]. However, subsequent studies employing more sensitive methods for detecting AG-induced ototoxicity (eg. brainstem auditory evoked response, pure tone audiometry, electronystagmography) have reported subclinical alterations in function in as many as 45% of patients treated with the drugs [35].

A complete review of the mechanisms of both auditory and vestibular toxicity of the AGs as well as a clinical and experimental comparison of the primary agents has been published by Prazma [36]. Briefly, the proposed mechanisms responsible for AG-induced ototoxicity include alterations in the electrical potential and intracelluar osmotic pressure within endolymph, as well as direct interaction with glucose transport and cellular metabolism. As a class, AGs can be divided into two groups with regard to their propensity to produce ototoxicity [2]. The predominantly vestibulotoxic compounds (eg. streptomycin, gentamicin, tobramycin) tend to selectively destroy type I hair cells of the crista ampullaris while those with predominant cochlear toxicity (eg. neomycin, kanamycin, amikacin) are actively translocated into the hair cells by a process believed to be analogous to that which regulates the accumulation of AGs into proximal renal tubular cells. The pattern of cochlear AG toxicity is characteristic of the agents which produce this injury with the initial production of lesions in the outer hair cells of the basal turn. As drug accumulation continues consequent to both the AG dose and duration of exposure, the lesion extends apically and to the inner hair cells. While the damage to the outer hair cells produces ototoxicity which is generally reversible and is associated with high-frequency (ie. 4000–8000 Hz) hearing loss, tinnitus and a sensation of fullness, progression of the cochlear lesion with involvement of the hair cells of the apex may produce permanent or only partially reversible loss of lower frequencies with possible accompanying conversational hearing loss. Vestibular dysfunction is considered to be irreversible in most cases. It may be characterized by nausea, dizziness, vertigo and nystagmus and may parallel AG-induced cochlear damage. Finally, the more rapid perilymph clearance of gentamicin, tobramycin and amikacin relative to older AGs (eg. kanamycin, neomycin), may explain the lower incidence of clinical ototoxicity associated with these agents [36].

Risk factors for the development of AG-induced ototoxicity have been reviewed [2] and are summarized as follows: the intrinsic ototoxic potential of the drug, impaired renal function producing accumulation of AG concentrations in the serum, concomitant administration of other drugs which may produce and/or facilitate the development of vestibular or cochlear injury (eg. loop diuretics, vancomycin), the cumulative AG dose, senescence and exposure to intense nosie. As with AG-associated nephrotoxicity, there is not complete agreement concerning the predictive ability of risk factors for ototoxicity; an assertion supported by previous studies in adults which found that plasma AG concentrations, AG type, furosemide use, diabetes, age, gender, renal function, initial auditory acuity, hematocrit and presence of shock did not enable accurate prediction [37].

Previously espoused clinical dogma has indicated that high peak serum AG concentrations predispose patients to AG-associated ototoxicity while high trough concentrations increase the risk for drug-induced nephrotoxicity. Despite the fact that anecdotal case reports implicate high serum AG concentrations in the production of ototoxicity, a review of several controlled clinical trials has refuted this relationship [27]. This is also supported by specific studies in patients with CF. An early study of tobramycin toxicity in 53 patients with CF who had normal renal function and received repeated courses of high dose therapy, evaluated cochlear and vestibular function and found a transient, bilateral high tone of loss at 8000 Hz in only one patient [38]. A more recent controlled study [39] which used high-frequency, pure tone audiometry to evaluate 22 patients with CF who had been treated with multiple courses of AGs (ie. either gentamicin, tobramycin, amikacin or netilmicin) demonstrated statistically significant reductions in cochlear function only at frequencies higher than 16000 Hz in patients with CF who were younger than 20 years and who had received AGs. In 13 patients with CF who had never received AGs, audiometry results were not significantly different than observed in 38 control subjects without CF and a history of AG therapy.

As is true of AG-associated nephrotoxicity, the clinical evaluation and detection of ototoxicity may be problematic. Lack of standardization in the definition of drug-induced ototoxicity based on audiometric and electronystagmorgraphic evaluations, failure to select a proper testing environment (ie. a noisy patient care unit vs a suitable chamber), lack of patient acceptance for procedures which are time-consuming, require accurate responses and/or are unpleasant (eg. caloric testing for vestibular function) and absence of specific monitoring guidelines for the detection and longitudinal evaluation of AG-induced ototoxicity [5, 19] all contribute to the lack of clinical vigilance in the prospective evaluation of this specific adverse drug effect. Certainly, the apparent low incidence of AG-induced ototoxicity in patients with CF would appear to support the use of pharmacokinetic-based, individualized dose regimen selection coupled with therapeutic drug monitoring [19, 27] in lieu of scheduled, specific evaluations of auditory and vestibular function. However, these tests should be used if clinical symptoms are apparent and/or a specific risk factor is identified to be of concern. Finally, the selection of agents with a lower propensity to produce vestibular and/or cochlear damage (eg. aztreonam, ceftazidime, ciprofloxacin) [33] may represent important therapeutic alternatives for either the avoidance of AG-induced ototoxicity and/or the treatment of patients who manifest symptoms consistent with this adverse effect.

Neuromuscular Blockade

Neuromuscular blockade is a relatively rare adverse effect of the AG [2] and is believed to be caused by inhibition of acetylcholine release at the presynaptic cholinergic junction [40]. The onset of this adverse reaction is most often characterized by respiratory failure or muscle weakness that is not readily and fully explained by the attendant pathology. Factors which can predispose patients to AG-associated neuromuscular blockade include: i) rapid intravenous administration of high doses and/or unrecognized accumulation of the drug in patients with impaired renal drug clearance, ii) concomitant adminstration of AG with neuromuscular blockers or in the presence of hypermagnesemia or hypocalcemia and iii) patients with underlying cholinergic dysfunction such as myasthenia gravis or botulism [2, 41]. Of the most commonly used AGs in patients with CF (ie. tobramycin, amikacin and gentamicin), there appears to be little difference with respect to their propensity to produce and/or augment neuromuscular blockade [42]. While this particular side effect may rarely be of clinical concern, it must be considered in patients who, because of severe illness and/or possibly, the receipt of an organ transplant, may require prolonged mechanical ventilation and concomitant aggressive antibiotic therapy. Since AG-associated neuromuscular blockade is completely reversible upon clearance of the offending agent and modification of predisposing therapies and/or conditions (ie. selection of alternative paralytic agents and/or correction of electrolyte abnormalities), its prompt recognition and treatment in the patient with CF may prevent potentially serious morbidity or mortality.

Colistin

The increasing occurrence of pulmonary exacerbations associated with strains of *Pseudomonas aeruginosa* that are resistant to multiple antibiotics has prompted the use of colistin, both by the aerosol [43] and intravenous [44] routes. Colistin is an antibacterial cationic cyclic polypeptide belonging to the polymyxin group of antibacterial agents which acts by altering the functional integrity of bacterial cell membranes through its detergent action on phospholipid constituents. Adverse reactions to parenteral colistin have been reported to occur in approximately 36% of patients and for the most part, appear to be completely reversible [45]. The major toxicities of this agent have included the production of acute tubular necrosis in approximately 20% of patients who receive normal doses of the drug and also, neuromuscular blockade [45, 46]. However, in a more recent study [44], the evaluation of 21 courses of intravenous colistin therapy in 19 patients with CF demonstrated discernable nephrotoxicity in only one patient and neurotoxicity (characterized by perioral paresthesia, ataxia, or both) in six patients. These authors concluded that the incidence of serious toxicity associated with colistin in patients with CF may be lower than previously reported and that the intravenous form of the drug can be considered as a viable therapeutic alternative in patients with resistant strains of *Pseudomonas* sp.

Vancomycin

Vancomycin is occasionally used in CF patients to provide anti-staphylococcal coverage. Early reports of a high rate of toxicity associated with vancomycin use have not been reproduced with the use of more purified vancomycin preparations. Currently, the most common adverse effects associated with vancomycin use are dermatologic, with rashes occurring in 2–6% of treated patients. However, there have been rare reports of an exfoliative dermatitis associated with its use (47).

Infusion-Related Complications

Several different adverse effects have been associated with the infusion of vancomycin. A histamine mediated "red-neck" or "red-man syndrome" is not an infrequent complication and consists of fever, chills, pruritus, erythema on the upper trunk and neck and occasionally hypotension [48, 49]. Other infusion-related phenomena include hypotension alone, thrombophlebitis and the "pain and spasm syndrome," consisting of chest pain and parasternal muscle spasm [49]. These reactions resolve when the infusion is discontinued. The incidence of these toxicities can be reduced with the use of more dilute vancomycin solutions and slower infusion rates [48].

Ototoxicity

Ototoxicity associated with vancomycin use was a frequent concern because two of the earliest reported trials of this agent found that 40% of patients experienced some form of this adverse effect [50, 51]. However, subsequent reports have not reproduced these findings, possibly due to the availability of a more purified form of vancomycin [52]. Since 1983 there has been one reported case of vancomycin-associated ototoxicity identified only by audiogram [53]. In most reports of ototoxicity, patients had received other potentially ototoxic drugs such as aminoglycosides or erythromycin, the ototoxicity was not clinically apparent (being noted on audiogram only), and resolved with discontinuation of the drug [54, 55]. Ototoxicity appears to be very rare in children, with one reported case which did not describe how ototoxicity was identified in a child (a six week old infant) who had also received kanamycin and erythromycin [56].

Nephrotoxicity

Vancomycin-associated nephrotoxicity is another frequent clinical concern. This complication typically occurs in less than 5–8% of patients treated with vancomycin alone but increases to between 20% and 35% in patients concomitantly receiving an aminoglycoside [53, 58–61]. The incidence of this adverse effect appears to be particularly low in pediatric patients with the combined incidence of approximately 3% based on data from seven studies involving 225 patients between 1960 and 1989, some of whom were also treated with aminoglycosides [56, 62–67].

Quinolones

Quinolones are valuable agents in the management of patients with CF because they are orally administered agents with excellent activity against *Pseudomonas* species. Much of the experience gained with these drugs has been in adult patients, as concern over the potential for quinolone-associated arthropathies has limited their use in the pediatric population.

Quinolones are generally well tolerated with the overall rate of adverse effects being 4–8% [68, 69]. Adverse drug reactions which require discontinuation of therapy occur in approximately 1–2% of treated patients [70]. Gastrointestinal effects are the most common, occurring in 5–9% of children [68–71]. Less common reactions occurring in 2–5% of patients include neurologic, dermatologic and non-specific complaints (malaise, chills). Neurotoxic symptoms typically include headache, dizziness, agitation and sleep disturbances [72]. Seizures have been rarely reported, possibly as a result of quinolone binding at the GABA receptor site [72, 73]. In one case of ciprofloxacin-related partial complex seizures, there were no predisposing risk factors (such as a known seizure disorder, concomitant use of other neurotoxic agents or central nervous system abnormalities) and the seizures recurred when the patient was re-exposed to the drug [73]. Dermatologic effects typically include rash and pruritus although toxic epidermal necrolysis, an idiosyncratic, exfoliative dermatitis, has been rarely associated with ciprofloxacin use [72, 74]. Hypersensitivity reactions have also occurred with quinolone therapy [72, 75].

Quinolone-Associated Arthropathy

Quinolone use in pediatric patients has been limited because of the potential risk for associated arthropathies. When quinolones were given to young dogs, erosions of the articular surfaces of the weight bearing joints have been noted [76]. However, in an evaluation of thirteen prepubertal children treated with ciprofloxacin for three months, no changes of the articular cartilage were noted by magnetic resonance imaging, although none of these children had been symptomatic [70]. Nalidixic acid, a structural analog of the quinolones, also produces extensive cartilage damage in young animals, a finding which has not been reproduced in pediatric patients treated with this drug [69]. Thus, the arthropathy related to quinolone use observed in laboratory animals may be species specific and may not occur to a great degree in children during episodic, therapeutic use of these drugs.

Current clinical experience suggests that there is a low risk of quinolone-associated arthropathy in children, although ciprofloxacin is the only quinolone to be extensively evaluated. In a report of 202 children treated with ciprofloxacin, the overall incidence of arthralgia alone was 2.5%, occurring only in patients with CF and resolving with discontinuation of quinolone therapy [71]. In another review of the safety of ciprofloxacin in 634 children [71], arthralgia alone was reported in eight patients (1.3%), all of whom were females with CF, age two to 17 years [68]. Again, the arthralgia resolved with discontinuation of therapy. The incidence of arthralgias was much higher in a third study of CF patients treated with ciprofloxacin, with eight of 30 children (27%) developing this adverse effect which resolved with discontinuation of therapy [77]. Thus, there appears to be a small but significant risk of reversible arthralgia in CF patients treated with ciprofloxacin.

Arthralgias have not been reported with the same frequency in other groups of patients. As reviewed by Kubin [78], over 300 patients without CF have been treated with ciprofloxacin with no reports of arthritis or arthralgia. It remains to be resolved whether CF patients are at greater risk for this toxic reaction or, with more extensive use of ciprofloxacin, the incidence will be the same in all groups of pediatric patients. The incidence of arthropathy in these patients is difficult to interpret because of the presence of immune-mediated arthropathies and/or hypertrophic pulmonary osteoarthropathies which occur in 7–8% of adolescents and adults with CF [79].

Thus, the limited information concerning quinolone use in children would indicate that arthropathies are an infrequent complication and, when present, consist of an apparently mild, reversible arthralgia. Whether the adverse drug reaction data for ciprofloxacin, the most extensively evaluated quinolone in children, can be generalized to other quinolones in patients with CF requires further study.

Beta-Lactam Antibiotics

Some beta-lactam antibiotics are regularly used in the management of acute pulmonary exacerbations in CF patients because of their activity against *P. aeruginosa* [80]. These include the extended spectrum peni-

Table 2. Beta-lactam antibiotics minor adverse drug reactions

Gastrointestinal Irritation	1–3%
Dermatologic Reactions	2–3%
Laboratory Abnormalities	3–7%
Hepatic Transaminase	2–7%
Leucopenia	1–3%

Table 3. Beta-lactam antibiotics serious adverse drug reactions

	Allergic reactions	Bleeding	Seizures
Ticarcillin (carboxypenicillin)	+ + +	+ +	—
Piperacillin (ureidopenicillin)	+ + +	—	—
Ceftazidime (cephalosporin)	+ +	—	—
Imipenem (carbapenem)	+	—	+ + +
Aztreonam (monobactam)	+	—	—

+ + + greatest risk; + + possible complication; + rare complication; — not reported.

cillins such as the carboxypenicillins (carbenicillin, ticarcillin) and the ureidopenicillins (piperacillin, mezlocillin), anti-pseudomonal cephalosporins (examplified by ceftazidime), carbapenems (imipenem) and monobactams (aztreonam).

Although beta-lactam antibiotics represent a diverse group of drugs, they share similar adverse drug reaction profiles, as described in Tables 2 and 3. The overall rate of all possible side effects is approximatley 6% [31, 32, 81–88]. These drugs are generally regarded as safe, with few serious toxicities associated with their use.

Hypersensitivity Reactions and Immunogenic Cross-Reactivity

Hypersensitivity reactions cause most concern. Allergic reactions to penicillin have been reported in up to 10% of the general population and are the most frequent reported cause of drug-related anaphylaxis [1, 89]. In CF patients, allergic reactions associated with the use of anti-pseudomonal penicillins occurred in 11% of patients [90]. With repeated exposures, the incidence of hypersensitivity reactions appears to increase with one study finding that 62% of 121 cystic fibrosis patients eventually developed hypersensitivity reactions to at least one beta-lactam antibiotic [91]. Since these patients frequently require repeated courses of therapy with beta-lactams, hypersensitivity reactions can become particularly problematic, limiting therapeutic options.

The incidence of allergic reactions to different beta-lactam antibiotics in the general population varies widely although these reactions are most commonly reported with penicillins. Aztreonam and imipenem appear to be weakly immunogenic with allergic reactions occurring in less than 2% to 3% of exposed patients [85, 88]. Cephalosporin-related allergic reactions are also infrequent, occurring in less than 2% of treated patients, and more commonly with the first generation cephalosporins as opposed to the third generation cephalosporins [1, 92, 93]. A similar trend among the different beta-lactam antibiotics has been noted in CF patients. In these patients, Koch and coworkers [91] found that piperacillin had the highest rate of hypersensitivity reactions (51%), followed by carbenicillin and azlocillin (21–24%) and the anti-pseudomonal cephalosporins, cefsulodin and ceftazidime (13–17%). Aztreonam and imipenem had the lowest rates of allergic reactions (4–6%).

There is concern that exposure to one beta-lactam could result in the development of cross reactivity to other beta-lactams. For example, in patients without CF, there appears to be a high degree of cross-reactivity with imipenem in penicillin-allergic patients, with 50% of those with positive penicillin skin testing also demonstrating positive skin tests to imipenem [94]. Cross-reactivity occurred much less often with aztreonam but was still present [95, 96]. However, since CF patients receive many courses of different beta-lactam antibiotics and can become sensitized to the individual drugs, it is difficult to determine the exact incidence with which cross-reactivity develops.

Abnormalities of Hemostasis

Beta-lactam antibiotics can interfere with normal hemostasis through two different mechanisms: interference with the generation of coagulation factors, and interference with platelet aggregation [87, 97]. Hypoprothrombinemia occurs more commonly with cephalosporins, particularly moxalactam, cefamandole and cefoperazone, and is secondary to interference with the synthesis of vitamin K dependent coagulation factors [97]. These compounds share a 3-methylthiotetrazole substituent on the cephem ring which can dissociate from the antibiotic and interfere with the activity of vitamin K dependent carboxylase [93, 97]. Therapy with ceftriaxone, which has a similar side chain, has occasionally increased prothrombin times [97], while the use of ceftazidime, which lacks such a side chain, has not been associated with clinically significant hypoprothrombinemia [81, 82].

Abnormal hemostasis associated with beta-lactam use can also be secondary to impaired platelet aggregation. This adverse effect is most pronounced with carboxypenicillins (carbenicillin, ticarcillin) and moxalactam [92, 93]. While the exact mechanism is unknown, this adverse effect is most prominent in beta-lactam antibiotics with an alpha-carboxyl configuration [97]. There is a concentration–response relationship associated with this effect, which is most prominent in patients receiving high drug doses and/or having impaired elimination secondary to renal insufficiency [87, 97]. *In vitro* studies using concentrations of aztreonam and ureido-penicillins which are much higher than those attained clinically have demonstrated an anti-platelet effect [87, 88]. However, clinically significant hypoprothrombinemia and platelet abnormalities have not been observed in patients treated with ceftazidime, aztreonam, the ureidopenicillins (piperacillin, mezlocillin, azlocillin) or imipenem [81, 85, 86, 88].

Seizures

Seizures have occasionally been reported in association with the use of beta-lactam antibiotics. This appears to be a concentration-related phenomenon, as predisposing factors are renal impairment resulting in drug accumulation, and high dose therapy [98, 99]. Laboratory evidence suggests that penicillin-associated seizures result from an interaction between the intact beta-lactam ring and the GABA receptor [98]. Although benzylpenicillin appears to have the greatest *in vitro* seizure potential, other beta-lactams, including the antipseudomonal penicillins and some cephalosporins have been associated with this adverse effect [87, 92, 98]. There have been no reports of seizures with aztreonam [88].

There is considerable concern that seizures may occur more commonly in patients treated with imipenem. Calandra and coworkers [85] found that 1.5% of patients treated with imipenem experienced seizures. However, in a retrospective review of a similar group of patients treated with other antibiotics, the incidence of seizures was 1.6% [85]. Therefore, while it appears that imipenem may be associated with a higher risk of seizures compared to other beta-lactam antibiotics, it is difficult to define the risk of this adverse effect in patients with normal imipenem pharmacokinetics.

Factors Influencing Antimicrobial Pharmacotoxicity in Cystic Fibrosis Patients

In view of the fact that many adverse drug reactions occur consequent to the accumulation of drugs in the plasma and tissues, it is generally appreciated that decrements in function of those organs responsible for either drug metabolism or excretion could predispose patients to concentration-related toxicity. However, in most patients with CF, alterations in hepatic and/or renal functions capable of reducing drug clearance do not routinely occur. In contrast, both the renal and hepatic clearance of many antimicrobial agents have been reported to be increased in patients with CF as a result of disease-specific alterations in the processes which govern cellular drug transport and/or substrate-specific steps in drug biotransformation [21, 100–103]. Despite this apparent disparity, the clinician should be vigilant to the possibility of both overt and subclinical alterations in organ function which may alter disposition of a drug. Prompt recognition of altered pharmacokinetics will allow timely dosing changes, thereby minimizing the risk of drug-induced toxicity. This is especially important given that the longer lifespan of patients with CF [20] increases the chances of organ dysfunction due to the effect of disease progression on extrapulmonary organs.

In additon to disease effects on drug disposition and action, development changes in pharmacokinetics must be considered in the evaluation of both the efficacy and toxicity of antimicrobial therapy [104]. As demonstrated in pharmacokinetic studies of ticarcillin–clavulanic acid, the developmental patterns which govern the renal clearance and apparent volume of distribution of this drug in normal children were indeed present in patients with CF [105]. Consequently, the clinician must consider the influence of development on drug disposition when individualizing drug therapy or evaluating drug safety and efficacy in CF patients.

Finally, the impact of drug interactions on the pharmacotoxicity of antimicrobial agents in patients with CF must be considered. As recently reviewed [106], drug–drug interactions based on inhibition or induction of the cytochrome P450 system may produce significant alterations in pharmacokinetics, possibly leading to pharmacodynamic consequences which demand alteration of therapy. Examples which may be relevant to antimicrobial therapy in CF include potentially significant drug interactions with the fluoroquinolones (eg. in combination with oral anticoagulants, cimetidine, cyclosporine and theophylline), the macrolides (eg. in combination with oral anticoagulants, carbamazepine, cyclosporine, digoxin, terfenadine, astemizole, triazolam and methylprednisolone) and the sulfonamides (eg. in combination with cyclosporine and oral anticoagulants) [106]. Because of the propensity of polypharmacy to result in increased incidence of drug–drug interactions, especially with drugs which are either metabolized by the liver or are highly protein bound, drug regimens in patients with CF should be reviewed carefully to identify potentially significant drug interactions and modify therapy appropriately.

Conclusions

This chapter represents an overview of the pharmacotoxicity of antimicrobial agents which are commonly used in patients with CF, with the data summarized in Table 4. It is beyond the scope of this chapter to provide the reader with a compendium of all adverse effects associated

Table 4. Comparison of serious drug-related toxicities

	Nephrotoxicity	Ototoxicity	Arthropathy	Neurotoxicity*	Bleeding	Allergic reactions
Aminoglycosides						
Amikacin	++	+++	–	–	–	+
Gentamicin	+++	+++	–	–	–	+
Tobramycin	+++	++	–	–	–	+
Netilmicin	++	++	–	–	–	+
Colistin						
Vancomycin	++	+	–	–	–	+
Quinolones	–	–	++	+	–	+
Beta-Lactams						
Carboxypenicillins	–	–	–	–	+++	+++
Ureidopenicillins	–	–	–	–	–	+++
Ceftazidime	–	–	–	–	–	++
Imipenem	–	–	–	+++	–	+
Aztreonam	–	–	–	–	–	+

+++ greatest risk; ++ possible complication; + rare complication; – not reported; *neurotoxicity includes seizures, paresthesias, ataxia.

with antimicrobial agents. It is our hope that the information provided, both factual and theoretical, will enable the reader to identify what is common and to use inductive reasoning coupled with available data to formulate a rational basis for the prospective evaluation of antimicrobial therapy which will minimize the risk of drug-induced toxicity. It is the development of a sound therapeutic "plan" which will enable the clinician to carefully and critically evaluate the toxicity of both new antimicrobial agents in patients with CF and older agents recruited once again for introduction into therapy. Finally, it is important for the clinician to understand (and embrace) that the true incidence of any drug-related toxicity can only be discovered through vigilance and proper reporting of adverse effects. It is this knowledge which will serve as the cornerstone for the development of safer and more effective treatments for all patients with CF.

Acknowledgements

The inspiration and guidance provided by Drs. Bettina Hilman, John Wilson, Jeffrey Blumer, Robert Warren, George Mallory, Jr. and Karl Karlson, Jr. is gratefully acknowledged.

References

1. Anderson JA. Allergic reactions to drugs and biological agents. JAMA 1992; 268: 2845–2857.
2. Steele RW, Kearns GL. Antimicrobial therapy for pediatric patients. Pediatr Clin North Am 1989; 36: 1321–1349.
3. Whelton A. Therapeutic initiatives for the avoidance of aminoglycoside toxicity. J Clin Pharmacol 1985; 25: 67–81.
4. Zaske DE. Aminoglycosides, in Applied Pharmacokinetics: Principles of Therapeutic Drug Monitoring, second edition, In: Evans WE, Schentag JJ, Jusko WJ (eds.), Applied Therapeutics Inc., Spokane 1986; 331–381.
5. Garrison MW, Zaske DE, Rotschafer JC. Aminoglycosides: another perspective. DICP Ann Pharmacother 1990; 24: 267–272.
6. Kaloyanides GJ, Pastoriza-Munoz E. Aminoglycoside nephrotoxicity. Kidney Int 1980; 18: 571–582.
7. Luft FC, Rankin LI, Sloan RS, Yum MN. Recovery from aminoglycoside nephrotoxicity with continued drug administration. Antimicrob Ag Chemother 1978; 14: 284–287.
8. Bennett WM. Aminoglycoside nephrotoxicity. Nephron 1983; 35: 73–77.
9. Walker RJ, Duggin GG. Drug nephrotoxicity. Ann Rev Pharmacol Toxicol 1988; 28: 331–345.
10. Humes DH, Weinberg JM, Knauss TC. Clinical and pathophysiologic aspects of aminoglycoside nephrotoxicity. Am J Kidney Dis 1982; 2: 5–29.
11. Schentag JJ, Plaut ME, Cerra FB, et al. Aminoglycoside nephrotoxicity in critically ill surgical patients. J Surg Res 1979; 26: 270–279.
12. Gordon JA, Dillingham MA, Guggenheim SJ, et al. The renal concentrating defect after gentamicin administration in the rat. J Lab Clin Med 1983; 101: 903–910.
13. Reed MD, Vermeulen MW, Stern RC, et al. Are measurements of urine enzymes useful during aminoglycoside therapy? Pediatr Res 1981; 15: 1234–1239.
14. Kearns GL, Berry PL, Boochini JA Jr., Hilman BC, Wilson JT. Renal handling of beta-microglobulin in patients with cystic fibrosis. DICP Ann Pharmacother 1989; 23: 1013–1017.

15. Kahlmeter G, Dahlager JI. Aminoglycoside toxicity – a review of clinical studies published between 1975 and 1982. J Antimicrob Chemother 1984; 13 (A): 9–22.
16. Burkle WS. Comparative evaluation of the aminoglycoside antibiotics for systemic use. Drug Intell Clin Pharm 1981; 15: 847–862.
17. Smith CR, Lipsky JJ, Laskin OL, Hellman DB, Mellits ED, Longstreth J, Lietman PS. Double-blind comparison of nephrotoxicity and auditory toxicity of gentamicin and tobramycin. N Engl J Med 1980; 302: 1106–1109.
18. Burkle WS. Is tobramycin less nephrotoxic than gentamicin? Clin Pharm 1986; 5: 514–516.
19. Lindsay CA, Bosso JA. Optimisation of antibiotic therapy in cystic fibrosis patients: pharmacokinetic considerations. Clin Pharmacokinet 1993; 24: 496–506.
20. Wallace CS, Hall M, Kuhn RJ. Pharmacologic management of cystic fibrosis. Clin Pharm 1993; 12: 657–674.
21. Prandota J. Drug disposition in cystic fibrosis: progress in understanding pathophysiology and pharmacokinetics. Pediatr Infect Dis J 1987; 6: 1111–1126.
22. Delage G, Desautels L, Legault S, Lasalle R, Lapierre JG, Lamarre A, Masson P, Spier S. Individualized aminoglycoside dosage regimens in patients with cystic fibrosis. Drug Intell Clin Pharm 1988; 22: 386–389.
23. Horrevorts AM, Degener JE, Dzoljic-Danilovic G, Michel MF, Kerrebijn KF, Driessen O, Hermans J.Pharmacokinetics of tobramycin in patients with cystic fibrosis: implications for the dosing interval. Chest 1985; 88: 260–264.
24. Touw DM, Vinks AATMM, Heijerman HGM, Hermans J, Bakker W. Suggestions for the optimization of the initial tobramycin dose in adolescent and adult patients with cystic fibrosis. Ther Drug Monitor 1994; 16: 125–131.
25. Moore RD, Smith CR, Lipsky JJ, Mellits ED, Lietman PS. Risk factors for nephrotoxicity in patients treated with aminoglycosides. Ann Intern Med 1984; 100: 352–357.
26. Bertino JS, Jr., Booker LA, Franck PA, Jenkins PL, Franck KR, Nafziger AN. Incidence of and significant risk factors for aminoglycoside-associated nephrotoxicity in patients dosed by using individualized pharmacokinetic monitoring. J Infect Dis 1993; 167: 173–179.
27. Bertino JS, Rodvold KA, Destache CJ. Cost considerations in therapeutic drug monitoring of aminoglycosides. Clin Pharmacokinet 1994; 26: 71–81.
28. McCormack JP, Jewesson PJ, A critical re-evaluation of the therapeutic range of aminoglycosides. Clin Infect Dis 1992; 14: 320–339.
29. Hustinx WNM, Hoepelman IM. Aminoglycoside dosage regimens: is once a day enough? Clin Pharmacokinet 1993; 25: 427–432.
30. Gilbert DN. Once-daily aminoglycoside therapy. Antimicrob Ag Chemother 1991; 35: 399–405.
31. Brewer NS, Hellinger WC. The monobactams. Mayo Clin Proc 1991; 66: 1152–1157.
32. Childs SJ, Bodey GP. Aztreonam. Pharmacother 1986; 6: 138–152.
33. Moore RD, Lerner SA, Levine DP. Nephrotoxicity and ototoxicity of aztreonam versus aminoglycoside therapy in seriously ill non-neutropenic patients. J Infect Dis 1992; 165: 683–688.
34. Jackson GG, Arcieri G. Ototoxicity of gentamicin in man: a survey and controlled analysis of clinical experience in the United States. J Infect Dis 1971; 124(Suppl): S130.
35. Tablan OC, Molagros PR. Renal and auditory toxicity of high-dose, prolonged therapy with gentamicin and tobramycin in *Pseudomonas* endocarditis. J Infect Dis 1984; 149: 257–263.
36. Prazma J. Ototoxity of aminoglycoside antibiotics. In Brown RD, Daigneault EA (eds.), Pharmacology of Hearing: Experimental and Clinical Bases. New York: John Wiley and Sons, Inc., 1981: 154–195.
37. Moore RD, Smith CR, Lietman PS. Risk factors for the development of auditory toxicity in patients receiving aminoglycosides. J Infect Dis 1984; 149: 23–30.
38. Thomsen J, Friis B, Jensen K, Bak-Pedersen K, Kildegard, Larsen P. Tobramycin ototoxicity. Repeated courses of high dosage treatment in children with cystic fibrosis. J Antimicrob Chemother 1979; 5: 257–260.
39. McRorie TI, Bosso J, Randolph L. Aminoglycoside ototoxicity in cystic fibrosis. Am J Dis Child 1989; 143: 1328–1332.

40. Brazil OV, Prado-Francheshi J. The nature of neuromuscular block produced by neomycin and gentamicin. Arch Int Pharmacodyn Ther 1969; 1: 179.
41. L'Hommedieu CS, Nicholas D, Armes DA, Jones P, Nelson T, Pickering LK. Potentiation of magnesium sulfate-induced neuromuscular weakness by gentamicin, tobramycin and amikacin. J Pediatr 1983; 102: 629–631.
42. Scheife RT, Barza M: Aminoglycosides. In: Handbook of Drug Therapy, Miller RP, Greenblatt DG, editors. New York: Elsevier 1979: pp. 84–120.
43. Jensen T, Pedersen SS, Garne S, et al. Colistin inhalation therapy in cystic fibrosis patients with chronic *Pseudomonas aeruginosa* lung infection. J Antimicrob Chemother 1987; 19: 831–838.
44. Bosso JA, Liptak CA, Seiheimer DK, Harrison GM. Toxicity of colistin in cystic fibrosis patients. DICP Ann Pharmacother 1991; 25: 1168–1170.
45. Koch-Weser J, Sidel VW, Federman EB, et al. Adverse effects of sodium colistimethate. Manifestations and specific reaction rates during 317 courses of therapy. Ann Int Med 1970; 72: 857–868.
46. McQuillen MP, Cantor HE, O'Rourke JR. Myasthenic syndrome associated with antibiotics. Arch Neurol 1968; 18: 402–415.
47. Forrence EA, Goldman MP. Vancomycin-associated exfoliative dermatitis. Ann Pharmacother 1990; 24: 369–371.
48. Cunha BA, Ristuccia AM. Clinical usefulness of vancomycin. Clin Pharm 1983; 417–424.
49. Levine JF. Vancomycin: a reveiw. Med Clin North Am 1987; 71: 1135–1145.
50. Dutton AAC, Elmes PC. Vancomycin: report on treatment of patients with severe staphylococcal infections. Brit Med J 1959: 1144–1149.
51. Geraci JE, Heilman FR, Nichols DR, Wellman WE. Antibiotic therapy of bacterial endocarditis VII. Vancomycin for acute micrococcal endocarditis. Staff Meet Mayo Clin 1958; 33: 172–181.
52. Griffiths RS. Vancomycin use – an historical review. J Antimicrob Chem 1984; 14: 1–5 (D).
53. Wang L, Liu C, Wang F, Fung C, Chiu Z, Cheng D. Chromatographically purified vancomycin: therapy of serious infections caused by *Staphylococcus aureus* and other gram-positive bacteria. Clin Ther 1988; 10: 574–584.
54. Bailie GR, Neal D. Vancomycin ototoxicity and nephrotoxicity: a review. Med Toxicol 1988; 3: 376–386.
55. Brummet RE, Fox KE. Vancomycin and erythromycin-induced hearing loss in humans. Antimicrob Ag Chemother 1989; 33: 791–796.
56. Riley HD, Ryan NJ. Treatment of severe staphylococcal infections in infancy and childhood with vancomycin. Antibiot Ann 1960; 908–916.
57. Katz SM, Krueger LJ, Falkner B. Microscopic nephrocalcinosis in cystic fibrosis. N Engl J Med 1988; 319: 263–266.
58. Farber BF, Moellering RC. Retrospective study of the toxicity of preparations of vancomycin from 1974 to 1981. Antimicrob Ag Chem 1983; 23: 138–141.
59. Downs NJ, Neihart RE, Dolezal JM, Hodges GR. Mild nephrotoxicity associated with vancomycin use. Arch Intern Med 1989; 149: 1777–1781.
60. Rybak MJ, Albrecht LM, Boike SC, Chandrasekar PH. Nephrotoxicity of vancomycin, alone and with an aminoglycoside. J Antimicrob Chem 1990; 25: 679–687.
61. Pauly DJ, Musa DM, Lestico MR, Lindstrom MJ, Hetsko CM. Risk of nephrotoxicity with combination vancomycin-aminoglycoside antibiotic therapy. Pharmacother 1990; 10: 378–382.
62. Schaad UB, Nelson JD, McCracken GH. Pharmacology and efficacy of vancomycin for staphylococcal infections in children. Rev Infect Dis 1981; 3: S282–S288 (suppl.).
63. Odio C, McCracken GH, Nelson JD. Nephrotoxicity associated with vancomycin–aminoglycoside therapy in four children. J Pediatr 1984; 105: 491–494.
64. Swinney VR, Rudd CC. Nephrotoxicity of vancomycin–gentamcin therapy in pediatric patients. J Pediatr 1987; 110: 497–498.
65. Nahata MC. Lack of Nephrotoxicity in pediatric patients receiving concurrent vancomycin and aminoglycoside therapy. Chemother 1987; 33: 302–304.
66. Goren MP, Baker DK, Shenep JL. Vancomycin does not enhance amikacin-induced tubular nephrotoxicity in children. Pediatr Infect Dis J 1989; 8: 278–282.

67. Leonard MB, Koren G, Stevenson DK, Prober CG. Vancomycin pharmacokinetics in very low birth weight neonates. Pediatr Infect Dis J 1989; 8: 282–286.
68. Chysky V, Kapila K, Hullman R, Arcieri G, Schacht P, Echols R. Safety of ciprofloxacin in children: worldwide clinical experience based on compassionate use; emphasis on joint evaluation. Infection 1991; 19: 289–296.
69. Douidar SM, Snodgrass WR. Potential role of fluoroquinolones in pediatric infections. Rev Infect Dis 1989; 11: 878–889.
70. Schaad UB. Use of the quinolones in paediatrics. Drugs 1993; 45(3): 37–41.
71. Black A, Redmond AOB, Steen HJ, Oborska IT. Tolerance and safety of ciprofloxacin in paediatric patients. J Antimicrob Chem 1990; 26(F): 25–29.
72. Hooper DC, Wolfson JS. Fluoroquinolone antimicrobial agents. New Engl J Med 1991; 324: 384–394.
73. Isaacson SH, Carr J, Rowan AJ. Ciprofloxacin-induced complex partial status epilepticus manifesting as an acute confusional state. Neurology 1993; 43: 1619–1621.
74. Moshfeghi M, Mandler HD. Ciprofloxacin-induced toxic epidermal necrolysis. Ann Pharmacother 1993; 27: 1467–1469.
75. Walker RC, Wright AJ. The fluoroquinolones. Mayo Clin Proc 1991; 66: 1249–1259.
76. Norrby SR, Lietman PS. Safety and tolerability of fluoroquinolones. Drugs 1993; 45: 59–64 (suppl 3).
77. Hoiby N, Pedersen SS, Jensen T, Valerius NH, Koch C. Fluoroquinolones in the treatment of cystic fibrosis. Drugs 1993; 45(3): 98–101.
78. Kubin R. Safety and efficacy of ciprofloxacin in paediatric patients: review. Infection 1993; 21: 413–421.
79. Phillips BM, David TJ. Pathogenesis and management of arthropathy in cystic fibrosis. J Royal Soc Med 1986; 72(12): 44–50.
80. Wallace CS, Kuhn RJ. Pharmacologic management of cystic fibrosis. Clin Pharm 1993; 12: 657–674.
81. Gentry LO. Antimicrobial activity, pharmacokinetics, therapeutic indications and adverse reactions of ceftazidime. Pharmacother 1985; 5: 254–267.
82. Moellering RC. Ceftazidime: a new broad spectrum cephalosporin. Pediatr Infect Dis J 1985; 4: 390–393.
83. Russo J, Russo ME. Comparative review of two new wide-spectrum penicillins: mezlocillin and piperacillin. Clin Pharm 1982; 1: 207–216.
84. Brodgen RN, Heel RC, Speight TM, Avery GS. Ticarcillin: a review of its pharmacological properties and therapeutic efficacy. Drugs 1980; 20: 325–352.
85. Calandra GB, Brown KR, Grad LC, Ahonkhai VI, Wang C, Aziz MA. Review of adverse experiences and tolerability in the first 2516 patients treated with imipenem/cilastatin. Amer J Med 1985; 78(6A): 73–78.
86. Pastel DA. Imipenem–cilastatin sodium, a broad-spectrum carbapenem antibiotic combination. Clin Pharm 1986; 5: 719–736.
87. Donowitz GR, Mandell GL. Beta-lactam antibiotics. New Engl J Med 1988; 318: 419–426.
88. Chartrand SA. Safety and toxicity profile of aztreonam. Pediatr Infect Dis J. 1989; 8: S120–S123.
89. Kent EK. Penicillin Allergy. Amer J Asthma Allergy 1988; 1: 214–220.
90. Moss RB, Babin S, Hsu YP, Blessing-Moore J, Lewiston NJ. Allergy to semisynthetic penicillins in cystic fibrosis. J Pediatr 1984; 104: 460–466.
91. Koch, C, Hjelt K, Pedersen SS, et al. Retrospective clinical study of hypersensitivity reactions to aztreonam and six other beta-lactam antibiotics in cystic fibrosis patients receiving multiple treatment courses. Rev Infect Dis 1991; 13(7): S608–S611.
92. Donowitz GR, Mandell GL. Beta-lactam antibiotics. New Engl J Med 1988; 318: 490–500.
93. Gustaferro CA, Steckelberg JM. Cephalosporin antimicrobial agents and related compounds. Mayo Clin Proc 1991; 66: 1064–1073.
94. Saxon A, Adelman DC, Patel A, Hajdu R, Calandra GB. Imipenem cross-reactivity with penicillin in humans. J Allergy Clin Immunol 1988; 82: 213–217.
95. Moss RB, McClelland E, Williams RR, Hilman BC, Rubio T, Adkinson NF. Evaluation of the immunologic cross-reactivity of aztreonam in patients with cystic fibrosis who are allergic to penicillin and/or cephalosporin antibiotics. Rev Infect Dis 1991; 13(7): S598–S607.

96. Jensen T, Pedersen SS, Hoiby N, Koch C. Safety of aztreonam in patients with cystic fibrosis and allergy to beta-lactam antibiotics. Rev Infect Dis 1991; 13(7): S594–S597.

97. Sattler FR, Weitekamp MR, Ballard JO. Potential for bleeding with the new beta-lactam antibiotics. Ann Intern Med 1986; 105: 924–931.

98. Barrons RW, Murray KM, Richey RM. Populations at risk for penicillin-induced seizures. Ann Pharmacother 1992; 26: 26–29.

99. Nicholls PJ. Neurotoxicity of penicillin. J Antimicr Chem 1980; 6: 161–172.

100. Kearns GL. Hepatic drug metabolism in cystic fibrosis: recent developments and future directions. Ann Pharmacother 1993; 27: 74–79.

101. de Groot R, Smith AL. Antibiotic pharmacokinetics in cystic fibrosis: differences and clinical significance. Clin Pharmacokinet 1987; 13: 228–253.

102. Spino M. Pharmacokinetics of drugs in cystic fibrosis. Clin Rev Allergy 1991; 9: 169–210.

103. Kearns GL, Reed MD. Clinical pharmacokinetics in infants and children: a reappraisal. Clin Pharmacokinet 1989; 17(1): 29–67.

104. Kearns GL, Trang JM. Introduction to pharmacokinetics: aminoglycosides in cystic fibrosis as a prototype. J Pediatr 1986; 108 (suppl): 847–853.

105. Jacobs RF, Trang JM, Kearns GL, et al. Ticarcillin/clavulanic acid disposition in children with cystic fibrosis. J Pediatr 1985; 106: 1001–1006.

106. Gillum JG, Israel DS, Polk RE. Pharmacokinetic drug interactions with antimicrobial agents. Clin Pharmacokinet 1993; 25: 450–482.

Cystic Fibrosis Pulmonary Infections:
Lessons from Around the World
ed. by A. Bauernfeind, M. I. Marks and B. Strandvik
© 1996 Birkhäuser Verlag Basel/Switzerland

CHAPTER 4
Microbial Resistance

Lisa Saiman and Alice Prince

College of Physicians and Surgeons, Columbia University, New York, NY 10032, USA

Introduction

The availability of effective anti-*Pseudomonas* antibiotics has contributed to the increased longevity for patients with cystic fibrosis. Unfortunately, clinicians and microbiologists caring for CF patients have been all too familiar with the consequences of prolonged courses of antibiotics, that is the selection of multiply resistant organisms within the lungs of these patients. With seeming predictability, *P. aeruginosa* becomes progressively resistant to several classes of antimicrobial agents including β-lactam antibiotics, aminoglycosides, and the fluoroquinolones [1].

The CF Patient Registry's 1992 Annual Report noted that 58% of all American CF patients and 85% of patients 28 years or older are infected with *P. aeruginosa*. In addition to *P. aeruginosa*, other multiply resistant gram-negative organisms may be recovered from CF patients. A small proportion of patients, 2.8%, harbor *Burkholderia* (*Pseudomonas*) cepacia, 1.9% are colonized/infected with *Stenotrophomonas* (*Pseudomonas*) *maltophilia* and 2.3% of patients harbor other *Pseudomonas* species. The prevalence and perhaps the clinical significance of these rarer multiply resistant organisms remains unknown and presents a therepeutic dilemma to CF physicians.

The average life expectancy of CF patients has increased during the past three decades from five years of age to 28 years and it is estimated that a child born with CF today will survive into the fifth decade of life [2, 3]. It is likely that multiply resistant pathogens will be isolated with increasing frequency in the upcoming decade. Thus an understanding of the mechanisms of resistance is critical to optimize antibiotic selection for CF patients.

Mechanisms of Resistance

General Principles

Gram-negative organisms in general and *P. aeruginosa* in particular are successful opportunistic pathogens which develop resistance to antimicrobial agents using a number of different strategies. The organisms may become resistant to an entire class of antibiotics via a single genetic event, they may acquire genes which specifically target a single drug, or a combination of factors may result in clinically significant resistance. There are three basic mechanisms of resistance to the commonly used antimicrobial agents. These include: (1) alteration of permeability, ex. the agent cannot get into the microorganism or is pumped out via an efflux pump; (ii) production of enzymes which destroy the antibiotic or render it inactive or (iii) mutations in the affinity of the target for the antibiotic. The CF lung contains a large population of organisms that are chronically exposed to sub-therapeutic levels of antimicrobials and thus represents an optimal environment for the selection of strains that are resistant to multiple classes of antibiotics.

The structure of Gram-negative organisms presents many impediments to antibiotics prior to reaching their site of action (Figure 1). An antimicrobial agent gains access to *P. aeruginosa* by first traversing the outer cell wall which is composed primarily of lipopolysaccharides. For most agents this is accomplished by entry via porins, water filled channels which are relatively large (mw > 35 000) [4], but usually

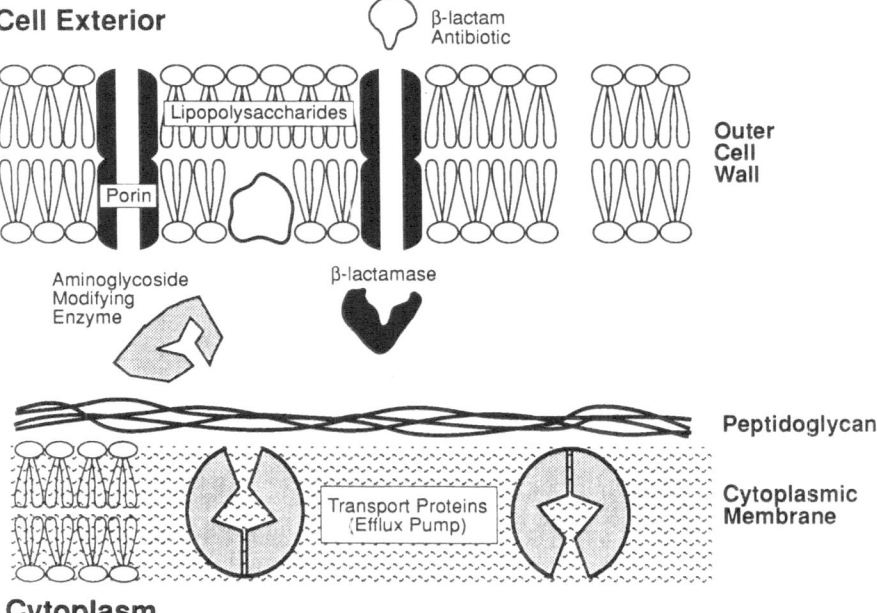

Figure 1. The structure of the cell wall of a Gram-negative organism. The components of the cell wall are shown and includes the outer cell wall with porins, the periplasm with β-lactamases and aminoglycoside modifying enzymes, and the cytoplasmic membrane with efflux pumps.

Table 1. Mechanism of action of the major classes of antibiotics

Antibiotic	Major target	Mechanism
β-lactams		
penicillins	PBP's*	interfere
cephalosporins		with cell wall
monobactams	PBP 3	synthesis
carbapenems	PBP 2	
aminoglycosides	30S ribosomal subunit	interfere with
tetracyclines		protein
		synthesis
fluoroquinolones	DNA gyrase	interfere with
		DNA
		transcription
trimethoprim/	dihydrofolate reductase	inhibition of
sulfamethoxazole	dihydropteroate synthetase	folic acid
		synthesis

*Penicillin binding protein.

closed. Once across the outer membrane, the drug encounters the periplasm where β-lactamases and aminoglycoside modifying enzymes are strategically located to encounter antibiotics as they enter the cell. Drugs which must enter the cytoplasm to reach their site of action must then traverse a second lipid bilayer, the cytoplasmic membrane which may contain transport proteins that function as efflux pumps to remove antimicrobials. The site of action of the major classes of antibiotics is shown in Table 1 and Figure 2.

Resistance to β-Lactam Antibiotics

β-lactam antibiotics, penicillins and cephalosporins, with anti-*Pseudomonas* activity are used widely in CF patients. There has been an increasing variety of agents in this class ranging from carbenicillin produced in the 1960s to piperacillin paired with the β-lactamase inhibitor tazobactam (Zosyn[R]) introduced in 1994 (Figure 2). However with prolonged use of β-lactam antibiotics, resistance can develop secondary to a wide variety of mechanisms.

All *P. aeruginosa* can express a Bush group 1 chromosomal β-lactamase in response to β-lactam antibiotics in clinical usage [5]. Ticarcillin is a weak inducer of β-lactamase, whereas imipenem is a potent inducer of this enzyme [6]. The chromosomal β-lactamase of *P. aeruginosa* primarily has cephalosporinase activity and can hydrolyze the β-lactam ring of first and second generation cephalosporins, although piperacillin

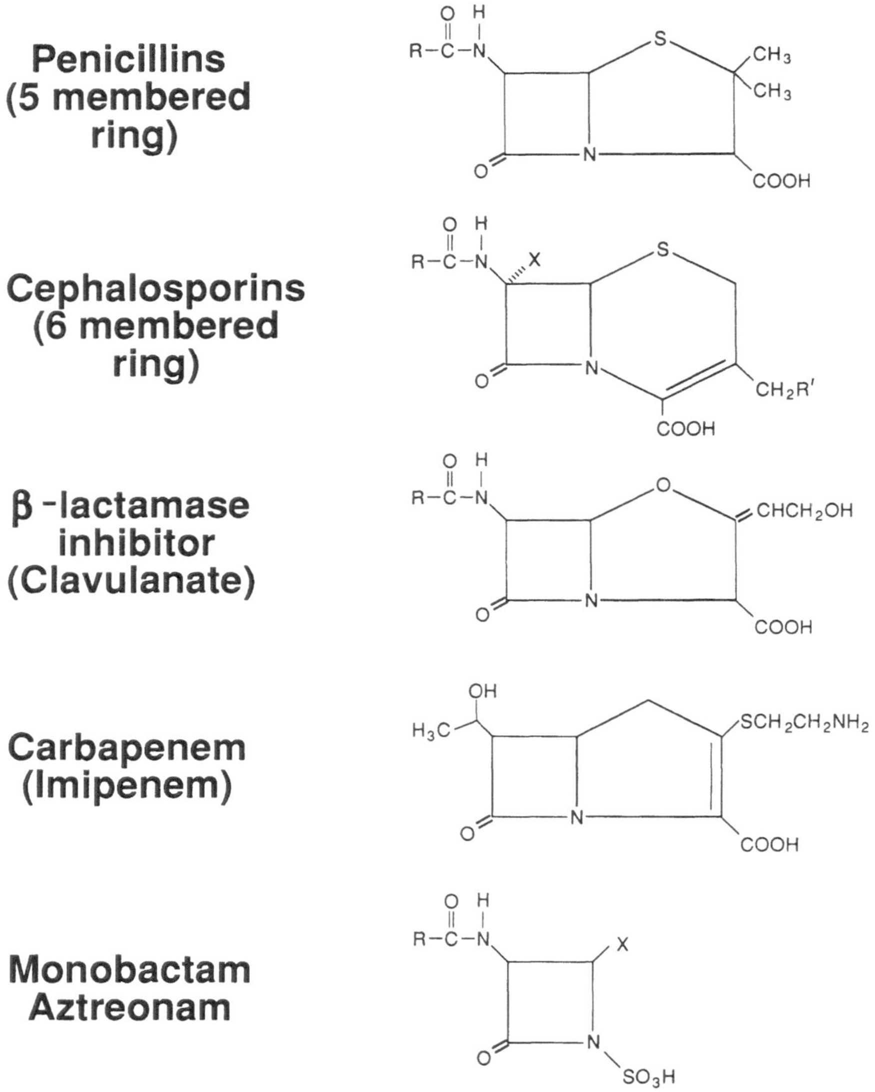
Penicillins (5 membered ring)
Cephalosporins (6 membered ring)
β-lactamase inhibitor (Clavulanate)
Carbapenem (Imipenem)
Monobactam Aztreonam
R–C–N
CH3
COOH
CH2R′
CHCH2OH
H3C
OH
SCH2CH2NH2
SO3H

Figure 2. The chemical structures of β-lactam antibiotics and structurally related compounds. All five compounds have the β-lactam ring in common and vary by the structure of the adjacent ring and side chains. Different antimicrobials have modifications in side chains that occur at sites designated R and X.

can also be destroyed by this enzyme [5]. The carbapenem, imipenem and the monobactam, aztreonam are not hydrolyzed by this β-lactamase [6]. Inducible β-lactamase expression in *P. aeruginosa*, as has been described in other Enterobacteriaceae, is highly regulated and involves several genes [7, 8]. These genes include the structural gene for the

β-lactamase enzyme, *ampC* [9], a sensor–transducer system which promotes β-lactamase expression in response to the presence of β-lactam compounds, as well as positive and negative regulatory elements [10, 11].

Expression of the chromosomal β-lactamase can be constitutive whereby copious amounts of enzyme are produced even in the absence of an antibiotic inducer. Constitutive expression of β-lactamase is thought to be due to mutations in regulatory genes such as *ampD* [11]. In the large population of organisms within the CF lung, mutants with constitutive expression (stable derepression) of β-lactamase production arise spontaneously and with some frequency. Treatment with β-lactam antibiotics can lead to the selection of these stably derepressed mutants which subsequently become the dominant population.

Plasmid mediated β-lactamases have been common in *P. aeruginosa* since the 1970s when reports of the "R" factors responsible for resistance to carbenicillin were first noted. Approximately 20% of multiply resistant *P. aeruginosa* strains isolated from CF patients express plasmid encoded β-lactamases in addition to the chromosomal enzyme (L. Saiman, unpublished data). Now there are over 20 different β-lactamases described and many have extended spectrums of activity with wide substrate profiles. These newer enzymes can hydrolyze third generation cephalosporins such as ceftazidime, cefoperazone and cefsulodin as well as aztreonam and imipenem [12, 13].

The β-lactamase inhibitors have been developed to overcome resistance mediated by the β-lactamases, but these agents appear to have a limited role in the treatment of *Pseudomonas* infection in CF. The chromosomal β-lactamase of *P. aeruginosa* is not inhibited by clavulanate or sulbactam [14]. Thus ticarcillin/clavulanate (Timentin) does not have increased activity against this enzyme when compared to ticarcillin alone. However clavulanate and sulbactam can inhibit some of the plasmid mediated β-lactamases with penicillinase activity. Tazobactam is a newer β-lactamase inhibitor with activity against the *P. aeruginosa* chromosomal β-lactamase and potentially can expand the activity of piperacillin [15]. However tazobactam does not enhance the activity of piperacillin against highly resistant strains of *P. aeruginosa* (L. Saiman, unpublished data), presumably because of either constitutive β-lactamase production or permeability mutations or the combined effect of both mechanisms.

Permeability mutations are very important mechanisms of resistance in *P. aeruginosa* and may be secondary to innate characteristics of the organisms, or may be acquired in response to the selective pressure exerted by antibiotics. *P. aeruginosa* is intrinsically resistant to many β-lactam antibiotics because of the inherent low-permeability of its outer membrane [16]. Organisms may further limit the amount of drug entering the cell by mutations that lead to loss of specific bacterial porins. Resistance to imipenem occurs via this mechanism; loss of porin D2, the channel that imipenem utilizes to traverse the outer membrane of *P. aeruginosa*, is the best described means of acquiring resistance to this carbapenem antimicrobial [17]. Outer membrane impermeability and β-lactamases are frequently present together and appear to mediate additive or even synergistic resistance.

Active efflux of antibiotics is also a potent mechanism of resistance for *Pseudomonas* [16]. Recent work has described a membrane-associated multi-drug transporter that confers resistance to chloramphenicol, tetracycline, β-lactams, and fluoroquinolones [18]. It is possible that this mechanism is responsible for a large part of the intrinsic resistance of *P. aeruginosa* and works in concert with the lack of permeability of the outer membrane [18].

The targets for the action of β-lactam antibiotics are penicillin binding proteins which are enzymes that are involved with cell wall biosynthesis. The penicillin binding proteins may mutate to generate resistance by developing decreased affinity for β-lactam antibiotics. It is not known how frequently this mechanism of resistance occurs in clinical isolates obtained from CF patients.

Resistance to Aminoglycosides by P. aeruginosa

Aminoglycoside uptake by microorganisms is complex and occurs in two steps. These antibiotics must traverse both the outer cell wall as well as the lipid bilayer of the cytoplasmic membrane to reach their targets on the bacterial ribosome. An initial passive energy-independent step begins the process as ionic binding of the cationic aminoglycoside to the negatively charged lipopolysaccharides causes displacement of the cations Ca^{2+} and Mg^{2+} [19]. This disrupts the stability of the outer membrane and facilitates further entry of aminoglycoside molecules across the cytoplasmic membrane. Subsequent transport of the drug across the cytoplasmic membrane is an energy-dependent process and is thought to involve an anionic transporter. The aminoglycosides are then transferred from the cytoplasmic transporter to specific binding sites on the ribosomes.

Mutations that lead to permeability changes, also called accumulation-deficiency mutants, appear to be common among isolates from CF patients [20]. Approximately two-thirds of the multiply resistant clinical CF isolates studied expressed permeability mutations. The mechanism by which decreased uptake occurs is not understood as these mutants do not demonstrate detectable changes in outer membrane proteins or lipopolysaccharides.

Resistance to aminoglycoside antibiotics also occurs by acquisition of aminoglycoside modifying enzymes [19, 21, 22]. These plasmid mediated enzymes modify and inactivate the aminoglycoside molecules. These enzymes are encoded by transposons which facilitate their dissemination among Gram-negative organisms. The nomenclature of the aminoglycoside modifying enzymes describes the biochemical reaction (N-acetylation, O-nucleotidylation, or O-phosphorylation, Figure 3) and the molecular site on the aminoglycoside where the enzymatic modification occurs. In general *P. aeruginosa* preferentially acquires specific enzymes which include: APH(3')-I and APH(3')-III which inactivate kanamycin and kanamycin/amikacin respectively; AAC(3)-I and AAC(3)-III, IV, V which inactivate gentamicin and tobramycin; and AAC(6') which inactivates kanamycin and tobramycin [20, 23, 24]. Among *P. aeruginosa* isolates obtained from CF patients AAC(3)-I and AAC (6') are the most common aminoglycoside modifying enzymes [20]. The former confers conventional low level resistance to tobramycin (MICs less than 16 μg/ml) and the latter enzyme leads to high level resistance (MICs greater than 100 μg/ml) (L. Saiman, unpublished data).

The biochemical modification of these agents has two consequences. The altered aminoglycoside does not bind avidly to the ribosome and therefore fails to terminate protein synthesis. In addition, unlike the modified compound, the structurally altered agent fails to induce the entry of further aminoglycoside molecules across the cytoplasmic membrane.

Resistance due to mutations at the target of aminoglycoside action, the ribosome, may also occur. However this is probably a less significant mechanism among strains of *P. aeruginosa*.

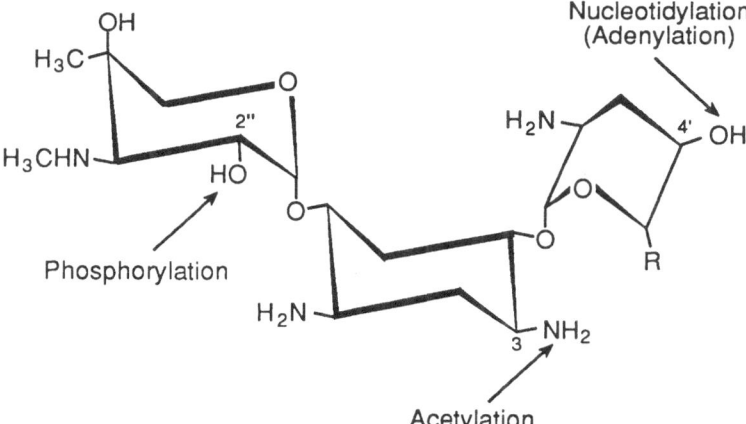

Figure 3. The basic structure of an aminoglycoside. The three 6-membered carbon rings are shown. The activity of an aminoglycoside depends on the position of the –OH and –NH₂ groups and modifications in side chains. Aminoglycosides modifying enzymes can acetylate, adenylate, or phosphorylate the aminoglycoside molecules. Examples of the sites of enzymatic action are shown.

Adaptive resistance to aminoglycosides has also been described. Down-regulation of aminoglycoside uptake occurs in the *P. aeruginosa* that survive in the continuing presence of aminoglycosides [25]. This phenomenon is unstable and reverses when the aminoglycoside is removed. The mechanism by which this down-regulated uptake occurs is unknown, but changes in lipopolysaccharides, loss of a transport protein, or a collapse in electrical potential driving aminoglycoside uptake have been offered as possible explanations.

Finally "functional" resistance to aminoglycosides can occur whereby the activity of the antibiotic is impaired due to specific biologic conditions present in the host [26]. The CF lung possesses many of these biologic conditions which include an anaerobic environment, high ionic concentrations, an acid pH, and inflammatory exudate which may bind the aminoglycoside. Thus despite the potential *in vitro* susceptibility of *P. aeruginosa* to aminoglycosides, the activity of these agents may be substantially reduced in the environment of the CF lung.

Resistance to Fluoroquinolones by *P. aeruginosa*

With the introduction of fluoroquinolone antibiotics, there is finally an effective oral anti-*Pseudomonas* agent. These agents have been in wide clinical use since the mid 1980s. While resistance to ciprofloxacin was described early on, it appears to be less frequent than resistance to the β-lactam agents and the aminoglycosides. Among a collection of multi-resistant *P. aeruginosa* strains from patients with CF, only about 25% are resistant to ciprofloxacin, despite widespread use of this agent (L. Saiman, unpublished data). The reasons for this observation are unclear, but reversion to a susceptible phenotype can occur with some frequency among CF patients when the fluoroquinolone is discontinued [26]. The clinical benefit is obvious as these agents can be utilized for future treatment. Resistance to one of the fluoroquinolone confers resistance to other drugs in this class. Thus there is no advantage in treating a patient with another quinolone if their organism is resistant to ciprofloxacin.

There are two major mechanisms of resistance to quinolones: mutations at the site of action and decreased access of these agents to the cytoplasm. The target of action of the fluoroquinolones in DNA gyrase, the enzyme responsible for nicking and uncoiling the DNA superhelix which allows transcription to occur. Mutations in DNA gyrase occur in *P. aeruginosa* and mutations in the *gyrA* subunit are far more common than mutations in *gyrB* subunit [27, 28].

Decreased access of fluoroquinolones to the gyrase target also occurs with some frequency in *P. aeruginosa* isolated from CF patients [27, 29]. The mechanism of decreased antimicrobial entry is still under investiga-

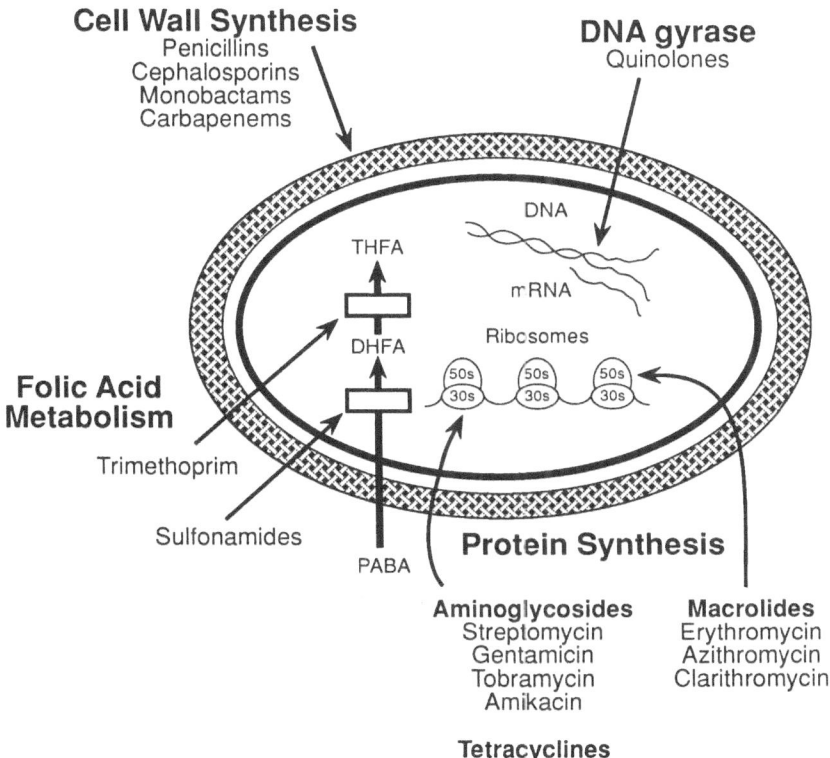

Cell Wall Synthesis
Penicillins
Cephalosporins
Monobactams
Carbapenems

DNA gyrase
Quinolones

DNA

THFA

mRNA

DHFA

Ribosomes

**Folic Acid
Metabolism**

Trimethoprim

Sulfonamides

PABA

Protein Synthesis

Aminoglycosides
Streptomycin
Gentamicin
Tobramycin
Amikacin

Macrolides
Erythromycin
Azithromycin
Clarithromycin

Tetracyclines

Figure 4. The sites of action of the anti-*Pseudomonas* antibiotics. The major targets of the classes of antibiotics with activity against *P. aeruginosa*, *B. cepacia*, and *X. maltophilia* are shown.

tion and most likely is secondary to several mechanisms. It has been suggested that loss of the outer membrane porin F leads to resistance to ciprofloxacin [30]. Approximately 14% of CF clinical isolates that are resistant to ciprofloxacin lack OmpF [31]. However decreased permeability has been shown to occur in the absence of detectable quantitative changes in outer membrane proteins suggesting that alterations in lipopolysaccharides may lead to decreased drug entry [29]. Most recently a chromosomally encoded efflux pump which normally functions to transport siderophore out of the organism has been shown to confer resistance to several classes of antimicrobials including the fluoroquinolones, tetracycline, chloramphenicol and β-lactam antibiotics [18]. It is likely that this mechanism is responsible for resistance to fluoroquinolones in a proportion of the clinical isolates from CF patients infected with multiply drug resistant strains.

Enzymatic modification of the fluoroquinolones by bacteria has not been shown as yet.

Resistance by Burkholderia cepacia

B. cepacia is more inherently resistant than *P. aeruginosa*. Among drugs that have been shown to be initially clinically useful are trimethoprim/sulfamethoxazole, chloramphenicol, and ciprofloxacin. β-lactam antibiotics are also occasionally useful. However, susceptible strains readily develop resistance and therapeutic options for CF patients infected with this pathogen are very limited.

Much of the resistance of *B. cepacia* is due to its intrinsic low outer membrane permeability [32]. In addition there appears to be expression of a drug efflux system similar to that of *P. aeruginosa* (J. Burns, personal communication). This efflux mechanism may also account for non-enzymatic resistance to chloramphenicol also observed in *B. cepacia*. Intrinsic resistance also confers resistance to aminoglycosides in that these agents cannot bind to the cationic sites on the lipopolysaccharides of *B. cepacia* [33].

In addition, *B. cepacia* is an organism of tremendous metabolic diversity and thus able to withstand further changes in its permeability due to porin loss. Decreased permeability via porin loss confers resistance to many classes of antibiotics. Loss of an outer membrane protein (27 000 mw) is associated with high levels of resistance to β-lactam agents [34].

B. capacia has two inducible chromosomal β-lactamases, both a cephalosporinase and a penicillinase [35]. The penicillinase, PenA has homology with the chromosomal β-lactamase of *P. aeruginosa* and is regulated by the transcriptional activator AmpR in a similar manner to other Enterobacteriaceae [36].

Many *B. cepacia* are initially susceptible to trimethoprim/sulfamethoxazole, but resistance frequently develops during treatment. It has been demonstrated that high level resistance to these agents is associated with production of a trimethoprim-resistant dihydrofolate reductase [37]. Thus this target enzyme is not inhibited by the antimicrobial trimethoprim.

There has been a great deal of interest in the development of antimicrobial agents with good activity against multiply drug resistant pathogens such as *B. cepacia*. New broad spectrum fluoroquinolones such as sparfloxacin [38] and clinafloxacin [39] and the carbapenem, meropenem appear to have more *in vitro* activity against *B. capacia* than ciprofloxacin and imipenem, respectively. However the clinical utility of these agents against multiply resistant pathogens may be limited as the microorganisms exhibit such a wide variety of resistance mechanisms and the ability to acquire foreign genes.

Resistance by X. maltophilia

Stenotrophomonas (Xanthomonas) maltophilia, previously known as *Pseudomonas maltophilia*, is generally a nosocomial pathogen isolated from immunocompromised patients as well as from hospital environmental surfaces such as sink drains and respirators [40]. *X. maltophilia* has been an increasingly common isolate from clinical specimens, including the sputum of CF patients, but its clinical relevance in CF remains unknown. *In vitro* susceptibility of 130 clinical isolates revealed that the most active compounds were minocycline, trimethoprim/sulfamethoxazole, and ticarcillin/clavulanate [41]. *X. maltophilia* are variably susceptible to ofloxacin and ciprofloxacin, and investigational quinolones appear to have good activity against this pathogen [38, 39]. Ceftazidime has poor activity against *X. maltophilia*.

Like *B. cepacia*, *X. maltophilia* is highly resistant to many antibiotics. This organism is inherently resistant to imipemen due to a combination of low permeability and hydrolysis by a β-lactamase [42, 43]. *X. maltophilia* expresses two inducible chromosomal β-lactamases, L1 and L2. L1 is a zinc-metaloenzyme which hydrolyses imipenem and meropenem. L2 is a cephalosporinase inhibited by clavulanate and sulbactam. There appears to be heterogeneity among the β-lactamases of clinical isolates as well [44].

Outer membrane proteins from quinolone resistant *X. maltophilia* display several distinct changes [45]. Alterations in drug entry has been hypothesized to account for resistance and some of the mutations not only conferred resistance to quinolones, but also lead to cross-resistance to chloramphenicol and frequently to doxycycline. It is possible that a multi-drug resistant efflux pump exists for this pathogen as well, but such studies have not been performed.

Post-antibiotic effect

A post-antibiotic effect occurs when, after an exposure to an antimicrobial agent, there is suppression of bacterial growth when the antibiotic is no longer detectable. A post-antibiotic effect for the anti-*Pseudomonas* antibiotics ceftazidime, ciprofloxacin, imipenem, piperacillin, and tobramycin has been noted among both susceptible and resistant *B. cepacia* isolated from cystic fibrosis patients [46]. The precise mechanism by which antimicrobial agents exert a post-antibiotic effect is not known nor is the clinical relevance of such an effect understood, but this effect may partially explain clinical improvement while on antibiotics to which the organisms are reportedly resistant.

Conclusion

Organisms isolated from CF patients have high levels of intrinsic resistance as well as acquired resistance to antimicrobial agents, due to a number of diverse genetic events. Decreased access of antibiotics to their target sites is an important mechanism of resistance which can occur as a result of inherently low permeability, further loss of porins, or expression of an active efflux pump. An efflux pump can confer resistance to several classes of antimicrobial agents including β-lactams, chloramphenicol, tetracycline, and fluoroquinolones and therefore can increase the potential development of multi-drug resistance. Decreased permeability, in combination with the strategically located β-lactamases and aminoglycoside modifying enzymes, provide an effective defense against much of the available therapeutic armamentarium. Pseudomonas frequently acquire new resistance genes and this contributes to the dissemination of resistance in CF pathogens. The growing diversity of plasmid encoded β-lactamases and aminoglycoside modifying enzymes will further limit the utility of the anti-*Pseudomonas* cephalosporin, ceftazidime as well as newer agents such as aztreonam and imipenem. Finally the unique environment of the CF lung no doubt contributes to resistance by providing a conducive environment for the persistence and selection of multi-resistant organisms.

References

1. Bosso JA, Allen JE, Matsen JM. Changing susceptibility of *Pseudomonas aeruginosa* isolates from cystic fibrosis patients with the clinical use of newer antibiotics. Antimicrob Agents Chemother 1989; 33: 526-8.
2. FitzSimmons SC. The changing epidemiology of cystic fibrosis. J Pediatr 1993; 122: 1-9.
3. Collins FS. Cystic fibrosis: molecular biology and therapeutic implications. Science 1992; 256: 774-9.
4. Nikaido H. Porins and specific channels of bacterial outer membranes. Mol Microbiol 1992; 6: 435-42.
5. Lindberg F, Normark S. Contribution of chromosomal β-lactamases to β-lactam resistance. Rev Inf Dis 1988; 8: S292-304.
6. Kropp H, Gerckens L, Sundelof JG, Kahan FM. Antibacterial activity of imipenem: the first thienamycin antibiotic. Rev Inf Dis 1985; 7: S389-410.
7. Lindberg F, Normark S. Common mechanism of *ampC* β-lactamase induction in enterobacteria: regulation of the cloned *Enterobacter cloacae* P99 β-lactamase gene. J Bacteriol 1987; 169: 758-63.
8. Lindquist S, Galleni M, Lindberg F, Normark S. Signalling proteins in enterobacterial AmpC β-lactamase expression. Mol Microbiol 1989; 3: 1091-1102.
9. Lodge JM, Michin SD, Piddock LJV, Busby SJ. Cloning, sequencing, and analysis of the structural gene and regulatory region of the *Pseudomonas aeruginosa* chromosomal *ampC* β-lactamase. Biochem J 1990; 272: 627-31.
10. Lindquist S, Lindberg F, Normark S. Binding of the *Citrobacter freundii* AmpR regulator to a single DNA site provides both autoregulation and activation of the inducible *ampC* β-lactamase gene. J Bacteriol 1989; 171: 3746-53.
11. Tuomanen E, Lindquist S, Sande S, Galleni M, Light K, Gage D, Normark S. Coordinate regulation of β-lactamase induction and peptidoglycan composition by the amp operon. Science 1991; 251: 201-4.
12. Sanders CC. β-lactamases of gram-negative bacteria: new challenges for new drugs. Clin Inf Dis 1992; 14: 1089-99.
13. Nordmann P, Naas T. Sequence analysis of PER-1 extended-spectrum β-lactamase from *Pseudomonas aeruginosa* and comparison with class A β-lactamases. Antimicrob Agents Chemother 1994; 38: 104-14.

14. Cullman W. Interaction of β-lactamase inhibitors with various β-lactamases. Chemother 1990; 36: 200–8.
15. Bush K, Macalintal C, Rasmussen BA, Lee VJ, Yang Y. Kinetic interactions of tazobactam with β-lactamases from all major structural classes. Antimicrob Agents Chemother 1993; 37: 851–8.
16. Nikaido H. Prevention of drug access to bacterial targets: permeability barriers and active efflux. Science 1994; 264: 382–7.
17. Quinn JP, Dudek EJ, DiVincenzo CA, Lucks DA, Lerner SA. Emergence of resistance to imipenem during therapy for *Pseudomonas aeruginosa* infections. J Infect Dis 1986; 154: 289–94.
18. Pooke K, Krebes K, McNally C, Neshat S. Multiple antibiotic resistance in *Pseudomonas aeruginosa*: evidence for involvement of an efflux operon. J Bacteriol 1993; 175: 7363–72.
19. Bryan LE. Aminoglycoside resistance. In: LE Bryan, editor. Antimicrobial drug resistance. Orlando: Academic Press, 1984: 242–77.
20. Saiman L, Niu WW, New HC, Prince A. Antibiotic strategies to treat multi-resistant *Pseudomonas aeruginosa*. Pediatr Pulm 1992; S8: 286–7.
21. Shaw KJ, Cramer CA, Rizzio M, et al. Isolation, characterization, and DNA sequence analysis of an AAC(6')-II gene from *Pseudomonas aeruginosa*. Antimicrob Agents Chemother 1989; 33: 2052–62.
22. Davies JE. Resistance to aminoglycosides: mechanisms and frequency. Rev Infect Dis 1983; 5: 1324–8.
23. Shimizu K, Kumada T, Hsieh WC, et al. Comparison of aminoglycoside resistance patterns in Japan, Formosa and Korea, Chile and the United States. Antimicrob Agents Chemother 1985; 28: 282–8.
24. Shaw KJ, Hare RS, Sabatelli FJ, et al. Correlation between aminoglycoside resistance profiles and DNA hybridization of clinical isolates. Antimicrob Agents Chemother 1991; 35: 2253–61.
25. Daikos GL, Jackson GG, Lolans VT, Livermore DM. Adaptive resistance to aminoglycoside antibiotics from first-exposure down-regulation. J Infect Dis 1990; 162: 414–20.
26. Diver JM, Schollaardt T, Rabin HR, Thorson C, Bryan LE. Persistence mechanisms in *Pseudomonas aeruginosa* from cystic fibrosis patients undergoing ciprofloxacin therapy. Antimicrob Agents Chemother 1991; 35: 1538–46.
27. Wolfson JS, Hooper DC. Bacterial resistance to quinolones: mechanisms and clinical importance. Rev Infect Dis 1989; 11: S960–8.
28. Inoue Y, Sato K, Fujji T, et al. Some properties of subunits of DNA gyrase from *Pseudomonas aeruginosa* PAO1 and its nalidixic acid-resistant mutant. J Bacteriol 1989; 169: 2322–5.
29. Kaatz GW, Seo SM. Mechanisms of ciprofloxacin resistance in *Pseudomonas aeruginosa*. J Infect Dis 1988; 158: 537–41.
30. Daikos GL, Lolans VT, Jackson GG. Alterations in outer membrane proteins of *Pseudomonas aeruginosa* associated with selective resistance to quinolones. Antimicrob Agents Chemother 1988; 32: 785–787.
31. Saiman L, Niu WW, Neu HC, Prince A. Omp F expression and susceptibility to fluoroquinolones in multi-resistant *Pseudomonas aeruginosa*. Proceedings of the 33rd Interscience Conference on Antimicrobial Agents and Chemotherapy; 1993 Oct 17–20; New Orleans (LA).
32. Parr TR, Moore RA, Moore LV, Hancock REW. Role of porins in intrinsic antibiotic resistance of *Pseudomonas cepacia*. Antimicrob Agents Chemother 1987; 31: 121–3.
33. Moore RA, Hancock REW. Involvement of outer membrane *Pseudomonas cepacia* in aminoglycoside and polymyxin resistance. Antimicrob Agents Chemother 1986; 30: 923–6.
34. Aronoff SC. Outer membrane permeability in *Pseudomonas cepacia*: diminished porin content in a β-lactam-resistant mutant and in resistant cystic fibrosis isolates. Antimicrob Agents Chemother 1988; 32: 1636–1639.
35. Beckman W and Lessie TG. Response of *Pseudomonas cepacia* to antibiotics: utilization of penicillin G as the carbon source. J Bacteriol 1979; 140: 1126–8.
36. Proenca R, Niu WW, Cacalano G, Prince A. The *Pseudomonas cepacia* 249 chromosomal penicillinase is a member of the AmpC family of chromosomal β-lactamases. Antimicrob Agents Chemother 1993; 37: 667–74.

37. Burns JL, Lien DM, Hedin LA. Isolation and characterization of dihydrofolate reductase from trimethoprim-susceptible and trimethoprim-resistant *Pseudomonas cepacia*. Antimicrob Agents Chemother 1989; 33 1247–51.
38. Louie A, Baltch AL, Ritz WJ, Smith RP. Comparative in-vitro susceptibilities of *Pseudomonas aeruginosa*, *Xanthomonas maltophilia*, and *Pseudomonas* spp. to sparfloxacin (C1-978, AT-4140, PD131501) and reference antimicrobial agents. J Antimicrob Chemother 1991; 27: 793–9.
39. Ford AS, Baltch AL, Smith RP, Ritz W. *In vitro* susceptibilities of *Pseudomonas aeruginosa* and *Pseudomonas* spp. to the new fluoroquinolone clinafloxacin and PD 131628 and nine other antimicrobial agents. J Antimicrob Chemother 1993; 31: 523–32.
40. Khardori N, Elting L, Wong E, Schable B, Bodey GP. Nosocomial infections due to *Xanthomonas maltophilia (Pseudomonas maltophilia)* in patients with cancer. Rev Infect Dis 1990; 12: 997–1003.
41. Vartivarian S, Anaissie E, Bodey G, Sprigg, Rolston K. A changing pattern of susceptibility of *Xanthomonas maltophilia* to antimicrobial agents: implications for therapy. Antimicrob Agents Chemother 1994; 38: 624–7.
42. Saino Y, Kobayashi F, Inoue M, Mitsushashi S. Purification and properties inducible penicillin β-lactamase isolated from *Pseudomonas maltophilia*. Antimicrob Agents Chemotherap 1982; 22: 564–70.
43. Akova M, Bonfiglio G, Livermore DM. Susceptibility to β-lactam antibiotics of mutant strains of *Xanthomonas maltophilia* with high and low-level constitutive expression of L1 and L2 β-lactamases. J Med Microbiol 1991; 35: 208–213.
44. Payne DJ, Cramp R, Bateson J, Clarke G, Knowles DJC. Detection of metallo and serine β-lactamases from *Xanthomonas maltophilia*. Proceedings of the 33rd Interscience Conference on Antimicrobial Agents and Chemotherapy; 1993 Oct 17–20; New Orleans (LA).
45. Lecso-Bornet M, Pierre J, Sarkis-Karam D, Lubera S, and Bergogne-Berezin. Susceptibility to *Xanthomonas maltophilia* to six quinolones and study of outer membrane proteins in resistant mutants selected *in vitro*. Antimicrob Agents Chemother 1992; 36: 669–71.
46. Kumar S, Hay MB, Maier GA, Dyke JW. Post-antibiotic effect of ceftazidime, ciprofloxacin, imipenem, piperacillin and tobramycin for *Pseudomonas cepacia*. J Antimicrob Chemother 1992; 30: 597–602.

Cystic Fibrosis Pulmonary Infections:
Lessons from Around the World
ed. by A. Bauernfeind, M. I. Marks and B. Strandvik
© 1996 Birkhäuser Verlag Basel/Switzerland

CHAPTER 5
Microbial Virulence and Pathogenesis in Cystic Fibrosis

Eshwar Mahenthiralingam[1] and David P. Speert[1,2]

[1]Division of Infectious and Immunological Diseases, Department of Paediatrics and
the Canadian Bacterial Disease Network, University of British Columbia, Vancouver, Canada
[2]Department of Microbiology and Immunology, University of British Columbia, Vancouver,
Canada V5Z 4H4

Introduction

The abnormal airway conditions in patients with cystic fibrosis (CF) predisposes them to pulmonary infection with a number of bacterial species including *Staphylococcus aureus*, *Haemophilus influenzae*, *Pseudomonas aeruginosa*, *Pseudomonas cepacia*, *Xanthomonas* species and various non-tuberculous mycobacteria. Patients with CF may initially become infected with a number of bacterial species including *S. aureus* [1] and *H. influenzae* [2], however *Pseudomonas aeruginosa* is the principal respiratory tract pathogen leading to chronic infection in these patients [3]. Once CF patients are colonized with *P. aeruginosa*, the organism is rarely eradicated. Another species, *Pseudomonas cepacia*, is an evolving pathogen in CF infection [4, 5]; its resistance to many antibiotics, enhanced virulence in certain CF patients [6] and the capacity to spread from patient to patient [7] have introduced a new set of problems to CF caregivers.

A unifying explanation of why patients with CF are prone to lung infection with *P. aeruginosa* has not yet been provided, but several underlying mechanisms have been postulated in the literature. It has been suggested that tissue damage due to *S. aureus* infection in young CF patients may "prime" the lung for subsequent infection with *P. aeruginosa* [8] and although there is no direct evidence for this theory, *in vitro* experiments have shown that *P. aeruginosa* has a high avidity for damaged epithelial tissues [9]. Enhanced adhesion of *P. aeruginosa* to CF buccal epithelial cells (BEC) has been observed *in vitro* [10, 11] and increased numbers of receptors to which *P. aeruginosa* is able to

Correspondence address: Dr. Eshwar Mahenthiralingam & Dr. David P. Speert, Rm. 304, Research Centre, 950 West 28th Avenue, Vancouver, B.C., V5Z 4H4 Canada.

bind have been found on cultured CF nasal polyp cells [12] suggesting that *P. aeruginosa* has a propensity to colonize CF cell surfaces. The altered viscosity and "stickiness" of the respiratory mucus in CF may also create an ideal environment for *P. aeruginosa* colonization; the organism is highly mucinophilic [13] and is able to adhere *in vitro* to respiratory mucins [14].

Data from our laboratory suggest that the predilection for *P. aeruginosa* to colonize the CF lung may also be due to the unique dependency on the presence of glucose for efficient nonopsonic phagocytosis of the organism by macrophages [15]. Glucose is present in low concentrations in bronchial fluids [16] and macrophage-mediated clearance of *P. aeruginosa* from the lung may be limited as a result; this factor, together with the defective mucociliary clearance in CF [17], may be sufficient to allow colonization of the respiratory airway with *P. aeruginosa*.

Perhaps the success of *P. aeruginosa* as a pathogen in CF is due to a combination of host and bacterial factors described above. *P. aeruginosa* is tremendously versatile, enabling it to survive in a wide range of

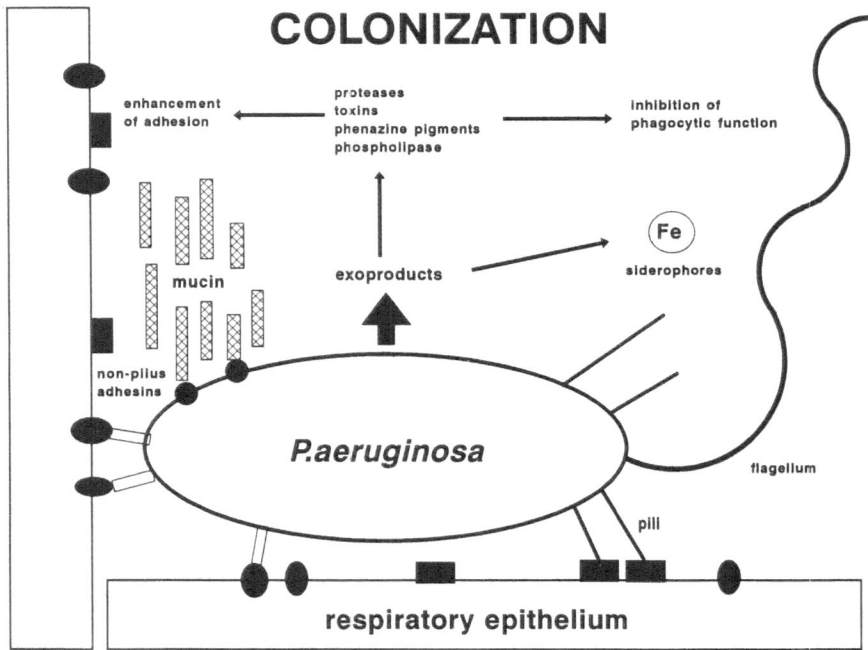

Figure 1. Diagrammatic illustration of *P. aeruginosa* virulence factors thought to be important for the establishment of respiratory infection in CF. Pili and non-pilus adhesins mediate binding to the respiratory epithelium. Non-pilus adhesins may also enable entrapment in the mucous secretions. Motility and chemotaxis towards mucin may aid the establishment of infection. *P. aeruginosa* also secretes a number of exoproducts which may (i) enhance adhesion by exposing sites to which the organism may bind and (ii) impair phagocytic cell function and aid colonization of the respiratory airway in CF.

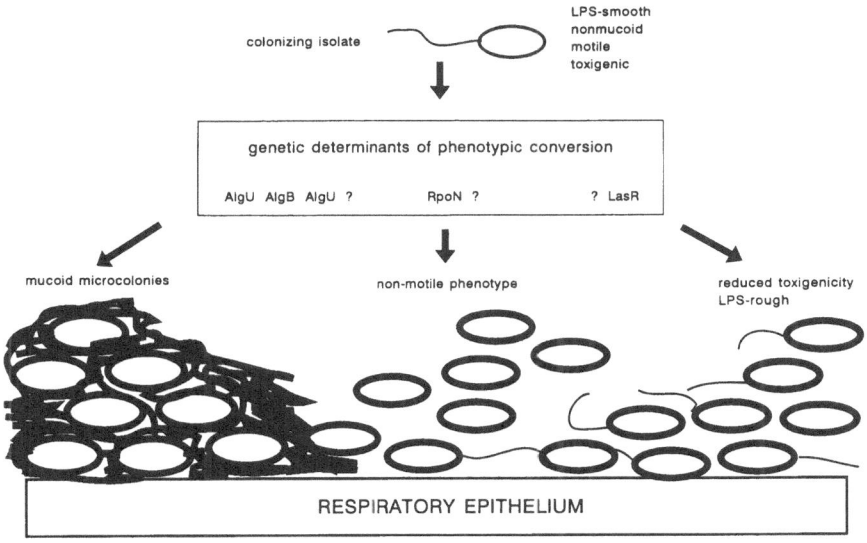

Figure 2. Diagrammatic illustration of the phenotypic conversion of *P. aeruginosa* during chronic colonization in CF. *P. aeruginosa* from chronic colonization are often LPS-rough, mucoid, non-motile and generally less toxigenic. Some of the genetic determinants implicated in facilitating these phenotypic changes are outlined.

environments and the CF lung unfortunately appears an ideal niche for its persistence. During the last decade, investigation of microbial pathogenesis in CF has focused on the mechanisms by which *P. aeruginosa* may cause infection in CF. Many *P. aeruginosa* virulence factors have been proposed to play a role in pathogenesis during CF infection, including mucoid exopolysaccharide (MEP), lipopolysaccharide (LPS), pili, exotoxins, proteases, lipases, siderophores and phenazine pigments. *P. aeruginosa* must be able to initially colonize the host and subsequently evade clearance by host defense mechanisms in order for successful chronic colonization. Our review will focus only on the salient virulence factors which have been implicated to play a role in (i) colonization of the respiratory airway (summarized in Figure 1) and (ii) survival of the organism during chronic infection (outlined in Figure 2). A brief discussion of our current knowledge of *P. cepacia* pathogenesis will also be provided in view of the emergence of this organism as a serious clinical problem in CF during the last decade.

P. aeruginosa: Adherence and Colonization Factors

The initial step of *P. aeruginosa* respiratory infection is thought to be adherence to the mucosal epithelial surface of the oropharynx. Binding of *P. aeruginosa* to surfaces has been studied using cultured epithelial cells, mucin binding models and animal models, resulting in several *P. aeruginosa* adhesions being characterized. Flagellar-mediated motility is also important for establishing contact between cell surfaces and infecting bacteria and for promoting the spread of infection. Adhesion-promoting and other determinants of *P. aeruginosa* that appear critical for establishing colonization are illustrated diagrammatically in Figure 1 and are discussed below in more detail.

Pili

Pili are perhaps the best characterized of all the *P. aeruginosa* adhesions. The polar pili of *P. aeruginosa* are filaments, approximately 2500 nm in length [18], composed of a single protein subunit, pilin, which generally has a molecular size of 15 kDa [19]. The structural genes of several *P. aeruginosa* pilins have now been cloned [20, 21, 22]. *P. aeruginosa* pili appear to mediate adherence to a number of respiratory cell types *in vitro*. Early studies indicated that *P. aeruginosa* used pili to bind to mammalian buccal epithelial cells *in vitro* [23] and that depletion of fibronectin from the surface of cells, a phenomenon associated with CF epithelia, may provide an explanation for the enhanced binding of *P. aeruginosa* to the respiratory tract of CF patients [11]. Acid-injured mouse tracheal epithelial cells (TEC; [24] and hamster TEC [25] have also been used as models for pilus-mediated adhesion in CF).

Recently, the use of genetically engineered strains of *P. aeruginosa* that lack only surface pili have clearly demonstrated that these structures are important for attachment to respiratory epithelial cells [26, 27]. Chi *et al.* [27] also demonstrated that *P. aeruginosa* strain PAK may invade and survive within cultured pneumocyte carcinoma cells in a pilus-dependent fashion, while internalized non-piliated mutants were rapidly killed by these epithelial cells, suggesting that pili may interfere with cellular killing mechanisms following endocytosis. However, the significance of this cellular invasion *in vivo* is uncertain since there have been no reports of intracellular bacteria in the respiratory tissues of chronically colonized CF patients.

A murine model of chronic mucosal colonization was used [28] to examine the role of *P. aeruginosa* colonization factors, including pili and flagella, whose expression is dependent on the alternate sigma factor of the RNA polymerase encoded by the *rpoN* gene (see section on motility and adhesion factors under the control of *RpoN* and [29]). Isogenic mutants of *P. aeruginosa* strain PAK which were pilin-deficient and *rponN*-deficient colonized the gastric mucosa of the experimental mice at 1–10% of the level of the parental wild-type strains, indicating the importance of pili and non-pilus adhesions (see next section) in mucosal colonization. Whether this gastrointestinal colonization model is relevant to respiratory colonization in CF is uncertain; however, these *in vivo* findings are consistent with data from *in vitro* experiments which have examined the role of these virulence factors in adherence of *P. aeruginosa* to mucins and respiratory epithelial cells [26, 27, 30, 31, 32].

Other studies have demonstrated that purified pili may competitively inhibit the attachment of *P. aeruginosa* to human respiratory epithelial cells and that the receptors blocked by individual pili are the same as those that mediate binding of the whole bacterium [33]. It has been shown that the C-terminal fragment of *P. aeruginosa* PAK pilin and synthetic peptides spanning this region can bind specifically to human epithelial cells, suggesting that the pilus binding adhesin lies within this region [34]. Monoclonal antibodies directed against epitopes in the C-terminal region of pilin block the adhesion of PAK to BEC [35], raising the possibility that vaccines able to prevent *P. aeruginosa* adherence may be developed.

Non-Pilus Adhesins

While pili on the surface of *P. aeruginosa* have been shown to be important mediators of attachment to epithelial cells, recent studies using pilin-deficient genetic mutants of *P. aeruginosa* have shown that pili play a minimal role in the attachment of bacteria to mucin [30]. Moreover, mutants of *P. aeruginosa* carrying a mutation in the regulatory gene, *rpoN*, and hence not expressing pili [29] are unable to bind to both mucins and epithelial cells [26, 27, 30] suggesting that *P. aeruginosa* possesses additional non-pilus epithelial cell specific adhesins. Simpson *et al.* [36] devised an elegant strategy to genetically characterize these RpoN-dependent non-pilus adhesins and their data suggested that *P. aeruginosa* expresses at least two adhesins, one able to attach to receptors present on both epithelial cells and mucins and the other recognizing mucin alone [36]. Although the exact nature of the *P. aeruginosa* adhesin for mucin remains poorly defined, several potential binding sites for *P. aeruginosa* in respiratory mucins have been demonstrated *in vitro* [32, 37, 38] which may play a role in entrapment of the organism in the mucous secretion during infection.

P. aeruginosa Mucoid Exopolysaccharide

P. aeruginosa secretes an extracellular polysaccharide composed of L-glucuronic and D-mannuronic acids [39], commonly known as mucoid exopolysaccharide (MEP) or alginate. MEP is characteristically produced by CF *P. aeruginosa* strains and is thought to play a critical role in CF pathogenesis [40]. It appears to facilitate adhesion to tracheal cell surfaces [25, 41, 42]. Adhesion of mucoid *P. aeruginosa* is increased when mouse tracheal cells are pretreated with acid; adhesion to untreated tracheas is poor [41]. Therefore the exact nature of alginate-mediated adherence remains unclear. Although secretion of MEP is primarily associated with *P. aeruginosa* from chronic CF infection, a small amount of alginate secretion is also associated with initially colonizing nonmucoid strains [43]; the role of a "partial mucoid capsule" early in the course of colonization remains to be determined.

Flagellar Mediated Motility and Chemotaxis

The possession of a polar flagellum is a defining taxonomic feature of *P. aeruginosa* [44]. Flagellar and motility have been shown to be major virulence factors of *P. aeruginosa* in animal models of burn infections [45, 46, 47]. Several studies have indicated that flagellar mediated motility and chemotaxis may also be important for the establishment of lung infection in CF.

P. *aeruginosa* strains representing the primary colonizing isolates from patients with CF were motile and chemotactic towards CF mucin and components of mucin, suggesting that these determinants of the bacterium were important during the initial stages of pulmonary colonization [13]. In a study comparing binding of *P. aeruginosa* strains of various phenotypes to bovine trachea epithelial cell monolayers, nonmotile strains of *P. aeruginosa* were found to adhere poorly [26] and the authors suggest that the lack of motility reduced the degree of bacteria–monolayer interaction and subsequent adherence. It was also demonstrated that *rpoN*-mutants of *P. aeruginosa* (non-pilated, non-flagellated and lacking non-pilus adhesions [28, 29] were less able to colonize mouse gastric tissue suggesting that strain motility might be important in the establishment of mucosal infection. The authors noted however that *rpoN*-deficient strains exhibit multiple defects, including glutamine auxotrophy [29] and the reduced levels of colonization may therefore be reflective of a lower *in vivo* growth rate.

Data from *P. aeruginosa* isolates recovered from CF respiratory infection also suggest a role for motility during the early course of infection. *P. aeruginosa* strains isolated from CF patients in good clinical condition were generally motile and possessed functional flagella whereas isolates collected from patients in poor clincal condition often lacked flagella; these observations suggest that flagellation and motility are primarily linked with early colonization and not chronic infection in CF patients [48]. Recently we also demonstrated that primary CF isolates were highly motile, flagellated and piliated; however, after chronic colonization is established, we found *P. aeruginosa* strains deficient in these factors may predominate in certain CF patients [49].

Exotoxins, Proteases, and Secretory Products of P. aeruginosa

P. aeruginosa secretes a large number of exoproducts including exotoxin A, exoenzyme S, alkaline proteases, elastase, alkaline phosphatase, lipase, phospholipases, siderophores and phenazine pigments. The role many of these exoproducts play in the pathogenesis of *P. aeruginosa* during CF infection has been extensively reviewed elsewhere [50, 51, 52, 53]; those thought to play a role in colonization are described below.

Exotoxins. Two protein toxins of *P. aeruginosa*, exotoxin A (ETA) and exoenzyme S (exo-S), have been well characterized. Both may enter and poison eukaryotic cells by adenosine-diphosphate-ribosylation of cellular proteins [53, 54]. The role ETA plays in virulence during lung infection remains unclear; the toxin is produced by *P. aeruginosa* during experimental lung infection of rats [55] but the virulence of nontoxigenic mutants may vary, depending on the animal model used [50].

Proteases. *P. aeruginosa* secretes a variety of proteases of which two potent enzymes, elastase and alkaline protease, have been studied extensively. Alkaline protease is encoded by the *arpH* gene and is exported and secreted without modification, as a 48 kilodalton protein [56]. Complete elastolytic activity, on the other hand, requires the expression of two genes in *P. aeruginosa*: *lasA* and *lasB*. *LasA* encodes an enzyme, LasA, with proteolytic activity [57]. *LasB*, is the structural elastase gene [58] encoding an elastase precursor, which after proteolytic processing is released as mature elastase, LasB. Peters and Galloway [59] demonstrated that purified LasA enhanced the elastolytic activity of mature elastase and suggested that LasA interacts with the elastin substrate rendering it more susceptible to proteolysis. Subsequently, characterization of *P. aeruginosa* strains in which the elastase structural gene, *lasB*, was inactivated, demonstrated that these mutants retained some elastolytic activity and suggested that LasA in fact may be a second elastase [60, 61]. Recently, Kessler *et al.* [62] clearly demonstrated that LasA was able to enhance elastolysis by cleaving glycine-glycine bonds in elastin and further showed that LasA was a staphylolytic protease. They postulated that the potent staphylolytic activity of LasA may play a role during colonization by aiding elimination of *S. aureus* and thereby faciliating *P. aeruginosa* colonization.

Both alkaline protease and elastase are present in the sputa of patients chronically colonized with *P. aeruginosa* [63] and stimulate an antibody response [64]. Extensive degradation of constituents of connective tissue such as collagen, elastin, laminin and fibronectin may be mediated by these proteases [65, 66], and it has been proposed that the resultant tissue damage may aid *P. aeruginosa* colonization by exposing sites to which the bacteria can adhere [55]. These *P. aeruginosa* proteases have also been shown to disrupt respiratory cilia *in vitro* [67] thereby impairing pulmonary clearance.

Other secretory products. P. *aeruginosa* secretes a number of phenazine pigments, of which pyocyanin is perhaps the best characterized. Pyocyanin can inhibit lymphocyte proliferation *in vitro* [68] and it may also stimulate or inhibit superoxide radical generation by polymorphonuclear leukocytes depending on its concentration [69]. Pyocyanin also disrupts mucociliary function *in vitro* [70].

In order for bacterial pathogens to survive and cause disease, they must compete for iron, which is efficiently trapped by the host iron-binding proteins, transferrin and lactoferrin. *P. aeruginosa* secretes a number of siderophores which can sequester iron from these host compounds and aid bacterial survival *in vivo* [71, 72, 73]. These iron-chelating pigments, pyoverdin and pyochelin, secreted by *P. aeruginosa*, have also been proposed to contribute to the massive oxidant-mediated injury to the lung observed in CF, by providing a source of catalytic iron for the generation of toxic oxygen intermediates.

P. aeruginosa: **Determinants of Chronic CF Infection**

Once *P. aeruginosa* has established infection in the CF lung, it undergoes various phenotypic changes which may enable it to persist during chronic infection (Figure 2). Expression of MEP, conversion of LPS phenotype from smooth to rough, and alterations in bacterial motility are phenotypic features characteristic of *P. aeruginosa* isolated during chronic colonization; these determinants of chronic CF infection are discussed below.

Mucoid Exopolysaccharide

Strains of *P. aeruginosa* isolated from the sputum of chronically colonized CF patients are often mucoid in colonial morphology and produce copious amounts of MEP. The presence of MEP reactive antibody in colonized CF patients [74, 75] and the immunofluorescent detection of polysaccharide in histological sections of CF lung [76] indicates that MEP is produced *in vivo* during infection. Since synthesis of MEP requires a considerable investment of energy and the channelling of metabolizable sugars into alginate, it seems unlikely that expression of MEP would occur *in vivo* unless it provided the bacterium with a substantial survival advantage.

The MEP "capsule" has been proposed to aid survival of *P. aeruginosa* during chronic infection by a number of mechanisms. Expression of MEP and formation of a glycocalyx around microcolonies of *P. aeruginosa* has been suggested to protect the bacteria from engulfment by phagocytic cells [77, 78]. Indeed, *in vitro* studies have demonstrated that mucoid strains are less susceptible to both opsonic [79] and non-opsonic phagocytosis [80, 81]. In fact, MEP has been shown *in vitro* to interfere with a number of other phagocytic cell functions (described in more detail below).

The local factors in the CF lung responsible for triggering production of MEP are not well defined. Prolonged static culture of non-mucoid *P. aeruginosa* under nutrient limitation may result in conversion to the "CF phenotype" (mucoid and LPS-rough; [82]). Recent studies examining the growth of *P. aeruginosa* in a chemostat demonstrated that conversion to the mucoid phenotype could be achieved under conditions of osmotic stress and general nutrient limitation [83]. High osmolarity causes an increase in the expression of the gene encoding GDP-mannose dehydrogenase [84], a key enzyme in the biosynthesis of alginate. Sputum from CF patients contains slightly elevated levels of sodium, chloride and calcium ions [85] which may increase the osmolarity of bronchial secretions, lending weight to the argument that osmotic stress may increase the level of alginate synthesis in CF. However, expression of mucoidy may be lost from both laboratory and clinical strains when they are grown on bacteriological media with high osmolarity [86]. Thus the local conditions in the CF lung triggering expression of mucoidy in *P. aeruginosa* remain undetermined.

Conversion of Lipopolysaccharide phenotype – Smooth to Rough

P. aeruginosa isolates from chronically colonized CF patients are frequently sensitive to the bactericidal effect of human serum and are endowed with a rough LPS that lacks the typical O-polysaccharide side chain [87]. Pier *et al.* [43] showed that non-mucoid *P. aeruginosa* isolates from patients early in the course of colonization were frequently typable and serum resistant in contrast to isolates from patients co-colonized with non-mucoid and mucoid strains, which were predominantly serum sensitive. They suggested that initial non-mucoid colonizing strains of *P. aeruginosa* produce a smooth LPS and that once mucoid isolates emerge, LPS-rough, serum sensitive organisms predominate, regardless of exopolysaccharide phenotype.

The mechanisms underlying this conversion of LPS phenotype from smooth to rough are poorly understood although it can be induced by nutrient limitation *in vitro* [82]. The transition from smooth to rough LPS may reflect a general survival mechanism of Gram-negative bacteria chronically residing in the endobronchial space where they are deprived of nutrients and do not require protection from the bactericidal factors present in serum. Indeed, CF patients rarely suffer bacteremia due to *P. aeruginosa*. A further explanation for the change in LPS phenotype may lie in the toxigenicity associated with the antigen.

LPS-rough strains are generally of low toxigenicity [88, 89]; this may explain why CF patients do not suffer toxic shock as a result of the extraordinarily high numbers of *P. aeruginosa* present in their lungs during chronic infection.

Evasion of Host Phagocytic Defenses

Polymorphonuclear leukocytes (PMNs) and pulmonary alveolar macrophages play a critical role in defending the lung against infection with *P. aeruginosa*. Although an intrinsic defect in CF phagocytic cell function has not yet been identified, *P. aeruginosa* and its products interfere with the functions of both PMNs and macrophages and may thereby compromise normal pulmonary antibacterial defenses in CF patients.

MEP inhibits neutophil chemotaxis [90], opsonic [79] and nonopsonic [80] phagocytosis. Proteases inhibit PMN function [91] and may create a ligand–receptor mismatch by degrading both complement receptors and activated opsonic complement [92, 93]. Exotoxin A [94] and "leukocidins" [95] intoxicate phagocytic cells thereby impeding their normal antibacterial functions. All these factors conspire to compromise the normal phagocytic activities in the infected CF lung.

The aforementioned antiphagocytic effects of *P. aeruginosa* probably impair its clearance from the lung but cannot explain why this bacterial species has a particular predilection for CF respiratory tract infection. We have observed recently that macrophages have a unique requirement for glucose for phagocytosis of unopsonized *P. aeruginosa* [15]; all other bacterial species we have studied are ingested equally well in the presence and absence of glucose [95a]. Glucose is present in diminishingly low concentrations in the respiratory airways [16] where *P. aeruginosa* establishes infection in CF patients. Thus *P. aeruginosa* may have a unique survival advantage in the CF lung because of its capacity to exploit the selective inability of lung macrophages to phagocytose this one bacterial species under the peculiar conditions present in the bronchoalveolar space.

Changes in P. aeruginosa Motility

During chronic CF infection, *P. aeruginosa* undergoes a number of phenotypic changes described above. Luzar *et al.* [48] also noted that strains from chronically colonized CF patients were frequently non-motile and non-flagellated, and that this phenotype was most often recovered from patients in poor clinical condition. In a longitudinal study of virulence factor expression during CF infection, Burke *et al.*

[89] also demonstrated that *P. aeruginosa* strains from chronically colonized patients were less motile than those recovered early in colonization. Moreover, they demonstrated that expression of secreted virulence factors such as proteases, elastase, phospholipase, heat-stable hemolysin and exotoxin A also decrease during infection, corroborating earlier findings that *P. aeruginosa* strains collected from chronically colonized CF patients were relatively avirulent [96].

Recently, we examined the changes in *P. aeruginosa* strain motility which occur during CF infection in an extensive study of sequential isolates collected over a period of up to 10 years, from 20 CF patients [49]. Of 1030 isolates examined, approximately 40% were non-motile; the prevalence of mucoid strains in the same group of isolates was 35%. Immunoblot examination of these non-motile isolates demonstrated that many did not express flagellin or pilin and were also unable to grow on minimal media without the addition of glutamine; these phenotypic traits are characteristic of *rpoN*-mutants of *P. aeruginosa* (see section on RpoN, below and [29]). Isolates of this phenotype were repeatedly recovered from one CF patient studied for 7 years suggesting that they were not at any survival disadvantage despite the fact they lacked several of the *P. aeruginosa* factors thought to be important for colonization.

Given the high prevalence of non-motile isolates, we hypothesize that the loss of motility by *P. aeruginosa* during CF infection may represent a further mechanism by which the organism is able to adapt to the CF lung and establish chronic infection. These non-motile strains appear less susceptible to phagocytic clearance [49] and substantial energy is conserved since the production of flagella requires the expression of over 40 genes. Both non-motile and non-chemotactic mutants of *P. aeruginosa* were able to attach to respiratory mucins [13]; therefore the ability of such strains to remain within the airways of chronically infected patients might not be impaired by this phenotypic adaption.

Phenotypic Versatility of *P. aeruginosa*: Aspects of Gene Regulation

"Versatility" and "adaptability" are excellent ways to describe why *P. aeruginosa* is uniquely adept at colonizing and surviving in the CF lung. The ability of *P. aeruginosa* to adapt to conditions present during CF infection is perhaps the feature most critical to its survival. The mechanisms controlling the expression of several virulence determinants of *P. aeruginosa* have now been elucidated in some detail. Much of their control occurs at a level of gene transcription. Transcriptional control may be achieved by several mechanisms, two of which have been demonstrated to play a role in *P. aeruginosa* virulence factor expression: (i) RNA-polymerase (RNApol) is a polymeric enzyme, the functional form of which consists of two alpha, two beta and a single sigma (σ) subunits; many bacteria possess several σ factors and these dictate which promoter type can be recognized by RNApol, and hence facilitate the expression of a given subset of genes with that target promoter [97]; (ii) Control of transcription may also be achieved by DNA-binding proteins, termed transcriptional activators, which bind DNA and enhance the recognition and transcription of given promoters.

Aspects of gene regulation involved in the expression of: (a) MEP, (b) elastase and other exoproduct virulence factors, and (c) motility and adhesion factors, illustrate the remarkable adaptability of *P. aeruginosa*.

Control of Mucoid Exopolysaccharide Expression

Production of MEP is under an elaborate network of regulatory controls. In mucoid strains, there is strong transcriptional activation of the *algD* gene, encoding GDPmannose dehydrogenase, a key biosynthetic enzyme [98]. Transcriptional activation of this gene has become a useful tool in uncovering the regulation of mucoidy. Several regulatory elements affect the expression of this gene. Two response regulator proteins [99] have been shown to be involved in expression of *algD*: AlgR and AlbB. Full activation of *algD* requires the binding of AlgR to upstream promoter regions [100]. AlgB, a member of the NtrC family of transcriptional activators [101], is also required for *algD* transcription though the exact nature of its binding site remains unclear [102]. The conformation of the *algD* promoter is also effected by histone-like elements [103].

Recently, a new gene, *algU*, which appears critical for expression of mucoidy was cloned [104] and found to share considerable homology with the alternative sigma factor, SpoOH, responsible for triggering sporulation in *Bacillus subtilis* [105]. Overall, activation of alginate synthesis involves the complex interaction of a number of regulators in response to environmental stimuli. Conditions in the CF lung may enhance differentiation of *P. aeruginosa* to the mucoid phenotype via one or more of these regulatory elements. A clearer understanding of the regulatory events leading to activation of alginate expression may provide potential targets for therapeutic interventions [106].

LasR – A Global Regulator of P. aeruginosa Exoproduct Expression

Recent investigations into the regulation of *P. areuginosa* elastase by environmental stimuli resulted in the isolation of *lasR*, which encodes the protein LasR, a transcriptional activator of elastase gene expression [107]. Further studies demonstrated that LasR was required for the transcription of the alkaline protease gene [108], the *lasA* gene, which encodes a second elastase [60], and could also enhance expression of exotoxin A [108]. All of these genes encode exoproducts of *P. aeruginosa* associated with pathogenesis suggesting that LasR may be a global regulator of virulence gene expression [108]. Expression of the virulence factors under the control of *lasR* (proteases and exotoxins) appears to decrease during chronic colonization [89] as *P. aeruginosa* changes to a less toxigenic phenotype.

This network of global control underwent a further regulatory twist when it was discovered that high expression of elastase required the expression of the *lasI* gene, which encoded a protein involved in the synthesis of a small diffusible molecule, termed *Pseudomonas* autoinducer [109]. Using these mechanisms *P. aeruginosa* appears able to sense its environment and modulate expression of virulence genes necessary for survival during chronic infection. The elucidation of these complex regulatory relationships not only provides an insight into the versatility of *P. aeruginosa* pathogenesis but also provides a target for new therapeutic approaches which may block *P. aeruginosa* virulence gene expression [109].

Motility and Adhesion Factors Under the Control of RpoN

Recently, Lory and colleagues demonstrated that the product of the *rpoN* gene (RpoN or σ^{54}), an alternative sigma factor, is required for the expression of a number of genes in *P. aeruginosa*, including the flagellin gene [29] and pilin gene [110]. Subsequently, they demonstrated that *P. aeruginosa* also expresses at least two non-pilus adhesions responsible for binding to epithelial cells and mucins which also require RpoN for their expression (see section on non-pilus adhesions and [26, 27, 30]). Totten *et al.* [29] postulated that RpoN may allow *P. aeruginosa* to coordinately control the expression of these important surface virulence factors in response to environmental signals via gene-specific positive effectors. The RpoN-dependent genes described to date in a number of other Gram-negative bacteria also require transcriptional activators for their expression and are not controlled by the levels of RpoN, which remain constant within the cell [101]. As described previously, motility, pili and non-pilus adhesins are important virulence factors, all of which have been implicated in the establishment of infection in CF. The ability of *P. aeruginosa* to coordinately control and amplify the expression of these genes via an alternative sigma factor and other positive activators may contribute to its pathogenesis in CF.

We have shown that once chronic colonization is established in CF, non-motile *P. aeruginosa* may be recovered which lack flagella or both flagella and pili [49]. We demonstrated that partial complementation of motility in some of these isolates could be achieved by introduction of plasmid-borne copies of the *rpoN* locus of *P. aeruginosa*, suggesting that RpoN may be involved in the appearance of the non-motile phenotype. These data suggest that alternative sigma factors may be important in the expression of the *P. aeruginosa* phenotype characteristic of CF patients.

Pseudomonas Cepacia: A New Threat

Despite its evolving role in CF lung infections, very little is known about the pathogenesis of *P. cepacia* infection. *P. cepacia* shares several virulence factors with *P. aeruginosa*, which may serve similar functions during infection but which are, however, biochemically distinct. Mucoid strains of *P. cepacia* may be isolated [111] but this phenotype is not associated with CF infection. A number of *P. cepacia* exoproducts have also recently been characterized and include a protease [112], a haemolysin and phospholipase C [113].

   P. cepacia may bind to and colonize the respiratory epithelia by mechanisms similar to those described for *P. aeruginosa*. Both organisms are motile, express a polar flagellum, and are piliated [114]. They also adhere to the same disaccharide moiety present in many asialoglycolipids [115]. *P. cepacia* isolated from patients with "*cepacia* syndrome" (4) bind to respiratory mucins with high affinity *in vitro* [116]. The mucous secretions within the lungs of patients with CF may provide an ideal environment for colonization for these mucin-binding pseudomonads. Adherence of *P. cepacia* to cultured respiratory epithelial cells is enhanced by the presence of *P. aeuginosa* and its exoproducts [117] and *in vitro* adherence to buccal epithelial cells may occur via both pilus-mediated and non-pilus adhesive mechanisms [118]. A number of virulence mechanisms have therefore been postulated for *P. cepacia* colonization, however very little is known about the factors responsible for the rapid and fatal deterioration seen in some CF patients infected with the organism.

Discussion

P. aeruginosa is the major respiratory pathogen in patients with CF. Isolates from early in the course of infection differ from those recovering during chronic colonization; the changes observed may reflect mechanisms of pathogenesis utilized for establishment and subsequent maintenance of disease. Colonizing isolates are motile, piliated, possess smooth-LPS and are non-mucoid; phenotypically resembling *P. aeruginosa* prevalent in the environment. During the initial colonization of the respiratory epithelium, adherence of *P. aeruginosa* is mediated by pili and non-pilus adhesins. Motility and chemotaxis towards mucin is important in the establishment of infection and secretion of proteases can enhance adhesion by exposing sites to which *P. aeruginosa* may bind. *P. aeruginosa* may evade phagocytic clearance by secretion of toxins and pigments which poison the host cells, and proteases which can cleave opsonins and phagocytic receptors. Phagocytosis of *P. aeruginosa* may also be precluded in the uninflamed lung because of the unique requirement for glucose for the nonopsonic ingestion of the organism by macrophages.

Once colonization of the CF lung has been established, *P. aeruginosa* utilizes a number of mechanisms to grow and persist; as a consequence its phenotype changes markedly. *P. aeruginosa* isolates from chronic CF infection express rough lipopolysaccharide, secrete copious amounts of MEP, often do not express flagella and pili, and are generally of low toxigenicity. With the exception of the secretion of MEP, *P. aeruginosa* appears to adapt to conditions prevalent in the CF lung by reducing or halting the expression of many of the putative virulence factors thought to be important for establishing infection. In so doing *P. aeruginosa* may be able to direct most of its available energy into evasion of host defenses and persistence.

While the phenotypic markers associated with *P. aeruginosa* infection in CF are well defined, an understanding of the gene regulation behind the expression of many of these virulence factors is only lately emerging. As we have illustrated, *P. aeruginosa* has regulatory mechanisms that enable it to control the expression of virulence factors in response to environmental stimuli; the adaption to the environment mediated by these regulatory control networks may be fundamental to its pathogenesis in CF. A better understanding of the mechanisms controlling pathogenesis may enable the development of novel therapeutic approaches to prevent chronic *P. aeruginosa* infection in CF. The pathogenesis of *P. cepacia* is not well defined, and the factors responsible for the rapid deterioration of certain patients infected with this organism remain to be identified.

Acknowledgements

Dr. Mahenthiralingam was funded by a postdoctural research fellowship from the Canadian Cystic Fibrosis Foundation. Research in the authors' laboratory was supported by grants from the Canadian Cystic Fibrosis Foundation, the Medical Research Council of Canada and the Canadian Bacterial Diseases Network.

References

1. Marks MI. Clinical significance of *Staphylococcus aureus* in cystic fibrosis. Infection 1990; 18: 53–56.

2. Greenberg DP, Stutman HR. Infection and Immunity to *Staphyloccocus aureus* and *Haemophilus influenzae*. In: Moss, RB editor. Cystic Fibrosis. Totowa, New Jersey. Humana Press. 1990; 75–86.

3. Doggett RG, Harrison GM, Stillwell RN, Wallis ES. An atypical *Pseudomonas aeruginosa* associated with cystic fibrosis of the pancreas. J Pediatr 1966; 68: 215–221.

4. Isles A, Maclusky I, Corey M, Gold R, Prober C, Fleming P. *Pseudomonas cepacia* infection in cystic fibrosis: An emerging problem. J Pediatr 1984; 104: 206–210.

5. Lewin LO, Byard PJ, Davis PB. Effect of *Pseudomonas cepacia* colonization on survival and pulmonary function of cystic fibrosis patients. J Clin Epidemiol 1990; 43: 125–131.

6. Tablan OC, Martone WJ, Doershuck CF, Stern RC, Thomassen MJ, Klinger JW, *et al.* Colonization of the respiratory tract with *Pseudomonas cepacia* in cystic fibrosis: risk factors and outcome. Chest 1987; 91: 527–532.

7. Govan JRW, Brown PH, Maddison J, Doherty CJ, Nelson JW, Dodd M *et al.* Evidence for transmission of *Pseudomonas cepacia* by social contact in cystic fibrosis. Lancet. 1993; 342: 15–19.

8. Govan JRW, Nelson JW. Microbiology of lung infection in cystic fibrosis. British Medical Bulletin. 1992; 48: 912–930.

9. Ramphal R, Pyle M. Adherence of mucoid and nonmucoid *Pseudomonas aeruginosa* to acid-injured tracheal epithelium. Infect Immun 1983; 41: 345–351.

10. Woods DE, Bass JA, Johanson WG, Straus DC. Role of adherence in the pathogenesis of *Pseudomonas aeruginosa* lung infection in cystic fibrosis patients. Infect Immun 1980; 30: 694–699.

11. Woods DE, Straus DC, Johanson WG, Bass JA. Role of fibronectin in the prevention of adherence of *Pseudomonas aeruginosa* to buccal cells. J Infect Dis 1981; 143: 784–790.

12. Saiman L, Cacalano G, Gruenert D, Prince A. Comparison of adherence of *Pseudomonas aeruginosa* to respiratory epithelial cells from cystic fibrosis patients and healthy subjects. Infect Immun 1992; 60: 2808–2814.

13. Nelson JW, Tredgett MW, Sheehan JK, Thorton DJ, Notman D, Govan JRW. Mucinophilic and chemotactic properties of *Pseudomonas aeruginosa* in relation to pulmonary colonization in cystic fibrosis. Infect Immun 1990; 58: 1489–1495.

14. Ramphal R, Pyle M. Evidence for mucins and sialic acid as receptors for *Pseudomonas aeruginosa* in the lower respiratory tract. Infect Immun 1983; 41: 339–344.

15. Speert DP, Gordon S. Phagocytosis of unoponized *Pseudomonas aeruginosa* by murine macrophages is a two-step process requiring glucose. J Clin Invest 1992; 90: 1085–1092.

16. Valeyre D, Soler P, Bassert G, Loiseau P, Pre J, Turbie P *et al.* Glucose, K$^+$, and albumin concentrations in the alveolar milieu of normal and pulmonary sarcoidosis patients. Am Rev Respir Dis 1991; 143: 1096–1101.

17. Sanchis J, Dolovich M, Roosman C, Wilson W, Newhouse M. Pulmonary mucociliary clearance in cystic fibrosis. N Engl J Med 1973; 288: 651–654.

18. Folklhard W, Marvin DA, Watts TH, Paranchych W. Structure of polar pili from *Pseudomonas aeruginosa* strains K and O. J Mol Biol 1981; 149: 79–93.

19. Frost LS, Paranchych W. Composition and molecular weight of pili purified from *Pseudomonas aeruginosa*. J Bacteriol 1977; 131: 259–269.

20. Pasloske BL, Finlay BB, Parachych. Cloning and sequencing of *Pseudomonas aeruginosa* PAK pilin gene. FEBS Lett 1985; 183: 408–412.

21. Johnson K, Parker ML, Lory S. Nucleotide sequence and transcriptional initiation site of two *Pseudomonas aeruginosa* pilin genes. J Biol Chem 1986; 261: 15703–15708.

22. Pasloske BL, Sastry PA, Finlay BB, Paranchych W. Two unusual pilin sequences from different isolates of *Pseudomonas aeruginosa*. J Bacteriol 1988; 170: 3738–3741.

23. Woods DE, Straus DC, Johanson WG Jr., Berry VK, Bass JA. Role of pili in adherence of *Pseudomonas aeruginosa* to mammalian buccal epithelial cells. Infect Immun 1980; 29: 1146–1151.

24. Ramphal R, Sadoff JC, Pyle M, Silipigni JD. Role of pili in the adherence of *Pseudomonas aeruginosa* to injured tracheal epithelium. Infect Immun 1984; 44: 38–40.

25. Marcus H, Baker NR. Quantitation of adherence of mucoid and nonmucoid *Pseudomonas aeruginosa* to hamster tracheal epithelium. Infect Immun 1985; 47: 723–729.

26. Saiman L, Ishimoto K, Lory S, Prince A. The effect of piliation and exoproduct expression on the adherence of *Pseudomonas aeruginosa* to respiratory epithelial monolayers. J Infect Dis 1990; 161: 541–548.

27. Chi E, Mehl T, Nunn D, Lory S. 1991. Interaction of *Pseudomonas aeruginosa* with A549 pneumocyte cells. Infect Immun 1991; 59: 822–828.

28. Pier GB, Meluleni G, Neuger E. A murine model of chronic mucosal colonization by *Pseudomonas aeruginosa*. Infect Immun 1992; 60: 4768–4776.

29. Totten PA, Lara JC, Lory S. The *rpoN* gene of product of *Pseudomonas aeruginosa* is required for the expression of diverse genes, including the flagelin gene. J Bacteriol 1990; 172: 389–396.

30. Ramphal R, Koo L, Ishimoto K, Totten P, Lara JC, Lory S. Adhesion of *Pseudomonas aeruginosa* pilin deficient mutants to mucin. Infect Immun 1991; 59: 1307–1311.

31. Sajjen US, Reisman J, Doig P, Irvin RT, Forstner G, Forstner J. Binding of nonmucoid *Pseudomonas aeruginosa* to normal human intestinal mucin and respiratory mucin from patients with cystic fibrosis. Infect Immun 1992; 60: 657–665.

32. Reddy MS. Human tracheobronchial mucin: purification and binding to *Pseudomonas aeruginosa*. Infect Immun 1992; 60: 1530–1535.

33. Doig P, Todd T, Sastry PA, Lee KK, Hodges RS, Paranchych W et al. Role of pili in the adhesion of *Pseudomonas aeruginosa* to human respiratory epithelial cells. Infect Immun 1988; 56: 1641–1646.

34. Irvin RT, Doig P, Lee KK, Sastry PA, Paranchych W, Tood T et al. Characterization of the *Pseudomonas aeruginosa* pilus adhesion: Confirmation that the pilin structural protein subunit contains a human epithelial cell binding domain. Infect Immun 1989; 57: 3720–3726.

35. Lee KK, Doig P, Irvin RT, Paranchych W, Hodges RS. Mapping the surface regions of *Pseudomonas aeruginosa* pili: The importance of the C-terminal region for adherence to human buccal epithelial cells. Molec Microbiol 1989; 3: 1493–1499.

36. Simpson DA, Ramphal R, Lory S. Genetic analysis of *Pseudomonas aeruginosa* adherence: distinct genetic loci control attachment to epithilial cells and mucins. Infect Immun 1992; 60: 3771–3779.

37. Ramphal R, Houdret L, Koo L, Lamblin G, Roussel P. Differences in adhesion of *Pseudomonas aeruginosa* to mucin glycopeptides from sputa patients with cystic fibrosis and chronic bronchitis. Infect Immun 1989; 57: 3066–3071.

38. Ramphal R, Carnoy C, Fievre S, Michalski JC, Houdret N, Lamblin G et al. *Pseudomonas aeruginosa* recognizes carbohydrate chains containing type 1 (Galβ1-3GlcNAc) or type 2 (Galβ1-4GlcNAc) disaccharide units. Infect Immun 1991; 59: 700–704.

39. Linker A, Jones RS. 1966. A new polysaccharide resembling alginic acid isolated from *Pseudomonas*. J Biol Chem 1966; 241: 3845–3851.

40. Høiby N, Rosendal K. Epidemiology of *Pseudomonas aeruginosa* infection in patients treated at a cystic fibrosis center. Acta Pathol Microbiol Scand Sect B 1980; 88: 125–131.

41. Ramphal R, Pier GB. Role of *Pseudomonas aeruginosa* mucoid exopolysaccharide in adherence of tracheal cells. Infect Immun 1985; 47: 1–4.

42. Doig P, Smith NR, Todd T, Irvin RT. Characterization of the binding of *Pseudomonas aeruginosa* to human epithelial cells. Infect Immun 1987; 55: 1517–1522.

43. Pier GB, DesJardin D, Aguilar T, Barnard M, Speert DP. Polysaccharide surface antigens expressed by nonmucoid isolates of *Pseudomonas aeruginosa* from cystic fibrosis patients. J Clin Microbiol 1986; 24: 189–196.

44. Gilardi GL. *Pseudomonas*. In: *Manual of Clinical Microbiology*. Lennette EH, editor. American Society for Microbiology, Washington D.C. 1985; pp. 350–372.

45. McManus AT, Moody EE, Mason AD. Bacterial motility: a component in experimental *Pseudomonas aeruginosa* burn wound species. Burns 1980; 6: 235–239.

46. Montie TC, Doyle-Huntzinger D, Craven R, Holder IA. Loss of virulence associated with absence of flagellum in an isogenic mutant of *Pseudomonas aeruginosa* in the burned mouse model. Infect Immun 1982; 38: 1296–1298.

47. Drake D, Montie TC. 1988. Flagella, motility and invasive virulence of *Pseudomonas aeruginosa*. J Gen Microbiol 1988; 134: 43–52.

48. Luzar MA, Thomassen MJ, Montie TC. Flagella and motility alterations in *Pseudomonas aeruginosa* strains from patients with cysitc fibrosis: relationship to patient clinical condition. Infect Immun 1985; 50: 577–582.

49. Mahenthiralingam E, Campbell ME, Speert DP. Non-motility and phagocytic resistance of *Pseudomonas aeruginosa* isolates from chronically colonized patients with cystic fibrosis. Infect Immun 1994; 62: 596–605.

50. Woods DE, Iglewski BH. Toxins of *Pseudomonas aeruginosa*: New perspectives. Rev Infect Dis 1983; 5: 715–722.
51. Speert DP. Host defenses in patients with cystic fibrosis: modulation by *Pseudomonas aeruginosa*. Surv Synth Path Res 1985; 4: 14–33.
52. Woods DE, Sokol PA. Role of *Pseudomonas aeruginosa* extracellular enzymes in lung disease. Clin Invest Med 1986; 9: 108–112.
53. Wick MJ, Frank DW, Storey DG, Iglewski BH. Structure, function and regulation of *Pseudmonas aeruginosa* exotoxin A Ann Rev Microbiol 1990; 44: 335–363.
54. Woods DE, To M, Sokol PA. 1989. *Pseudomonas aeruginosa* exoenzyme S as a pathogenic determinant in respiratory infection. Antibiot Chemother 1989; 44: 27–35.
55. Woods DE, Cryz SJ, Friedman RL, Iglewski BH. Contribution of toxin A and elastase to virulence of *Pseudomonas aeruginosa* in chronic lung infections of rats. Infect Immun 1982; 36: 1223–1228.
56. Guzzo J, Murgier M, Filloux A, Lazdunski A. Cloning of the *Pseudomonas aeruginosa* alkaline protease gene and secretion of the protease into the medium by *Escherichia coli*. J Bacteriol 1990; 172: 942–948.
57. Goldberg JB, Ohman DE. Cloning and transcriptional regulation of the elastase *lasA* gene in mucoid and non-mucoid *Pseudomonas aeruginosa*. J Bacteriol 1987; 169: 1349–1351.
58. Schad PA, Bever RA, Nicas TI, Leduc F, Hanne LF, Iglewski BH. Cloning and characterization of the elastase genes from *Pseudomonas aeruginosa*. J Bacteriol 1987; 169: 2691–2696.
59. Peters JE, Galloway DR. Purification and characterization of an active fragment of the LasA protein from *Pseudomonas aeruginosa*: enhancement of elastase activity. J Bacteriol 1990; 2236–2240.
60. Toder DS, Gambello MJ, Igelwski BH. *Pseudomonas aeruginosa* LasA: a second elastase under the transcriptional control of *lasR*. Mol Microbiol 1991; 5: 2003–2010.
61. Wolz C, Hellstern E, Haug M, Galloway DR, Vasil ML, Döring G. *Pseudomonas aeruginosa* lasB mutant constructed by insertional mutagenesis reveals elastolytic activity due to alkaline proteinase and LasA fragment. Mol Microbiol 1991; 5: 2125–2131.
62. Kessler E, Safrin M, Olson JC, Ohman DE. Secreted LasA of *Pseudomonas aeruginosa* is a staphylolytic protease. J Biol Chem 1993; 268: 7503–7508.
63. Döring G, Obernesser HJ, Bozenhardt K, Flehming B, Holly N, Hofmann A. Protease of *Pseudomonas aeruginosa* in patients with cystic fibrosis. J Infect Dis 1983; 147: 744–750.
64. Klinger JD, Straus DC, Hilton CB, Bass JA. Antibodies to proteases and exotoxin A of *Pseudomonas aeruginosa* in patients with cystic fibrosis: demonstration by radioimmunoassay. J Infect Dis 1978; 138: 49–58.
65. Heck LW, Morihara K, McRae WB, Miller EJ. Specific cleavage of human type III and IV collagens by *Pseudomonas aeruginonsa* elastase. Infect Immun 1986; 51: 115–118.
66. Heck LW, Morihara K, Abrahamson DR. Degradation of soluble laminin and depletion of tissue-associated basement membrane laminin by *Pseudomonas aeruginosa* elastase and alkaline protease. Infect Immun 1986; 54: 149–153.
67. Hinglay ST, Hastie AT, Kueppers F, Higgins LM. Disruption of respiratory cilia by proteases including those of *Pseudomonas aeruginosa*. Infect Immun 1986; 54: 379–385.
68. Sorensen RU, Klinger JD, Cash HA, Chase PA, Dearborn DG. *In vitro* inhibition of lymphocyte proliferation by *Pseudomonas aeruginosa* phenazine pigments. Infect Immun 1983; 41: 321–330.
69. Miller KM, Dearborn DG, Sorensen RU. *In vitro* effect of synthetic pyocyanine on neutrophil superoxide production. Infect Immun 1987; 55: 559–563.
70. Wilson R, Roberts D, Cole P. Effect of bacterial products on human ciliary function *in vitro*. Thorax 1985; 40: 125–131.
71. Sokol PA, Woods DE. Relationship of iron and extracellular virulence factors to *Pseudomonas aeruginosa* lung infections. J Med Microbiol 1984; 18: 125–133.
72. Ankenbauer R, Sriyosachati S, Cox CD. Effects of siderophores on the growth of *Pseudomonas aeruginosa* in human serum and transferrin. Infect Immun 1985; 49: 132–140.
73. Döring G, Pfestorf M, Botzenhardt K, Abdallah MA. Impact of proteases on iron uptake of *Pseudomonas aeruginosa* pyoverdin from transferrin and lactoferrin. Infect Immun 1988; 56: 291–293.

74. Pier GB, Saunders JM. Ames P, Edwards MS, Auerbac H, Goldfrab J *et al.* Opsonophagocytic killing antibody to *Pseudomonas aeruginosa* mucoid exopolysaccharide in older noncolonized patients with cystic fibrosis. N Engl J Med 1987; 317: 793–798.

75. Speert DP, Lawton D, Mutharia L. Antibody to *Pseudomonas aeruginosa* mucoid exopolysaccharide and to sodium alginate in cystic fibrosis serum. Pediatr Res 1984; 18: 431–433.

76. Speert DP, Dimmick JE, Pier GB, Saunders JM, Hancock REW, Kelly N. An immunohistological evaluation of *Pseudomonas aeruginosa* infection in two patients with cystic fibrosis. Pediatric Res 1987; 22: 743–747.

77. Lam J, Chan R, Lam K, Costerton JW. Production of mucoid microcolonies by *Pseudomonas aeruginosa* within infected lungs in cystic fibrosis. Infect Immun 1980; 28: 546–556.

78. Costerton JW, Cheng KJ, Geesey GG, Ladd TI, Nickel JC, Dasgupta M *et al.* Bacterial biofilms in nature and disease. Ann Rev Microbiol 1987; 41: 435–464.

79. Baltimore RS, Shedd DG. The role of complement in the opsonization of mucoid and non-mucoid strains of *Pseudomonas aeruginosa.* Paediatric Res 1983; 17: 952–958.

80. Cabral DA, Loh BA, Speert DP. Mucoid *Pseudomonas aeruginosa* resists nonopsonic phagocytosis by human neutrophils and macrophages. Paediatric Research 1987; 22: 429–431.

81. Krieg DP, Helmke RJ, German VF, Mangos JS. Resistance of mucoid *Pseudomonas aeruginosa* to nonopsonic phagocytosis by alveolar macrophages *in vitro.* Infect Immun 1988; 56: 3172–3179.

82. Speert DP, Farmer SW, Campbell ME, Musser JM, Selander RK, Kuo S. Conversion of *Pseudomonas aeruginosa* to the phenotype characteristic of strains from patients with cystic fibrosis. J Clin Microbiol 1990; 28: 188–194.

83. Terry JM, Pina SE, Mattingly SJ. Environmental conditions which influence mucoid conversion in *Pseudomonas aeruginosa* PA01. Infect Immun 1991; 59: 471–477.

84. Berry A, DeVault JD, Chakrabarty AM. High osmolarity is a signal for enhanced *algD* transcription in mucoid and nonmucoid *Pseudomonas aeruginosa.* J Bacteriol 1989; 171: 2312–2317.

85. Knowles MR, Stutts MJ, Spock A, Fischer N, Gatzy JT, Boucher RC. Abnormal ion permeation through cystic fibrosis respiratory epithelium. Science 1983; 221: 1067–1070.

86. Deretic V, Govan JRW, Konyecsni WM, Martin DW. Mucoid *Pseudomonas aeruginosa* in cystic fibrosis: mutations in the *muc* loci affect transcription of the *algR* and *algD* genes in response to environmental stimuli. Mol Microbiol 1990; 4: 189–196.

87. Hancock REW, Mutharia LM, Chan L, Darveau RP, Speert DP, Pier GB. *Pseudomonas aeruginosa* isolates from patients with cystic fibrosis: a class of serum-sensitive, non-typable strains deficient in lipopolysaccharide O side chains. Infect Immun 1983; 42: 170–177.

88. Fegan M, Francis P, Hayward AC, Davis GHG, Fuerst JA. Phenotypic conversion of *Pseudomonas aeruginosa* in cystic fibrosis. J Clin Microbiol 1990; 28: 1143–1146.

89. Burke V, Robinson JO, Richardson CJL, Bundell CS. Lonitudinal studies of virulence of *Pseudomonas aeruginosa* in cystic fibrosis. Pathology 1991; 23: 145–148.

90. Stiver HG, Zachidniak K, Speert DP. Inhibition of polymorphonuclear leukocyte chemotaxis by the mucoid exopolysaccharide of *Pseudomonas aeruginosa.* J Clin Invest Med. 1988; 11: 247–252.

91. Kharazmi A, Eriksen HO, Döring G, Goldstein W, Høiby N. Effect of *Pseudomonas aeruginosa* proteases on human leukocyte phagocytosis and bacterial activity. Acta Pathol Microbiol Immunol Scand Sect C 1986; 94: 175–179.

92. Berger M, Sorensen RU, Tosi MF, Dearborn DG, Döring G. Complement receptor expression on neutrophils at an inflammatory site. J Clin Invest 1989; 84: 1302–1313.

93. Tosi MF, Zakem H, Berger M. Neutrophil elastase cleaves C3bi on opsonized *Pseudomonas* as well as CR1 on neutrophils to create a functionally important opsonin receptor mismatch. J Clin Invest 1990; 86: 300–308.

94. Pollack M, Anderson SE Jr. Toxicity of *Pseudomonas aeruginosa* exotoxin A for human macrophages. Infect Immun 1978; 19: 1092–1096.

95. Scharmann W. Interaction of purified leukocidin from *Pseudomonas aeruginosa* with bovine polymorphonuclear leukocytes. Infect Immun 1976; 13: 1046–1053.

95a. Barghouthi S, Everett KDE, Speert DP. Nonopsonic phagocytosis of *Pseudomonas aeruginosa* requires facilitated transport of D-glucose by macrophages. J Immunol 1995; 154: 3420–3428.

96. Luzar MA, Montie TC. Avirulence and altered physiological properties of cystic fibrosis strains of *Pseudomonas aeruginosa*. Infect Immun 1985; 50: 572–576.

97. Helman J, Chamberlin MJ. Structure and function of bacterial sigma factors. Ann Rev Biochem 1988; 57: 839–872.

98. Deretic V, Gill JF, Chakrabarty AM. Gene *algD* for the GDP-mannose dehydrogenase is transcriptionally activated in mucoid *Pseudomonas aeruginosa*. J Bacteriol 1987; 169: 351–358.

99. Miller JF, Mekalanos JJ, Falkow S. Coordinate regulation and sensory transduction in the control of bacterial virulence. Science 1989; 243: 916–922.

100. Mohr CD, Hibler NS, Deretic V. AlgR, a response regulator controlling mucoidy in *Pseudomonas aeruginosa* binds to the FUS sites of the *algD* promoter located unusually far upstream from the mRNA start site. J Bacteriol 1991; 173: 5136–5143.

101. Kustu S, Santero E, Keener J, Popham D, Weiss D. Expression of σ^{54} (*ntrA*)-dependent genes is probably united by a common mechanism. Microbiol Revs 1989; 53: 367–376.

102. Wozniak DJ, Ohman DE. *Pseudomonas aeruginosa* AlgB, a two component response regulator of the NtrC family, is required for *algD*-transcription. J Bacteriol 1991; 173: 1406–1413.

103. Deretic V, Mohr CD, Martin DW. Mucoid *Pseudomonas aeruginosa* in cystic fibrosis: signal transduction and histone-like elements in the regulation of bacterial virulence. Mol Microbiol 1991; 5: 1577–1583.

104. Martin DW, Holloway BW, Deretic V. Characterization of a locus determining the mucoid status of *Pseudomonas aeruginosa*: AlgU shows sequence similarities with a *Bacillus* sigma factor. J Bacteriol 1993; 175: 1153–1164.

105. Dubnau E, Weir J, Nair G, Carter III L, Moran Jr. C, Smith I. Bacillus sporulation gene *spoOH* codes for σ^{30} (σ^{H}). J Bacteriol 1988; 170: 1054–1062.

106. Martin DW, Schurr MJ, Mudd MH, Deretic V. Differentiation of *Pseudomonas aeruginosa* into the alginate-producing form: inactivation of *mucB* causes conversion to mucoidy. Mol Microbiol 1993; 9: 497–506.

107. Gambello MJ, Iglewski BH. Cloning and characterization of the *Pseudomonas aeruginosa lasR* gene, a transcriptional activator of elastase expression. J Bacteriol 1991; 173: 3000–3009.

108. Gambello MJ, Kaye S, Iglewski BH. LasR of *Pseudomonas aeruginosa* is a transcriptional activator of the alkaline protease gene (*apr*) and an enhancer of exotoxin A expression. Infect Immun 1993; 61: 1180–1184.

109. Passador L, Cook JM, Gambello MJ, Rust L, Iglewski BH. Expression of *Pseudomonas aeruginosa* virulence genes requires cell-to-cell communication. Science 1993; 260: 1127–1130.

110. Ishimoto KS, Lory S. Formation of pilin in *Pseudomonas aeruginosa* requires the alternative σ factor (RpoN) of RNA polymerase. Proc Natl Acad Sci USA. 1989; 86: 1954–1957.

111. Sage A, Linker A, Evan LR, Lessie TG. Hexose-phosphate metabolism and exopolysaccharide formation in *Pseudomonas cepacia*. Can J Microbiol 1990; 20: 191–198.

112. McKevitt AI, Bajaksouzian S, Klinger JD, Woods DE. Purification and characterization of an extracellular protease of *Pseudomonas cepacia*. Infect Immun 1989; 57: 771–778.

113. Vasil ML, Krieg DP, Kuhns JS, Ogle JW, Shortidge VD, Ostroff RM *et al.* Molecular analysis of hemolytic and phospholipase C activities of *Pseudomonas cepacia*. Infect Immun 1990; 58: 4020–4029.

114. Kuehn A, Lent K, Haas J, Hagenzieker J, Cervin M, Smith A. Fimbriation of *Pseudomonas cepacia*. Infect Immun 1992; 60: 2002–2007.

115. Krivan HC, Roberts DD, Ginsburg V. Many pulmonary pathogenic bacteria bind specifically to the carbohydrate sequence GalNAcβ1-4Gal found in some glycolipids. Proc Natl Acad Sci USA 1988; 85: 6157–6161.

116. Sajjan US, Corey M, Karmali MA, Forstner JF. Binding of *Pseudomonas cepacia* to normal human intestinal mucin and respiratory mucin from patients with cystic fibrosis. J Clin Invest 1992; 89: 648–656.

117. Saiman L, Cacalano G, Prince A. *Pseudomonas cepacia* adherence to respiratory epithelial cells is enhanced by *Pseudomonas aeruginosa*. Infect Immun 1990; 58: 2578–2584.

118. Sajjan US, Forstner JF. Role of a 22-kilodalton pilin protein in binding of *Pseudomonas cepacia* to buccal epithelial cells. Infect Immun 1993; 61: 3157–3163.

Cystic Fibrosis Pulmonary Infections:
Lessons from Around the World
ed. by A. Bauernfeind, M. I. Marks and B. Strandvik

CHAPTER 6
Lung Transplantation

Brendan P. Madden[1] and Margaret E. Hodson[2]

[1]Department of Cardiological Sciences, St. George's Hospital, Tooting, London SW17 0QT, UK
[2]Department of Cystic Fibrosis, Royal Brompton National Heart & Lung Hospital, London SW3 6NP, UK

Introduction

Despite improvements in medical care, cystic fibrosis (CF) is a disease associated with significant morbidity and mortality. The major cause of death among adult CF patients is end-stage respiratory failure. It was against this background that the possibility of lung transplantation became a therapeutic option for the CF patient. Advances in post operative medical care have contributed significantly to the improved survival and quality of life after transplantation [1]. The first successful heart–lung transplants (HLT) for CF were performed in the United Kingdom in 1985 [2] and encouraging intermediate term ($5\frac{1}{2}$ year experience) results have been reported [3] which compare favorably with results of HLT performed for diseases other than CF [4].

HLT was traditionally the transplant procedure of choice for patients with CF. Cited advantages of this procedure included low post-operative incidence of both tracheal dehiscence and accelerated coronary artery disease [3]. However with increasing numbers of centres worldwide performing cardiac transplantation, the numbers of available heart–lung blocs for HLT are declining significantly and the indications for HLT are changing. Results of en-bloc double lung transplantation (DLT) for CF were initially poor largely due to tracheal anastomotic dehiscence [6] although recent reports are more encouraging [7]. Bilateral single lung transplantation (BSLT) for CF requires further evaluation.

There are advantages in transplanting patients with CF compared to other patients requiring transplantation for end-stage lung disease. CF patients are usually young and well motivated, they are used to taking regular medication, attending outpatients clinics and generally taking an active role in their management. Their parents and family are good at providing support, which is particularly important during the waiting period and after surgery. With the recent identification of the CF gene

[8] it would appear that the CF defect is located in the cells and not serum of the affected patient and therefore should not affect the transplanted lungs.

Although there have been significant advances in pre- and post-operative care and new developments in surgical technique, the shortage of available donor organs and obliterative bronchiolitis remain the two major obstacles to be overcome [3].

Indications for Transplantation

Since 1985 the indication for lung transplantation in CF has not changed. Patients should only be accepted into the transplant waiting list if they have deteriorating chronic respiratory failure with a severely impaired quality of life in spite of the best available medical treatment. These patients usually have a life expectancy of less than 18 months. The patients themselves must positively want a transplant. In practice the forced expiratory volume in one second (FEV_1) is usually less than 30% of the predicted value. It is most important that patients are only referred for transplant assessment if, with optimal conventional CF medical care, their condition has failed to improve.

It is possible to perform combined heart–lung and liver transplantation on patients with portal hypertension and to operate successfully on patients who are on ventilators pre-operatively [3]. Although it is a policy in many centres not to conventionally ventilate patients with CF who are in end-stage respiratory failure, nasal intermittent positive pressure ventilation may be used as a bridge to transplantation in selected patients [9]. This technique has a number of advantages. Firstly invasion of the airways with an endotracheal tube is avoided, thus minimizing the risk of pseudomonal toxaemia. Secondly it is possible to manage patients on the ward in familiar surroundings or even at home and thus avoid the need for management in the intensive care unit. Thirdly patients are able to adjust the ventilatory support delivered by the ventilator and thus feel to some degree in control of their situation.

New techniques to control haemostasis such as the use of aprotinin [10] and the argon coagulator have made it possible to operate successfully on many patients who have had previous thoracic surgery including surgical pleurodesis [3]. If patients have had a pleurodesis they usually require a lateral thoracotomy immediately prior to the transplant procedure to free adhesions.

Preoperative ventilation, previous thoracic surgery, surgical or chemical pleurodesis; or severe liver disease necessitating combined heart–lung and liver transplantation are not absolute contraindications for HLT. However patients with one or more of the above have significantly increased early (but not late) mortality after transplantation [3].

This is believed to reflect bleeding and multi-organ failure which is more commonly encountered in these patients during the peri-operative and early post-operative periods [3].

Contraindications to Transplantation

With increasing experience, the absolute contraindications to lung transplantation in CF are becoming fewer. They include pre-existing malignant disease, other end organ failure (unless this is also amenable to transplantation e.g. combined HLT and liver transplantation), active aspergillus or mycobacterial infection, infection with human immunodeficiency virus (HIV) or hepatitis B, prednisolone therapy in excess of 10 mg/day and non-compliance with treatment [3, 5, 11].

Active mycobacterial infection is an absolute contraindication to transplantation as, in the presence of immunosuppression, fatal post operative infection may occur. It is therefore essential that such infection be completely eradicated prior to surgery. For similar reasons patients with an aspergilloma are contraindicated. All patients who are being considered for lung transplantation and who produce sputum are carefully screened for *Aspergillus fumigatus*. If the organism is identified prior to transplantation a course of oral itraconazole together with amphotericin B by nebuliser is recommended in an attempt to clear the sputum [12]. Patients who have a persistently high count $\geq 10^3$ colony forming units/ml are not accepted onto the transplant waiting list [12]. If a patient has a low positive sputum count on sputum culture at the time of lung transplantation, oral itraconazole and amphotericin B by nebuliser are prescribed throughout the first post operative month [12]. Following the introduction of this protocol a recent study found no significant increase in mortality from invasive aspergillosis among CF lung transplant recipients when compared to patients who received lung transplantation for diseases other than CF [12].

Patients who are non-compliant with treatment or clinic attendance are also excluded. Lung transplantation has been successfully performed in patients taking prednisolone 10 mg/day pre-operatively without added complication. However patients with cushingoid features are usually excluded until these changes subside with reduction in steroid dose. There is concern that long-term steroid therapy may adversely affect tissue healing (particularly in the large airways) after transplantation.

Diabetes mellitus is not a contraindication to transplantation unless there are microvascular complications. Diabetic control usually becomes easier for the successfully transplanted CF patient as exercise capacity improves and respiratory infection is significantly reduced [1, 3, 11]. It is important that gross malnutrition is vigorously addressed.

Dietary calorie intake and pancreatic enzyme supplementation is maximized. Patients may require overnight gastrostomy or jejunostomy feeding [1].

Pre-Transplant Assessment

This normally involves admitting patients to hospital for approximately one week. During this time they are able to meet the staff, visit the surgical centre and talk with patients who have already been successfully transplanted.

In addition to a full history and physical examination (which includes height, weight and chest measurements) an assessment of the patient's quality of life and psychosocial suitability is undertaken. Patients will have detailed lung function tests and arterial blood gas analysis. The FEV_1 and forced vital capacity (FVC) are usually in the region of 30% predicted at the time of assessment with arterial oxygen saturation at rest between 80% and 90% (with marked desaturation on exercise). Chest radiography and CT scan of thorax are routine to document evidence of pleural thickening and adhesions. If adhesions are present it may be necessary to free them via a lateral thoracotomy immediately prior to the transplant procedure. A detailed dental and ear, nose and throat examination is made as chronically infected sinuses or teeth may become potential sources of post-operative infection [13].

A clinical evaluation of cardiac function is performed together with electrocardiography, two-dimensional echocardiography and 24 hour Holter monitor.

Routine haemotological and biochemical investigations (including bleeding and prothrombin times) are measured and abnormalities in hepatic and renal function addressed if possible. Serological investigations for cytomegalovirus (CMV), Epstein Barr virus, Australia antigen, toxoplasma, HIV and herpes simplex virus are performed.

Sputum is analysed for bacterial pathogens, acid fast bacilli and fungi. The majority of patients grow *Pseudomonas aeruginosa* in their sputum at the time of preoperative assessment. Patients with *Burkholderia cepacia* or methicillin-resistant *Staphylococcus aureus* have been successfully transplanted [8]. However some centres consider the presence of *B. cepacia* to be an absolute contraindication to transplantation on account of the high mortality and morbidity associated with this organism [14, 15].

Once on the transplant waiting list, patients have an unpredictable waiting period. Some wait a few days, others two to three years. The major criteria matching potential recipients with donor organs are blood group, size of thoracic cage and CMV antibody status [3, 4]. Thus it is not possible to predict accurately when patients will be transplanted. It is essential therefore that patients can be found at all times and some benefit from having an aircall bleep or a portable telephone so that they are not confined to their homes. Over the past few years the development of support groups to help patients on the transplant waiting list have been particularly helpful [11].

Surgical Options

Heart – Lung Transplantation (HLT)

This procedure involves right atrial, aortic and tracheal anastomoses. The coronary–bronchial collateral circulation (which provides an important blood supply to the trachea [16] remains intact and thus ischaemic complications of the large airways are uncommon. It may be possible to use the heart from a CF patient undergoing HLT for transplantation into a patient requiring cardiac transplantation who has moderate reversible elevation in pulmonary vascular resistance. The results of this procedure are encouraging with important psychological implications for both donor and recipient [17]. However with more centres now performing cardiac transplantation fewer heart–lung blocs are available and there has been a significant world-wide decline in HLT in recent years. Other options for successful lung transplantation in CF have therefore been developed.

Double-Lung Transplantation (DLT)

In this operation tracheal, pulmonary arterial, and pulmonary venous (to left atrium) anastomoses are performed. DLT allows the patient to retain his own heart but in so doing, healing of the airway anastomosis is put at risk as a result of ischaemia [18]. This can lead to dehiscence at the level of the airway anastomosis or to the development of granulation tissue formation. The latter can promote sputum retention and therefore facilitate the development of pulmonary infection which in itself can be a stimulus for further granulation tissue formation. However improved results of DLT for CF are being reported [6, 7]. Important factors which may contribute to these improvements include better organ preservation techniques, short ischaemic times and early extubation following lung transplantation.

Bilateral Sequential Lung Transplantation (BSLT)

In addition to pulmonary arterial and venous anastomoses, bi-bronchial anastomoses are performed in BSLT. This procedure is usually performed via a transverse thoracosternotomy ('clam shell' incision) and involves sequential replacement of the lungs. In some cases it can be performed without cardiopulmonary bypass. Intermediate term results of BSLT for CF are awaited although early experience is encouraging [19].

Single Lung Transplantation

Single lung transplantation is usually inappropriate for CF patients because of the risk of infecting the transplanted lung by sputum overspill from the remaining CF native lung.

Lobar Transplantation

Limited early experience is available with living related lobar transplants for CF [20]. Starnes has performed a lower lobectomy from each parent and, following bilateral pneumonectomy has transplanted each lower lobe into an offspring with CF. Early results with this procedure in CF patients are encouraging [20]. This raises important ethical considerations particularly in families in which there is more than one child with CF. In view of the shortage of donor organs undue pressure may be brought to bear on healthy siblings. Couteil has successfully performed lobar transplantation in CF patients using cadaveric donors. Further experience with lobar transplantation is awaited.

Post-Operative Management

General Management

It has become clear that, in addition to post-operative problems common to all lung transplant recipients (Table 1), CF patients may develop particular problems related to their multisystem disease [1] (Table 2).

Table 1. Common medical problems following lung transplantation

1. Acute rejection
2. Infection
3. Bleeding
4. Multiorgan failure
5. Airway anastomotic dehiscence or stenosis
6. Complications of immunosuppression
7. Grand mal seizures
8. Lymphoproliferative disorders
9. Obliterative bronchiolitis

Table 2. Specific problems in CF patients following lung transplantation

1. Persistent infection in upper respiratory tract
2. Malabsorption of cyclosporin A
3. Malnutrition
4. Liver disease
5. Meconium ileus equivalent
6. Diabetes mellitus
7. Salt loss

Table 3. Indications for bronchoscopy after lung transplantation

1. Routinely between the 7th and 10th post-operative day
2. Reduction in lung function tests
3. Abnormally on chest radiograph
4. Pyrexia of unknown origin
5. Unexplained cough
6. Reduction in exercise capacity

Patients are routinely immunosuppressed with azathioprine and cyclosporin A (CSA) after transplantation [3, 4]. Episodes of acute allograft rejection are treated with intravenous methylprednisolone. This may be supplemented with anti-thymocyte globulin.

Episodes of acute rejection are diagnosed according to clinical and radiological indices with respiratory function test and analysis of transbronchial lung biopsies specimens obtained at fibreoptic bronchoscopy.

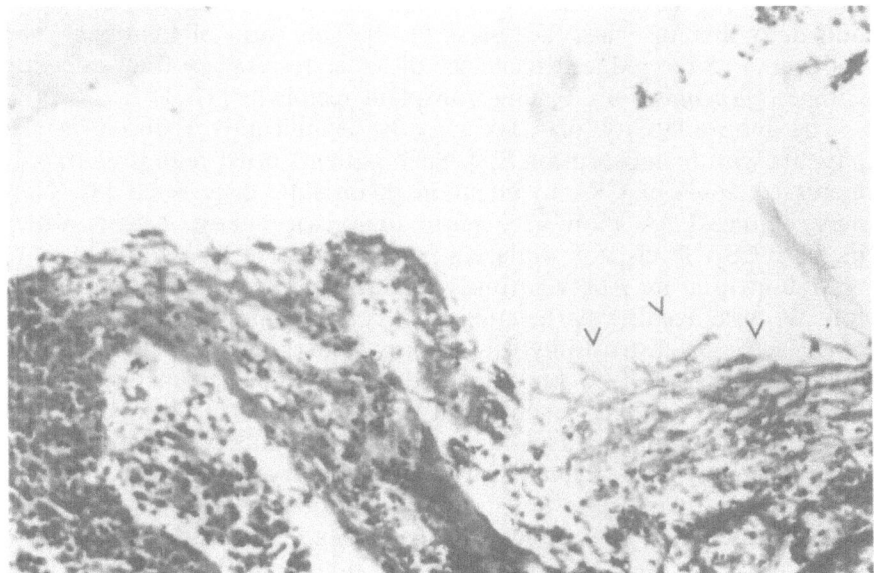

Figure 1. Transbronchial lung biopsy from a patient with invasive aspergillosis. The fungal hyphae are clearly seen (arrow). H and E, medium power.

This procedure is routinely performed at the end of the first post-operative week and thereafter if clinically indicated (Table 3). At broncho-scopy, the anastomosis is inspected and bronchoalveolar lavage speci-mens are taken for culture and sensitivity, opportunistic pathogen screen and immunocytochemistry. Transbronchial lung biopsy specimens are sent for histopathological examination and culture. The diagnosis of infection is made by a combination of clinical, serological and radiolog-ical findings together with examination of bronchoalveolar lavage fluid and transbronchial lung biopsy specimens (Figure 1). Episodes of infection are treated with appropriate antimicrobial agents. The com-mon medical problems encountered following lung transplantation are described elsewhere [1, 11].

Specific CF Management

Patients with CF commonly experience a complicated post-operative course [21]. As the upper airways and sinuses still maintain the CF defect and the newly transplanted lungs are denervated and have impaired ciliary beat frequency [22], infection in the sinuses may lead to infection in the allograft. It has been suggested that CF patients may benefit from maxillary sinus antrostomy and repeated sinus lavage following lung transplantation [13]. This is not usually necessary. It is our policy to prescribe life-long colistin sulphate (commencing at a dose of 1 mega unit twice daily for the first three post-operative months and thereafter 1 mega unit daily lifelong via a face mask [1, 3]. This form of treatment may contribute to the reduced incidence of lower respiratory tract infection with *P. aeruginosa* in CF lung transplant recipients [1, 3].

The bioavailability of CSA may be significantly reduced in CF patients with malabsorption [23]. Such patients often require markedly increased doses of CSA to maintain therapeutic drug levels [1]. They may require CSA more frequently than twice daily. Agents which increase CSA levels, e.g. diltiazem may be prescribed in addition.

Malnutrition may be vigorously addressed. The majority of patients tolerate oral feeding early after surgery when bowel sounds return. Nasogastric or gastrostomy/jejunostomy feeding may be required using high carbohydrate feed supplemented with medium chain triglycerides [1, 11]. Some patients benefit from the insertion of a feeding gastros-tomy tube after lung transplantation [1, 11]. If patients are intolerant of enteral feeding as a result of vagal nerve injury and impaired gastric motility, total parenteral nutrition is prescribed.

The presence of liver disease may necessitate modulation of azathio-prine and CSA dose, as both agents are potentially hepatotoxic.

Meconium ileus equivalent is treated conservatively in the first in-stance with N-acetylcysteine. Laparotomy is very rarely indicated.

In the early post-operative period diabetic patients may require insulin to control blood sugar. Thereafter diabetic control is often easier as patients exercise capacity improves and respiratory tract infection is less. Salt loss can be a particular problem in the early post-operative period when patients are in a warm environment and often receiving agents which enhance urinary sodium excretion e.g. diuretics and renal doses of dopamine. It is important that such patients have adequate salt replacement to avoid the complications of hyponatraemia.

Program of Long-Term Care

Following discharge from hospital patients are managed by the transplant unit in collaboration with the referring CF centre. Each patient receives a home microspirometer on discharge and is instructed to measure FEV_1 and FVC on a daily basis. If there is >15% reduction in lung function testing on two or more consecutive readings or if patients develop one or other of the parameters listed in Table 3, they must contact the transplant centre.

Outpatients visits are usually on a weekly basis to the transplant centre during the first month post-discharge but thereafter the frequency of appointments becomes less and eventually the majority of patients attend for review every six months. The referring centre is encouraged to play an active role in the management of the CF patient after transplantation. Indeed when patients develop problems the majority present to their local centre. In such instances early communication with the transplant centre is essential and, if necessary, prompt transfer.

Results

The largest experience in HLT for CF has been obtained in the United Kingdom [1, 2, 3]. The Brompton and Harefield group reported one and two year actuarial survival figures of 69% and 52% respectively in 79 CF HLT recipients. Twenty-three patients had one or more possible high risk factors and survival of these patients was 64% at one year and 52% at two years compared with 71% and 49% for the remaining patients. The difference between both groups was significant to three months ($p < 0.05$) but not thereafter [3]. The Papworth unit reported similar actuarial survival figures at 1 and 2 years (72% and 58% respectively) in 32 CF patients following HLT [2]. In both series the mean FEV_1 was approximately 70% of the predicted value by the third post-operative month. Improvements in lung function were maintained at three years post-transplantation [3]. In both series obliterative bronchiolitis was the most serious late complication and major cause of late mortality.

A North American group reported a 43% actuarial survival to one year after HLT with sepsis being the major cause of death [24]. The reasons for the difference in the North American and UK series may be multifactorial but it is noteworthy that 10 of the 14 centres performed two or fewer HLT for CF. This may imply that the surgical and particularly the medical team did not obtain sufficient experience in managing the complicated medical problems that these patients encounter after surgery.

A one year actuarial survival of 58% in 17 CF patients following BSLT was reported by the Toronto group [14]. The FEV_1 of transplant survivors had improved to 100% predicted value by the end of the first post-operative year. More recently the St Louis group described a one year actuarial survival of 80% following BSLT [25]. Further experience with lobar transplantation for CF is awaited.

Recurrence of Disease

In vivo measurements of airway potential difference after HLT has suggested that the CF membrane defect has not occurred in the donor lungs after two years follow-up [26].

Quality of Life

There is no doubt that the quality of life improves significantly for the successfully transplanted patient. Many patients have returned to school, work or higher education after surgery, some have married and others have gone on overseas holidays. Using the Nottingham Health Profile, HLT recipients have been shown to enjoy improved levels of social and emotional well-being [27, 28].

Challenges

The shortage of suitable donor organs remains a serious issue and continued efforts are necessary to ensure that the subject of organ donation is raised in a caring and compassionate way with relatives of potential donors fulfilling brainstem death criteria. National efforts should be made to maximise the use of all potential donor organs.

It is essential that patients are not referred too early for surgery as approximately 30% die during the first post-operative year. However a fine balance must be achieved as patients who are referred too late for transplant surgery may be too ill to be successfully transplanted or there may not be sufficient time to procure suitable donor organs.

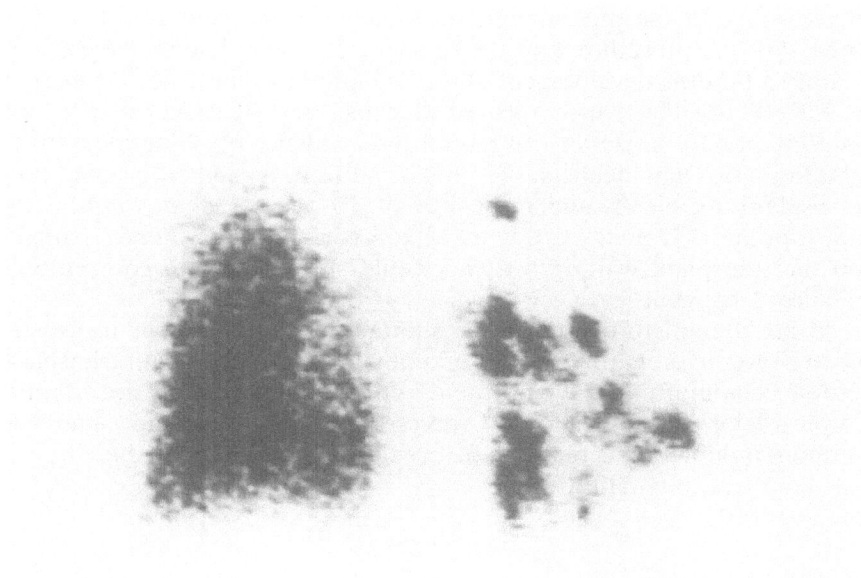

Figure 2. Technetium-99 mDTPA lung scan in a patient with obliterative bronchiolitis complicating left single lung transplantation for lymphangioleiomyomatosis. The patient subsequently had a right single lung transplant. Note patchy uptake and deposition of radio-isotope in the left lung, compared with the normal appearance on the right. (Permission to reproduce figure requested from Monaldi Archives of Chest Disease; ref 5).

Obliterative bronchiolitis remains the most serious late complication following lung transplantation, occurring in up to 40% of patients at 3 years [4]. It is a clinical diagnosis of progressive airflow obstruction. Chest radiography, transbronchial lung biopsy and DTPA scanning (Figure 2) may confirm the diagnosis. The incidence is higher in children under the age of 10 years [28]. There is evidence that it is an inevitable complication of lung transplantation [1]. The aetiology is unclear although it is suggested that obliterative bronchiolitis is a manifestation of chronic allograft rejection [29]. Other factors such as viral infection may also be involved [30] and it is possible that obliterative bronchiolitis is the end result from a variety of pulmonary injuries which include acute and chronic allograft rejection and infection [31].

For the majority of patients with obliterative bronchiolitis there is no effective cure. A minority will regain lost lung function with augmented immunosuppression [32]. However a significant proportion will deteriorate regardless until end-stage respiratory failure supervenes. For these patients the only remaining treatment option available is retransplantation [3, 4, 33]. Many centres are of the opinion that retransplantation is not justified at the present time on account of the poor results associated with the procedure and the shortage of available donor organs. It is hoped that the development of newer immunosuppressive agents such as FK506 together with improved diagnosis and treatment of rejection and pulmonary infection will reduce the incidence of obliterative bronchiolitis. As the incidence of this condition is higher among lung transplant recipients under the age of 10 years [28] it would seem appropriate that great care is taken to avoid putting younger patients on the transplant waiting list who would still respond to conventional medical treatment.

In an attempt to overcome the shortage of donor organs transplant centres are investigating the use of animal organs for human transplantation (xenografting). Hyperacute rejection leading to early graft failure is the major limiting factor to successful xenografting and significant immunomodulation is required before this becomes a therapeutic option for lung transplantation in CF.

References

1. Madden BP, Kamalvand K, Chan CM, Khaghani A, Hodson ME, Yacoub M. The medical management of patients with cystic fibrosis following heart–lung transplantation. Eur Resp J 1993; 6: 965–70.
2. Scott J, Higenbottam T, Hutter J et al. Heart–lung transplantation for cystic fibrosis. Lancet 1988; ii: 192–4.
3. Madden BP, Hodson ME, Tsang V, Radley-Smith R, Khaghani A, Yacoub MY. Intermediate-term results of heart–lung transplantation for cystic fibrosis. Lancet 1992; 339: 1583–7.
4. Madden B, Radley-Smith R, Hodson M, Khaghani A, Yacoub M. Medium term results of heart and lung transplantation. J Heart–Lung Transplant 1992; 11: S241–43.
5. Madden BP, Geddes DM. Which patients should receive lung transplants? Monaldi Arch Chest Dis 1993; 48(4): 346–352.
6. Patterson GA. Double lung transplantation. Pediatr Pulmonol 1989; 4: 56–7.
7. Egan TA. Overview of lung transplantation for cystic fibrosis. Paediatr Pulmonol 1992 (Suppl 8); 204–5.
8. Rommens JM, Ianuzzi MC, Kerrem B et al. Identification of the cystic fibrosis gene: chromosome walking and jumping. Science 1989; 245: 1059–1065.
9. Hodson ME, Madden BP, Steven MH, Tsang VT, Yacoub MH. Non-invasive mechanical ventilation for cystic fibrosis patients: a bridge to transplantation. Eur Respir J 1991; 4: 524–7.
10. Alajmo FR, Giancarlo C, Perna AM et al. High dose aprotinin haemostatic effects in open heart operations. Ann Thorac Surg 1989; 48: 536–9.
11. Madden B. Lung transplantation for cystic fibrosis. In: ME Hodson and DM Geddes, editors. Chapman and Hall, 1995; 329–346.
12. Madden BP, Chan CM, Kamalvand K, Siddiqi A, Vuddamalay P, Hodson ME. Aspergillus infection in patients with cystic fibrosis following lung transplantation. In: H. Escobar, F. Baquero and L. Suarez, editors: Clinical ecology of cystic fibrosis. Publ Excerpta Medica International Congress Series 1993; 189–94.
13. Lewiston N, King V, Umetsu D et al. Cystic fibrosis patients who have undergone heart-lung transplantation benefit from maxilary sinus antrostomy and repeated sinus lavage. Transplant Proc 1991; 23: 207–8.
14. Ramirez JC, Patterson GA, Winton TL et al. Bilateral lung transplantation for cystic fibrosis. J Thorac Cardiovasc Surg 1992; 103: 287–94.

15. Snell GI, de Hoyos A, Krajden M, Winton T, Maurer JR. *Pseudomonas cepacia* in lung transplant recipients with cystic fibrosis. Chest 1993; 103: 466–71.

16. Bonser RS, Jamieson SW. Heart–lung transplantation. Clin Chest Med 1990; 11: 235–246.

17. Wallis S. Domino cardiac transplantation. Paediatric Nursing 1993; 5: 24–26.

18. Patterson GA, Todd TR, Cooper JD *et al.* Airway complications after double lung transplantation. J Thorac Cardiovasc Surg 1990; 99: 14–21.

19. Pasque MK, Cooper JD, Kaiser LR *et al.* Improved technique for bilateral lung transplantation: rationale and initial clinical experience. Ann Thorac Surg 1990; 49: 785–91.

20. Starnes V. Living donor transplants: Medical and Ethical Implications. Presented at the 7th Annual North American Cystic Fibrosis Conference, Dallas, 1993.

21. Madden B, Hodson ME, Yacoub M. Heart–lung transplantation for cystic fibrosis. Br Med J 1992; 304: 835–6.

22. Shankar S, Fulsham L, Read R, Theodoroupoulos S, Cole P, Madden B, Yacoub M. Mucociliary function after lung transplantation. Trans Proc 1991; 23: 1222–1223.

23. Cooney GF, Fiel SB, Shaw LM, Cavarocchi NC. Cyclosporin bioavailability in heart–lung transplant candidates with cystic fibrosis. Transplantation 1990; 49: 821–3.

24. Frist WH, Fox PW, Campbell SB, Loyd JE, Merrill WH. Cystic fibrosis treated with heart–lung transplantation: North American results. Transplant Proc 1991; 23: 1205–6.

25. Cooper J. Lung Transplantation for Cystic Fibrosis. Presented at the 18th European Cystic Fibrosis Conference, Madrid, May 1993.

26. Alton EWFW, Khaghani A, Taylor RFH *et al.* Effect of heart–lung transplantation on airway potential difference in patients with and without cystic fibrosis. Eur Respir J 1991; 4: 5–9.

27. Caine N, Sharples LD, Smyth R *et al.* Survival and quality of life of cystic fibrosis patients before and after heart–lung transplantation. Transplant Proc 1991; 23: 1203–4.

28. Whitehead B, Helms P, Goodwin M *et al.* Heart–lung transplantation for cystic fibrosis. Outcome. Arch Dis Child 1991; 66: 1022–6.

29. Scott JP, Sharples L, Mullins P *et al.* Further studies on the natural history of obliterative bronchiolitis following heart–lung transplantation. Transplant Proc 1991; 23: 1201–2.

30. Griffith BP, Paradis IL, Zeevi A *et al.* Immunology mediated disease of the airways after pulmonary transplantation. Ann Surg 1988; 208: 371–9.

31. Madden BP, Siddiqi AJ, Burke M, Pomerance A. Possible aetiological factors in obliterative bronchiolitis following lung transplantation. Pediatr Pulmonol 1993; 9: 273.

32. Glanville AR, Baldwin JC, Burke CM, Theodore J, Robin ED. Obliterative bronchiolitis after heart–lung transplantation: apparent arrest by augmented immunosuppression. Ann Intern Med 1987; 107: 300–4.

33. Madden B, Khaghani A, Yacoub M. Successful retransplantation of the heart and lungs in an adult with cystic fibrosis. J Roy Soc Med 1991; 84: 561.

CHAPTER 7
The General Approach to Cystic Fibrosis-Related Pulmonary Infection in the United States

Harris R. Stutman

Director, Pediatric Infectious Disease, Memorial Miller Children's Hospital, Long Beach, California 90801, USA

Summary. The principal cause of morbidity and mortality in patients with cystic fibrosis remains pulmonary infection, resulting in progressive airway destruction, bronchiectasis, and pulmonary failure [1]. Endobronchial infection including pneumonia, with or without an appropriate inflammatory response, is nearly universal in cystic fibrosis patients. Our success at controlling albeit not curing, the pulmonary infection in cystic fibrosis has undoubtedly been a major cause of a remarkable improvement in median survival rates and quality of life seen in the U.S. over the past 20 years (Figure 1). This is also clearly related to coordinated management strategies disseminated by the U.S. CF Foundation, through their accredited clinical centers. This paper will focus on several aspects of the management of pulmonary infections that have been prioritized in the United States. First among these has been the development of new antibiotics and new antibiotic strategies to control acute bronchopulmonary exacerbations in cystic fibrosis. Second has been the development of appropriate strategies that may be useful in preventing progressive pulmonary infection. Third is the development of non-antimicrobial strategies, such as pulmonary clearance methods and anti-inflammatory therapies that may also prove useful in the control of progressive bronchopulmonary disease.

Pulmonary Infections in Cystic Fibrosis: Diagnosis

Distinctions between acute and chronic manifestations of bronchopulmonary infections in cystic fibrosis have long been problematic. Because CF patients are typically unable to eradicate bacterial pathogens from their airways, the criteria used to distinguish between acute and chronic bronchopulmonary disease, in other situations, do not apply. Therefore, a variety of definitions for acute exacerbations have been employed. Research studies are ongoing in the United States to more precisely explore this problem [2]. The acute symptoms of pulmonary infection are usually a result of an inflammatory response to ongoing endobronchial infection, sometimes related to the acquisition of new organisms or intercurrent respiratory, viral, or other (mycoplasma, legionella, mycobacterial) infection. Acute exacerbations are often

Correspondence address: Harris R. Stutman, Pediatric Infectious Disease, Memorial Miller Children's Hospital, 2801 Atlantic Avenue, Long Beach, CA 90801, USA.

Percent Survival

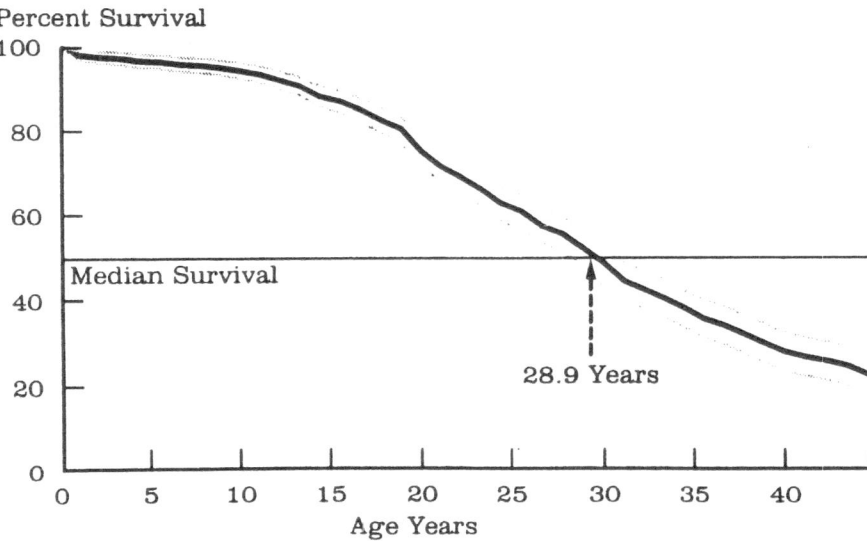

Figure 1. Median life expectancy for 19 220 patients included in the U.S. Data Registry, Cystic Fibrosis Foundation, for 1993.

characterized by an increased mucus secretion and airway obstruction, particularly of the small airways. Systemic manifestations of these acute exacerbations often include such features as fatigue, anorexia and weight loss, increased cough and sputum production, and fever. A change in pulmonary function is obviously the most objective measure of acute changes in obstructive airway disease, but is often absent even in patients who otherwise clearly have acute exacerbations. In patients over 5 years of age, forced expiratory volume at 1 second (FEV_1) and forced vital capacity (FVC) are typically the most useful measurements, both because of their ease of measurement and their reproducibility [3].

In studies in the United States and elsewhere, the microbiology of CF respiratory flora is unique (Figure 2) and there appears to be a common progression of pulmonary pathogens in cystic fibrosis. Typically, *Staphylococcus aureus* is the first organism to colonize and infect the bronchopulmonary tree [4]. Several recent studies have shown that this applies both to upper respiratory flora and to specimens obtained from the lower respiratory tract via flexible bronchoscopy [5]. Following some period of time, non-mucoid *Pseudomonas aeruginosa* and non-typable *Haemophilus influenzae* are the next organisms to emerge. Ultimately, non-mucoid phenotypes of *P. aeruginosa* are replaced by mucoid strains [6]. The mucoid (alginate) matrix provides a mechanical barrier to phagocytes and antibiotics, as well as serving anti-complement and anti-phagocytic functions. Once mucoid phenotypes of *P. aeruginosa* emerge, they typically persist. This makes the distinction of

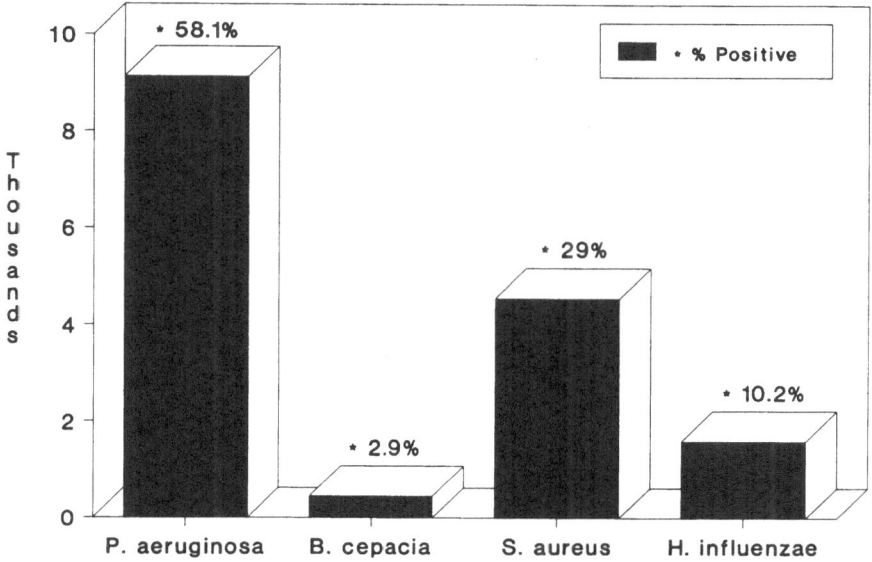

Figure 2. Relative distribution of bacterial pathogens isolated from respiratory tract cultures in 15 720 CF patients in the United States for 1993. Cystic Fibrosis Foundation Data Registry.

acute and chronic bronchopulmonary disease very difficult to base on microbiologic criteria.

As noted, the most objective laboratory measurement of pulmonary exacerbation is a decline in pulmonary function. Because the inherent variability of FEV_1 and FVC measurements is 5% to 10%, most clinicians expect greater declines when using these to diagnose bronchopulmonary exacerbation [7]. New infiltrates on chest radiography are also useful, but the chronic changes consistent with cystic fibrosis often make it difficult to interpret small differences as representing pneumonia. Sputum cultures when properly obtained, will identify bacterial pathogens that are colonizing the tracheobronchial tree. However, these are not available in younger patients because of the inability to expectorate and many physicians in the U.S. use upper respiratory specimens (throat culture) as a marker for lower airway colonization. Several studies have shown that the positive predictive value of throat culture for tracheobronchial colonization is 75% to 85% [8], suggesting that throat cultures positive for staphylococcus or pseudomonas are useful in directing antimicrobial therapy. Throat cultures negative for these pathogens do not, unfortunately, exclude these bacteria as causes of current pulmonary infection and some clinicians have advocated increased use of bronchoscopy for children unable to expectorate [9], before excluding the possibility of these bacteria as pathogens.

Although *P. aeruginosa* is the most common pathogen in cystic fibrosis secretions, many other bacteria and other organisms may play a role in an individual acute exacerbation. Most cystic fibrosis centers in the United States use selective media to enable *S. aureus*, *H. influenzae*, and other gram-negative bacilli (*B. cepacia*, *X. maltophilia*) to be detected [10]. These pathogens are difficult to detect on routine media when they co-exist with mucoid-producing *P. aeruginosa*. A typical media panel would be blood and MacConkey agars, mannitol salt agar (*S. aureus*), horse blood agar (*H. influenzae*), OFPBL or PC agars (*B. cepacia*) and Sabouraud agar [10]. When clinical, epidemiologic or geographic circumstances dictate, the search for etiologic pathogens of acute pulmonary exacerbations should also include respiratory viruses (especially RSV and influenza), mycoplasma, *Chlamydia pneumoniae*, legionella, and mycobacteria [11]. Most centers use mucolytic agents such as dithiothreiotol (sputalysin) to liquify sputum specimens and permit better characterization of individual bacterial isolates [12]. Quantitative cultures have not typically proven useful in providing more precise assessments.

Other inflammatory markers such as white blood cell count with differentials, erythrocyte sedimentation rate, C-reactive protein, and others are often elevated in patients with cystic fibrosis. Several authors have suggested that short-term increases may be useful in diagnosing acute exacerbations. However, without preceding measurement during periods without infection, these may be difficult to interpret [13]. A very interesting finding in cystic fibrosis-related pulmonary infection, given the pathogens involved, is the very rare phenomenon of bacterial dissemination. Cystic fibrosis patients are clearly not immunocompromised systemically, but rather suffering from a local phenomenon related to the endobronchial milieu and its effect on their inability to clear bacterial colonizers. Therefore, most U.S. physicians have adopted a pragmatic approach to the evaluation of CF-related pulmonary exacerbations. Studies such as chest radiography, blood and urine cultures, urinary antigen studies, and others are not typically obtained unless there is some specific clinical reason to do so.

Treatment of Pulmonary Infections: Antibiotic

Because of the variety of bacterial pathogens involved, and the fact that drug susceptibility patterns may differ widely among patients and among geographic areas, precise microbiology and susceptibility data are critical to the best use of antibiotics to treat acute bronchopulmonary infections. Clinicians in the United States rely heavily on annual reports from microbiology laboratories at their institutions to decide upon the best empiric approach to treat these infections. In younger patients where *S. aureus* may be a sole pathogen, antibiotics directed against this organism, such as nafcillin or cefazolin, are often used in the hospital setting. For milder infections that do not require hospitalization, such antibiotics as dicloxacillin and cephalexin are often useful for patients who are colonized only with *S. aureus*. Erythromycin has become less dependable over the years as resistance rates in the United States have increased (now typically >30%). For patients colonized with *S. aureus* and *H. influenzae*, second generation cephalosporins such as cefuroxime and betalactam-betalactamase inhibitor compounds such as ampicillin-sulbactam are often useful for hospitalized patients. Again, for milder infections not requiring hospitalization, oral equivalents such as cefuroxime, cefprozil, or amoxicillin-clavulanate have proven useful. Treatment courses are typically 2 to 3 weeks, although criteria for concluding therapy remain hopelessly empiric [14].

Pseudomonas aeruginosa can be much more problematic. Because of the presence of inducible beta-lactamases in most *P. aeruginosa* species, monotherapy with a beta-lactam is usually not used, for fear of the early emergence of resistance [15]. In the United States, patients colonized with non-mucoid or mucoid variants of *P. aeruginosa* are typically treated with beta-lactam plus aminoglycoside regimens for moderate to severe exacerbations. These regimens can be given in hospital or at home, if suitable nursing arrangements can be made [16]. In 1993, 16% of all U.S. CF patients received at least one course of IV antibiotic therapy at home. Appropriate management should also take into consideration other pathogens isolated from respiratory secretions. For example, the presence of staphylococcus in association with pseudomonas would suggest the addition of nafcillin to a regimen of anti-pseudomonal beta-lactam and an aminoglycoside, or perhaps the use of an aminoglycoside plus a beta-lactamase inhibitor-containing compound with activity against staphylococcus and pseudomonas (e.g. ticarcillin-clavulanate or piperacillin-tazobactam). We emphasize that these inhibitor compounds do not enhance activity of the putative beta-lactam for *P. aeruginosa*, however, and therefore attention to the susceptibility profile for each clinical isolate is mandatory.

For patients who have chronic pseudomonas colonization and are suffering from milder exacerbations not requiring inpatient or intravenous therapy, the availability of oral quinolones has been a major advance in the United States, and elsewhere. Many centers have found that short, repeated courses of ciprofloxacin or ofloxacin can be safely given to cystic fibrosis patients younger than 18 years of age, despite the concern over arthropathy described in immature, experimental animals. A number of papers, primarily from Europe, would tend to support this relative lack of toxicity by oral quinolones in younger patients with cystic fibrosis [17]. A major problem, however, as has been the case with beta-lactam monotherapy of *P. aeruginosa*, is the rapid emergence of bacterial resistance. In our hospital, for example, we have seen the

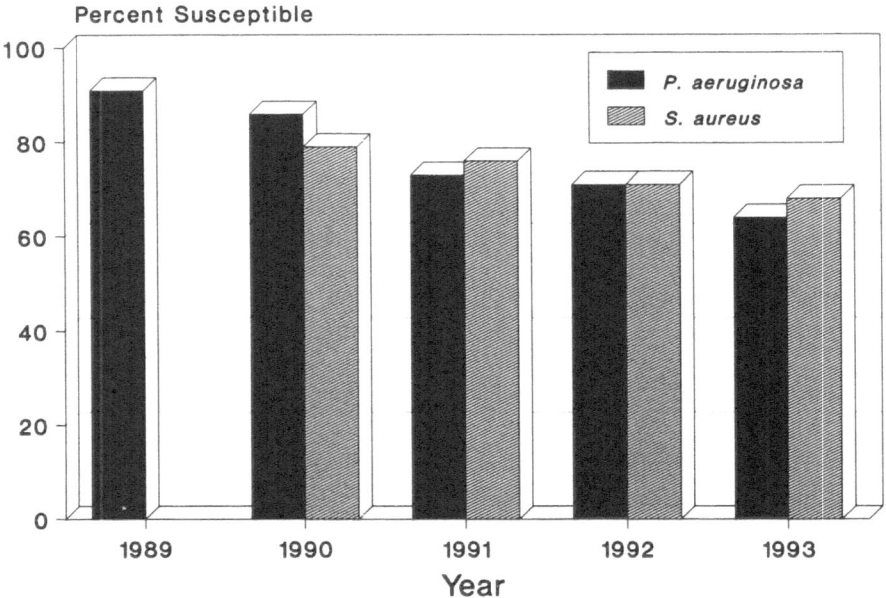

Figure 3. Percentage of susceptible isolates of *P. aeruginosa* and *S. aureus* to ciprofloxacin (CF and non-CF isolates) at the Long Beach (California) Memorial Medical Center from 1989 through 1993.

percentage of pseudomonas strains susceptible to ciprofloxacin decrease from 86% to 64% from 1990 to 1993 (Figure 3). Therefore, many cystic fibrosis clinicians in the United States combine oral ciprofloxacin with aerosolized tobramycin for the outpatient management of mild *P. aeruginosa*-related pulmonary exacerbations. It should be noted that a similar decline in the activity of quinolones against staphylococci have been noted over the last several years and, in patients with mixed flora including *S. aureus*, ciprofloxacin or ofloxacin should not automatically be assumed to be active against *S. aureus* (Figure 3). Similarly, it should be noted that although many of the aminoglycosides have some *in vitro* activity against *S. aureus* and *H. influenzae*, they have typically not been efficacious in the monotherapy of infections due to these organisms.

Burkholderia (*Pseudomonas*) *cepacia* has continued to be an indolent problem in the United States. The most recent data from the Cystic Fibrosis Foundation Data Registry indicate that approximately 3% of 16 000 cystic fibrosis patients in the U.S. are colonized with this organism (Figure 2), which unfortunately, is resistant to many antibiotics. Aminoglycosides, for example, are typically ineffective against this organism. Some beta-lactams do have activity against occasional strains, but trimethoprim-sulfamethoxazole is the most consistently active against this problem pathogen. The combination of trimethoprim-sulfamethoxazole is also typically the most active antibiotic combination against *X. maltophilia*, another non-fermenting Gram-negative bacillus that occasionally colonizes and infects cystic fibrosis patients. Fluoroquinolones also have some activity against *B. cepacia* and *X. maltophilia*.

Treatment of Pulmonary Infections: Aerosol Therapy

Many studies have confirmed that the amount of antibiotic that is delivered into the airway lumen when administered orally or intravenously is less than desirable to maximize antimicrobial effects. Recent studies have demonstrated that high dose aerosolized aminoglycoside (e.g. tobramycin) can achieve levels of intraluminal antibiotic activity consistent with greater antibacterial and, presumably, clinical effects. In a multicenter placebo-controlled study by Ramsey and colleagues, 4 week courses of aerosolized tobramycin therapy were associated with significant improvements in pulmonary function, and up to three log decreases in the sputum density of *P. aeruginosa* [18]. Importantly, the back diffusion of tobramycin given by this route into serum was minimal, suggesting that aminoglycoside-related ototoxicity or nephrotoxicity should not be of concern even when using doses as high as 600 mg, 3 times per day. In smaller studies, other investigators have also noted that inhaled colistin and amikacin may also have similar microbiologic effects, although the correlation with pulmonary function improvement is not as well demonstrated [19]. Therefore, many clinicians in the United States are using longer courses of aerosolized tobramycin, often combined with oral antibiotic therapy for patients with frequently recurrent or persistent *P. aeruginosa*-related pulmonary infections. The issue of combining aerosol and intravenous aminoglycoside therapy is not yet resolved, at least in the U.S. There has been one study published suggesting that there was no additional benefit with the combination of aminoglycoside therapy by multiple routes for acute exacerbations [20]. Therefore, most U.S. clinicians are not using aerosolized therapy in patients receiving aminoglycosides simultaneously, usually due to a concern over additive toxicities.

Chronic Therapy of Pulmonary Infections: Non-Antibiotic

The approach to mobilization of respiratory secretions in patients with cystic fibrosis is similar to that adopted in Western Europe and elsewhere. The thick and tenacious secretions characteristic of cystic fibrosis are directly related to the underlying pathophysiology. A variety of respiratory therapy methodologies have been used to facilitate the clearance of pulmonary secretions both for their beneficial mechanical effects, as well as for the postulated enhancement of antibiotic penetration into less viscous secretions. These techniques include chest percussion and postural drainage, airway vibration (using a flutter valve), positive expiratory pressure (PEP), and other forced expiratory techniques [21]. Although there has been an ongoing debate as to the ultimate benefit of these therapies, particularly because the more traditional methods such as chest physiotherapy require intensive time commitments and multiple care givers, recent studies have confirmed both short and long-term improvements in pulmonary function and general well being using these techniques. In a particularly helpful study, for patients with moderately severe cystic fibrosis who received forced expiratory therapies with or without conventional chest percussion and postural drainage, the rates of decline in pulmonary functions, particularly those reflecting small airway disease, were less in those patients receiving combined therapies [22]. These techniques have been traditionally used as part of an overall approach to the prevention (or perhaps, more appropriately, the delay) of chronic lung disease and progressive destruction of the airway in CF. At this point, there does not appear to be an overall consensus in the United States over which of these techniques is most efficacious. Nevertheless, the vast majority of CF clinicians in the U.S. are recommending that at least one of these therapies be commenced at the time of initial cystic fibrosis diagnosis and continued throughout the patient's lifetime. The availability of techniques such as PEP, autogenic drainage, and airway vibration (flutter valve) which do not require a second person are proving particularly useful as more and more cystic fibrosis patients reach adulthood and become independently responsible for their own medical management [23].

Airway reactivity and bronchospasm has long been a major component of the clinical presentation of cystic fibrosis. Several studies have suggested that as many as 50% of CF patients will have bronchial reactivity [24]. Although the data on the use of bronchodilators, particularly beta-andrenergics, have not been totally consistent, most clinicians in the United States have been using these therapies with success for many years. In the last several years, there has been an increasing realization of problems associated with the use of methylxanthines, particularly their propensity to increase gastroesophageal reflux, already a problem in many cystic fibrosis patients [25]. Therefore, there has been a substantial move away from the use of oral or intravenous theophylline and similar agents in CF. The use of anticholinergics, such as atropine and ipratropium, usually in combination with beta-andrenergics, such as albuterol, has increased substantially. Most U.S. clinicians combine aerosol and respiratory therapy modalities in all CF patients, unless aerosols are not tolerated or can be shown to be ineffective.

As is well known, there has long been a debate among cystic fibrosis clinicians concerning the relative effects of infection versus inflammation on progressive bronchopulmonary disease. Several investigations have suggested that the severity of pulmonary disease may be related more to the intensity of the host response, and that anti-inflammatory therapies might be very useful. A clinical study of alternate day prednisone conducted by Auerbach and colleagues seemed to support this hypothesis [26]. Unfortunately, a large multicenter study sponsored by the Cystic Fibrosis Foundation in the U.S. involving some 300 children with mild to moderate disease treated with alternate day prednisone did not yield encouraging results. Patients treated with high-dose therapy (2 mg/kg/day) had a significant increase in the frequency of steroid-related side effects such as growth retardation, glucose metabolism abnormalities, and cataracts. This study arm was terminated prematurely [27]. Final analysis of the placebo and low-dose (1 mg/kg/every other day) prednisone groups has not suggested a major beneficial effect for steroids and there is a suggestion that side effects such as glucose metabolism abnormalities and growth retardation are more common in the low dose steroid group [28]. A 4-year multicenter study of ibuprofen has recently been completed and the results suggest that this drug may be associated with small, but beneficial, effects on pulmonary function in patients less than 13 years of age. After 4 years of ibuprofen therapy, patients had a decrease of 2% in FVC and FEV, compared to 13% in the placebo group [29]. These studies strongly suggest the use of ibuprofen if anti-inflammatory therapy is given.

A final overview of preventive strategies must consider the use of drugs that affect the viscosity of pulmonary intraluminal secretions. Recombinant human deoxyribonuclease (DNAse), is now available in the United States for clinical use. In a large multicenter study involving over 900 patients, it appeared that regular use of this aerosolized compound was associated with a significant decrease in sputum viscosity and small, but significant, increases (averaging 5%) in forced vital capacity over a 6-month period [30]. There did not appear to be differences between once or twice daily therapy. This drug was licensed for use in the United States in early 1994 and post-marketing studies are presently being conducted. It remains to be seen what ultimate role this drug will have on the progressive pulmonary disease in CF, but standard recommendations in the United States would suggest that a trial of this therapy should be given to patients of more than 5 years of age with mild to moderate bronchopulmonary disease (FVC > 40%), to assess its effect on vital capacity and forced expiratory volume. If beneficial effects (an increase of 5% to 10% or greater) can be demonstrated, chronic therapy is probably appropriate. Preliminary results of a study of DNAse in patients with moderate to severe pulmonary disease (FVC < 40%) did not apparently yield statistically significant benefits (although analysis is incomplete) probably because of the fixed nature of the pulmonary disease in many of these patients [31]. Many CF clinicians in the U.S. are, therefore, cautious about recommending therapeutic use of this therapy in such patients. DNAse appears reasonably safe, with very few significant side effects, probably the most common being transient hoarseness or sore throat [30].

Other investigational drugs still being evaluated for their effect on decreasing the viscosity of CF sputum and perhaps enhancing the clearance of sputum are amiloride and nucleotides (UTP or ATP). Amiloride is a sodium channel blocker which appears to inhibit the absorption of sodium from cystic fibrosis airways. In small studies, this led to small, but statistically significant decreases in sputum viscosity. Other small studies have suggested that nucleotides such as ATP and UTP, which can increase chloride and water secretion even in cystic fibrosis, may synergistically enhance the hydration of airway secretions in CF. These are obviously not yet part of routine management strategies.

Chronic Therapy of Pulmonary Infections: Antibiotic

There is no general consensus on the chronic use of antibiotic therapy for cystic fibrosis-related pulmonary disease. Some CF clinicians continue to use drugs such as cephalexin, trimethoprim-sulfamethoxazole, or antistaphylococcal penicillins in an attempt to delay progressive bronchopulmonary disease. There are some data to suggest that attempts to intervene early with antistaphylococcal therapy may delay the progression to *P. aeruginosa*, bronchopulmonary colonization and its sequelae. A 6-year study of the hypothesis that early initiation of antistaphylococcal therapy will prevent or retard ongoing bronchopulmonary disease, has recently been completed [32]. Until the results of this study are available, most CF clinicians in the U.S. are not using chronic antibiotic therapy for cystic fibrosis patients, but rather managing acute exacerbations with vigorous antibiotic therapy and using non-antimicrobial strategies, including aerosol therapy, chest physiotherapy and other novel mechanisms of mobilizing respiratory secretions.

Discussion

As noted above, the long-term strategies for management of cystic fibrosis-related bronchopulmonary disease in the U.S. have traditionally focused on non-antimicrobial therapies, including chest physiotherapy, aerosol therapy, and now mucolytic agents. Although not the subject of this article, adjunctive therapies such as nutrition and hydration must not be ignored. These have been combined with vigorous antibiotic therapy for documented acute exacerbations of bronchopulmonary disease, using oral and/or aerosolized therapy for milder infections not requiring hospitalization or intravenous therapeutic interventions, and intravenous therapy, particularly beta-lactam and aminoglycoside combinations, for significant bronchopulmonary exacerbations. These strategies, when employed as part of a consistent management program at a CF center (accredited by, and following, CF Foundation guidelines [33]) have resulted in a progressive increase in life expectancy and well documented improvement in the quality of life for CF patients in the United States. Although U.S. data are sparse, the European experience would strongly support this emphasis on centralizing cystic fibrosis care [34, 35]. Additional information on the use of prophylactic antistaphylococcal antibiotics, aerosolized antibiotics, anti-inflammatory therapies, and sputum mobilization techniques, are awaited with great interest and may well be included in the overall approach to cystic fibrosis-related pulmonary disease within the next several years.

References

1. Stutman HR, Marks MI. Pulmonary infections in children with cystic fibrosis. Seminars in Respiratory Infection 1987; 2: 166–76.
2. Ramsey BW, Pepe M, Warren JW. Pulmonary exacerbation (PE): How do we define it? Eighth Annual North American Cystic Fibrosis Conference; 1994 Oct 20–23; Orlando (FL); New York: Wiley-Liss.
3. Cooper PJ, Robertson CF, Hudson IL, Phelan PD. Variability of pulmonary tests in cystic fibrosis. Pediatr Pulmonol 1990; 8: 16–22.
4. Hudson VL, Wielinski CL, Regelmann WE. Prognostic implications of initial oropharyngeal bacterial flora in patients with cystic fibrosis diagnosed before the age of two years. J Pediatr 1993; 122(6): 854–60.
5. Schwab UE, Wold AE, Carson JL, Leigh MW, Cheng PW, Gilligan PH, et al. Increased adherence of Staphylococcus aureus from cystic fibrosis lungs airway epithelial cells. Am Rev Resp Dis 1993; 148(2): 365–9.
6. Kerem E, Corey M, Stein R, Gold R, Levison H. Risk factors for Pseudomonas aeruginosa colonization in cystic fibrosis patients. Pediatr Infect Dis J 1990; 9: 494–8.
7. Smith AL, Redding G, Doershuk C, Goldmann D, Gore E, Hilman B, et al. Sputum changes associated with therapy for endobronchial exacerbation in cystic fibrosis. J Pediatr 1988; 112(4): 547–54.
8. Gilljam H, Malborg A, Strandvik B. Conformity of bacterial growth in sputum and contamination free endobronchial samples in patients with cystic fibrosis. Thorax 1986; 41: 641–6.
9. Accurso FJ, Sokol RJ, Hammond KB, Abman SH. Early respiratory course in infants with cystic fibrosis: Relevance to newborn screening. Pediatr Pulmonol 1991; 7(suppl): 42–5.
10. Gilligan PH. The role of the clinical microbiology laboratory in management of chronic lung infections in patients with cystic fibrosis. Rev Clin Microbiol 1991; 4: 35–51.
11. Pribble CG, Black PG, Bosso JA, Turner RB. Clinical manifestations of exacerbations of cystic fibrosis associated with non-bacterial infections. J Pediatr 1990; 117(2): 200–4.
12. Maduri-Traczewski M, L'Heureux C, Escalona L, Macone A, Goldmann D. Facilitated detection of antibiotic-resistant pseudomonas in cystic fibrosis sputum using homogenized specimens and antibiotic-containing media. Diagn Microbiol Infect Dis 1986; 5: 299–305.

13. Raynar RJ, Wiseman MS, Cordon SM, Norman D, Hiller EJ, Shale DJ. Inflammatory markers in cystic fibrosis. Resp Med 1991; 85(2): 139-45.
14. Marks MI. Clinical significance of *Staphylococcus aureus* in cystic fibrosis. Infect 1990; 18: 53-6.
15. Giwercman B, Lambert PA, Rosdahl VT, Shand GH, Hoiby N. Rapid emergence of resistance in *Pseudomonas aeruginosa* in cystic fibrosis patients due to *in vivo* selection of stable partially depressed β-lactamase producing strains. J Antimicrob Chemother 1990; 26: 247-259.
16. Donati MA, Guenette G, Auerbach H. Prospective controlled study of home and hospital therapy of cystic fibrosis pulmonary disease. J Pediatr 1987 Jul; 111(1): 28-33.
17. Schaad UB. Role of the new quinolones in pediatric practice. Pediatr Infect Dis 1992; 11: 1043-6.
18. Ramsey BW, Dorkin HL, Eisenberg JD, Schidlow DV, Wilmott RW, Astley SJ, et al. Efficacy of aerosolized tobramycin in patients with cystic fibrosis. N Engl J Med 1993; 328(24): 1740-6.
19. Valerius NH, Koch C, Hoiby N. Prevention of chronic *Pseudomonas aeruginosa* colonization in cystic fibrosis by early treatment. Lancet 1991; 338: 725-6.
20. Schaad UB, Wedgwood-Krucko J, Sutter S, Kraemer R. Efficacy of inhaled amikacin as adjunct to intravenous combination therapy (ceftazidime and amikacin) in cystic fibrosis. J Pediatr 1987; 111(4): 599-605.
21. Morton S, Gilbert J, Littlewood JM. The current physical therapy regimens of 108 consecutive patients attending a regional cystic fibrosis unit. Scand J Gastroenterol 1988; 23(suppl): 110-3.
22. Reisman JJ, Rivington-Law B, Corey M, Marcotte J, Wannamaker E, Harcourt D, et al. Role of conventional physiotherapy in cystic fibrosis. J Pediatr 1988; 113(4): 632-6.
23. Lapin CD. Conventional postural drainage and percussion: Is this still the gold standard? – Eighth Annual North American Cystic Fibrosis Conference; 1994 Oct 20-23; Orlando (FL); New York: Wiley-Liss.
24. Hiatt P, Eigen H, Yu P, Tepper R. Bronchodilator responsiveness in infants and young children with cystic fibrosis. Am Rev Resp Dis 1988; 137: 119-22.
25. Ruzkowski CJ, Sanowski RA, Austin J, Rohwedder JJ, Warring JP. The effects on inhaled albuterol and oral theophylline on gastroesophageal reflux in patients with gastroesophageal reflux disease and obstructive lung disease. Arch Intern Med 1992; 152(4): 783-5.
26. Auerbach HS, Williams M, Kirkpatrick JA, et al. Alternate-day prednisone reduces morbidity and improves pulmonary function in cystic fibrosis. Lancet 1985; 2: 686-8.
27. Rosenstein BJ, Eigen H. Risks of alternate-day prednisone in patients with cystic fibrosis. Pediatr 1991; 87(2): 245-6.
28. Engen H, Rosenstein BJ, FitzSimmons S, Schidlow DV and the Cystic Fibrosis Foundation Prednisone Trial Group. A multicenter study of alternate-day prednisone therapy in patients with cystic fibrosis. J Pediatr 1995; 126: 515-523.
29. Konstan MW, Davis PB, Byard PJ, Hoppel CL. Effect of high-dose ibuprofen in patients with cystic fibrosis. N Engl J Med 1995; 332: 848-854.
30. Fuchs HJ, Borowitz DS, Christiansen DH, Morris EM, Nash ML, Ramsey BW, *et al.* Effect of aerosolized recombinant human DNAse on exacerbations of respiratory symptoms and on pulmonary function in patients with cystic fibrosis. N Engl J Med 1984; 331(10): 637-42.
31. Johnson MB. A multi-center, double-blind, placebo-controlled study to evaluate the safety and efficacy of aerosolized rhDNAse therapy in patients with cystic fibrosis who have advanced lung disease. Eighth Annual North American Cystic Fibrosis Conference; 1994 Oct 20-23; Orlando (FL); New York: Wiley-Liss.
32. Stutman HR, Marks MI. Antibiotic Prophylaxis Study Group. Cephalexin prophylaxis in newly diagnosed infants with cystic fibrosis. Sixth Annual North American Cystic Fibrosis Conference; 1992 Oct 15-18; Washington (DC).
33. The Cystic Fibrosis Foundation Center Committee and Guidelines Subcommittee. Cystic fibrosis foundation guidelines for patient services, evaluation, and monitoring in cystic fibrosis centers. Am J Dis Childr 1990; 144: 1311-2.
34. Nielsen OH, Thomsen BL, Green A, Andersen PK, Hauge M, Schiotz PO. Cystic fibrosis in Denmark 1945 to 1985. Acta Pediatr Scand 1988; 77: 836-41.
35. Hill DJS, Martin AJ, Davidson GP, Smith GS. Survival of cystic fibrosis patients in South Australia. Med J Australia 1985; 143: 230-2.

Cystic Fibrosis Pulmonary Infections:
Lessons from Around the World
ed. by A. Bauernfeind, M. I. Marks and B. Strandvik
© 1996 Birkhäuser Verlag Basel/Switzerland

CHAPTER 8
The General Approach to Cystic Fibrosis Pulmonary Infection in Canada

Noni MacDonald[1], Mary Corey[2] and Rod Morrison[3]

[1]*Chair, Clinic Subcommittee,* [2]*Consultant Biostatistician,* [3]*Director, Policy Development and Medical/Scientific Program, Canadian Cystic Fibrosis Foundation, Toronto, Ontario, Canada M4S 2B4*

Introduction

In 1965, the Canadian Cystic Fibrosis Foundation (CCFF) put forward a strategic plan which called for the development of a national network of clinics specializing in care of patients with cystic fibrosis [1]. Seven clinics were accredited in 1968 and each received a small incentive grant from the Foundation to facilitate the development of their CF care programs. The clinic network now includes 33 clinics, stretches from coast to coast, and provides care for more than 90% of all cystic fibrosis patients in Canada. As part of the annual incentive grant application, each clinic provides a yearly update of changes in its CF care program as well as data for the Canadian patient data registry at the CCFF. Every five years each clinic receives a site visit by members of the CCFF Clinic Subcommittee to review the clinical program, personnel, and physical resources.

Overview

While the approach to CF pulmonary infection, both prevention and treatment, are not identical across the country, there are many common threads. Most clinics see patients at least every three months for assessment. This usually includes a careful history and physical examination which focuses on respiratory and gastrointestinal symptoms and signs as well as accurate measurements of height and weight, and in some clinics more complete anthropometric measurements. Pulmonary function testing is usually done at least every six months for children old enough to perform the manoeuvers. Chest X-rays are done yearly and more often if indicated. Respiratory secretions – preferably sputum, but, if not, a throat swab – are tested according to guidelines developed by the Clinic Subcommittee of the CCFF [2]. These guidelines were developed in collaboration with the Canadian Association of Medical Microbiologists and recommend the appropriate laboratory procedures required to isolate *Staphylococcus aureus*, *Haemophilus influenzae*, *Pseudomonas aeruginosa*, and *Burkholderia cepacia* (formerly *Pseudomonas cepacia*), as well as other less common organisms. Recommendations for infection control of patients colonized with *B. cepacia* were also developed under the auspices of the Clinic Subcommittee [3].

In most clinics, patients are encouraged to follow a pulmonary maintenance program which includes chest physiotherapy and antibiotic treatment for infectious episodes, as well as routine antibiotic therapy for some patients. For the majority of patients, chest physiotherapy usually involves classical postural drainage with percussion and directed coughing. Some clinics also utilize other techniques such as the positive expiratory pressure technique (PEP), autogenic drainage, and exercise for certain patients. While the value of chest physiotherapy has been questioned, studies at both the Montreal Children's Hospital and The Hospital for Sick Children in Toronto have shown that there is definite benefit in both the short and the long term [4, 5].

With respect to routine antibiotic therapy, the approaches used across the country are quite varied. Many clinics provide antistaphylococcal therapy for infants and young children. Some clinics continue this on a regular basis, while others use it only intermittently (e.g. if the child has a cold or sputum cultures are positive for *S. aureus*). Some clinics utilize cotrimoxazole and/or inhaled tobramycin or colistin, either long-term or intermittently, for patients with more advanced disease. Very few clinics utilize the more intensive treatment programs suggested by the Scandinavians consisting of a regular (i.e. every 3–4 months) antipseudomonas chemotherapeutic regimen [6]. Currently, several adult cystic fibrosis clinics have come together to determine if a daily regimen involving cycling of inhaled tobramycin and ciprofloxacin is advantageous [7].

Viral infections are also well recognized as important contributing factors to pulmonary deterioration in patients with cystic fibrosis [8, 9]. In terms of prevention of viral illness, all patients with cystic fibrosis in Canada are encouraged to receive measles, mumps, and rubella immunization as well as yearly influenza virus vaccine. Avoidance of exposure to respiratory syncytial virus and varicella are much more problematic.

Treatment of acute exacerbations has undergone some alteration in recent years. The concerns about transmission of *B. cepacia* among inpatients [10], and the increased interest in home intravenous antibiotic therapy as well as inhaled antibiotic therapy, has led many clinics to substantially decrease the number of hospitalizations for cystic fibrosis patients. Patients with more severe disease and/or more acute serious exacerbations may be hospitalized for intravenous antibiotic therapy as well as more aggressive chest physiotherapy. Selection of antibiotics for these patients is usually based upon sensitivities of the organisms isolated from sputum cultures and most clinics utilize combination rather than monotherapy. Frequent combinations include tobramycin and ceftazidime, ciprofloxacin and tobramycin, ticarcillin and tobramycin. The recent work from Calgary suggests that even when the quantity of organisms in the sputum does not decrease with intensive intravenous antibiotic therapy, the quantity of exoenzyme expression does decrease [11]. This is associated with a decrease in inflammation and clinical improvement.

Unusual organisms such as mycobacteria and aspergillus have not been major problems for the majority of patients with cystic fibrosis in Canada. Therefore, standardized protocols for the management of these types of infections have not been developed.

Good nutrition is also an important component of the Canadian CF pulmonary program. Comparison of survival, growth and pulmonary function in patients with cystic fibrosis in Boston and Toronto has shown that the Toronto emphasis on a high calorie/high fat diet pays dividends not only in terms of normal growth but also in terms of increased survival [12]. The majority of CF clinics across Canada place particular emphasis on good nutrition. Patients who fail to grow well with the high calorie/high fat diet with pancreatic enzymes (if pancreatic insufficiency is present) are encouraged to take additional nutritional supplements. If this is still not successful in achieving normal growth/ nutrition, then an enteral feeding program is often utilized [13–15].

Outcome of Pulmonary Care Program

The CCFF Canadian Patient Data Registry (CPDR) provides an overview of the results of the CF care program in Canada. Median survival age increased steadily in the 1980s after appearing to have stabilized at around 23 years of age during the 1970s. Figure 1 shows the survival curve for the 5 year period 1988–92, in which median survival age was 33 years [16]. Males continue to have consistently better survival than females at all ages; current median survival ages are 36 years for males and 29 years for females. The sex difference is similar to that reported in American patients [17], but the Canadian medians are about 5 years higher. Improved survival has resulted in a steadily growing population of CF adults, with the proportion of patients over age 18 increasing from 7% in 1970 to 37% in 1992.

Early diagnosis is common in the Canadian CF population. Since 1970 when the CPDR began prospectively recording newly-diagnosed patients, 48% have been diagnosed in the first 6 months of life, and the patterns of diagnosis are similar for males and females. Relating early

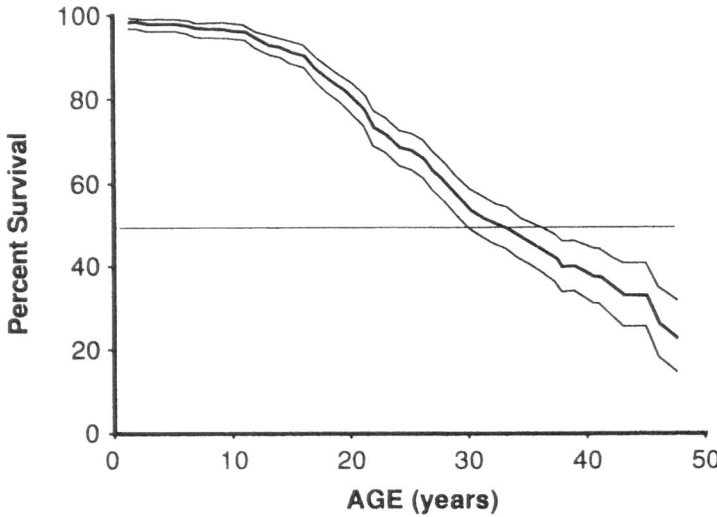

Figure 1. Survival curve, with 95% confidence limits, for the Canadian CF population, based on age-specific death rates observed in the five year period 1988–92.

diagnosis to outcome is complicated because patients diagnosed at older ages include those with mild disease as well as those in whom misdiagnosis of typical symptoms has delayed initiation of specific CF treatment. Survival regression analysis of the CPDR data show that those diagnosed between 6 months and 2 years of age had a poorer survival course than those diagnosed before 6 months, whereas those diagnosed at older ages had better survival [18]. If we assume that diagnosis in late infancy generally reflects delayed diagnosis, while diagnosis in late childhood or adulthood often reflects milder disease, these results confirm the wisely held belief that early diagnosis has positive prognostic value.

The results of an aggressive approach to nutrition in Canadian clinics are apparent in the anthropometric data which are compared to National Center for Health Statistics (NCHS) standards for weight and height [19] in Figure 2. A comparable figure appears in a report of the American CF population [17], showing 40% of American CF patients are below the 5th percentile for height and 36% below the 5th percentile for weight. The respective figures for the Canadian population are 16% and 17%. Regional analysis of the Canadian data shows that improved anthropometric data and survival were temporally associated with the initiation of an unrestricted high calorie diet and aggressive nutritional support programs [18].

Table 1 shows average pulmonary function results by age and sex in 1992. These values are similar to those in the comparative study of Boston and Toronto patients [12], and in particular show no differences

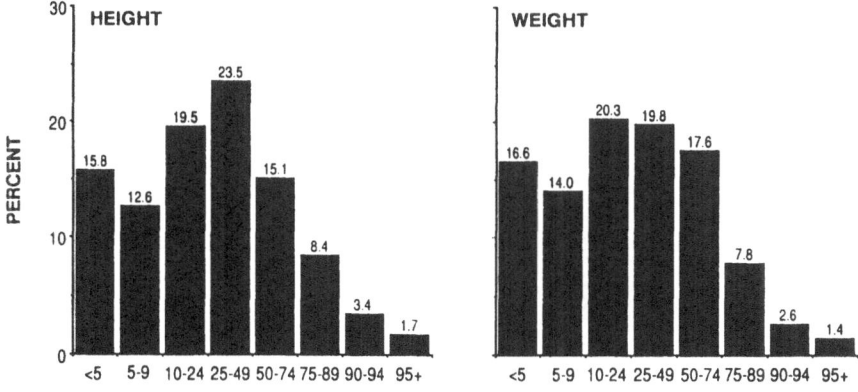

NCHS/CDC Percentile

Figure 2. Distribution of height and weight in the Canadian CF population in 1992, using the percentile standards of the National Center for Health Statistics/Centers for Disease Control [19]. Height percentile mean = 35, median = 29. Weight percentile mean = 33, median = 27.

between males and females. However, the larger number of males in the oldest age group shows the effects of greater female mortality. These patterns of pulmonary function by age and sex are similar throughout the eight years for which data have been recorded.

Table 2 gives estimates of the prevalence of the organisms most often cultured in CF sputum samples. These are point estimates relating to the first sputum culture of the year for each patient and are therefore minimal estimates of chronic colonization or annual prevalence. Besides the frequency of patients positive for each organism in each year since 1985, the data are also shown for four east-to-west regions of the country. There appears to be an increase in the prevalence of *S. aureus* over the eight year period, but this reflects an increase only in the region of lowest prevalence. The prevalence of *H. influenzae* has steadily decreased in region 1 and increased in region 2. Otherwise there are no

Table 1. Percent of predicted pulmonary function for male and female patients in Canada, by age group, in 1992. Data are presented as mean and standard deviation

Age (yrs)	Sex	N	FVC % pred.		FEV$_1$ % pred.	
			Mean	STD	Mean	STD
00–09	F	238	88	21	89	25
	M	267	89	19	87	21
10–19	F	449	86	20	78	24
	M	473	85	20	76	24
20–53	F	303	79	25	64	27
	M	409	78	25	61	28

Table 2. Point prevalence of sputum colonization in the Canadian CF population and in four regions (1 to 4). Data presented are the percentages of patients whose sputum was positive for the organism on the first sputum culture of the year

Calendar year	85	86	87	88	89	90	91	92
S. aureus	24.0	25.4	27.4	28.2	27.4	30.9	31.0	33.2
region 1	28.6	24.8	25.0	23.5	26.6	29.6	25.5	28.6
region 2	27.9	28.7	27.7	27.1	25.8	29.2	27.6	30.6
region 3	11.3	12.4	16.8	20.2	21.8	22.2	24.8	26.2
region 4	41.5	40.0	43.2	42.2	37.0	44.7	44.9	47.2
P. aeruginosa	48.1	45.7	46.4	51.1	47.3	47.5	46.3	47.2
region 1	22.9	26.1	27.2	24.3	20.3	19.3	21.7	23.8
region 2	42.6	37.2	39.2	47.6	44.2	46.9	43.4	48.1
region 3	59.2	56.2	57.8	57.8	56.2	52.8	51.6	51.9
region 4	47.1	49.5	47.8	57.4	51.0	52.9	53.2	49.1
B. cepacia	10.2	8.1	10.2	10.1	10.3	11.1	10.7	10.5
region 1	10.3	11.5	17.7	13.6	17.6	21.2	18.5	20.4
region 2	1.1	0.8	1.1	0.4	0.4	0.6	0.8	1.4
region 3	20.9	18.5	21.7	23.3	23.7	23.3	21.9	21.2
region 4	3.8	1.1	2.2	2.2	2.0	4.2	5.3	4.3
H. influenzae	14.5	15.3	13.8	17.1	14.3	14.0	13.0	15.1
region 1	32.0	31.9	17.7	15.2	10.9	10.2	10.1	5.6
region 2	4.4	6.3	6.0	12.1	10.5	15.5	12.0	13.5
region 3	15.9	15.3	15.9	22.0	18.3	17.4	17.0	20.2
region 4	21.0	19.4	19.6	16.9	15.1	9.2	10.6	14.4

remarkable trends over the eight years, particularly in *Pseudomonas* and *Burkholderia* which are thought to be associated with most CF morbidity. The regional discrepancies in *P. aeruginosa* and *B. cepacia* prevalence are notable but they are not associated with differential pulmonary function or mortality. Survival curves in the four regions are similar during this period.

Implications

The Canadian experience suggests that countries embarking on the development of a cystic fibrosis care program may do well to focus initially on the basics, namely timely diagnosis, aggressive support of nutrition with appropriate use of pancreatic enzymes, daily routine chest physiotherapy, and the judicious use of antibiotics. The development of a national network of cystic fibrosis clinics where the cystic fibrosis teams develop expertise in the management of these patients also appears to contribute to improved survival. The Canadian data also suggest that focusing attention, not only on the lungs but also on nutritional status, can improve survival. Increasing the availability of pancreatic enzyme supplements for cystic fibrosis patients in less developed countries as well as encouraging high calorie/high fat diets and teaching chest physiotherapy techniques may help improve the survival of patients in these countries.

References

1. Canadian Cystic Fibrosis Foundation: Thirty Year Retrospective. Canadian Cystic Fibrosis Foundation 1990. Toronto, Canada.
2. Clinic Subcommittee of the Medical/Scientific Advisory Committee of the Canadian Cystic Fibrosis Foundation (Principal Author: N. MacDonald): Microbiological processing of respiratory specimens from patients with cystic fibrosis. Can J Infect Dis 1993; 4: 166–169.
3. Medical/Scientific Advisory Committee Canadian Cystic Fibrosis Foundation: Epidemiology of *Pseudomonas cepacia* in cystic fibrosis. Can J Infect Dis 1993; 4: 163–166.
4. Desmond KJ, Schwenk WF, Thomas E, Beaudry PH, Coates AL et al. Immediate and long-term effects of chest physiotherapy in patients with cystic fibrosis. J Pediatr 1983; 103: 538–542.
5. Reisman JJ, Rivington-Law B, Corey M, Marcotte J, Wannamaker E, Harcourt D et al. Role of conventional physiotherapy in cystic fibrosis. J Pediatr 1988; 113: 632–636.
6. Pedersen SS, Jensen T, Hoiby, Koch C, Flensborg EW et al. Management of *Pseudomonas aeruginosa* lung infection in Danish cystic fibrosis patients. Acta Pediatr Scand 1987; 76: 955–961.
7. Rabin HR, Hegi CE, Brown D, Storey DG, Bryan LE, Woods DE et al. Chronic sequential oral ciprofloxacin and inhalational tobramycin (CSOCIT) in adult patients with cystic fibrosis – A pilot study. Pediatr Pulmonol 1993; Supplement (9): 224.
8. Wang EEL, Prober CG, Manson B, Corey M, Levison H et al. Association of respiratory viral infection with pulmonary deterioration in patients with cystic fibrosis. N Engl J Med 1984; 311: 1653–1658.
9. Abman SH, Ogle JW, Butler-Smith N, Rumack CM, Accurso FJ et al. Role of respiratory syncytial virus in early hospitalization for respiratory distress of young infants with cystic fibrosis. J Pediatr 1988; 113: 826–830.
10. Gold R. Frequent hospitalization and *P. cepacia*. In: *Pseudomonas cepacia* in Cystic Fibrosis Workshop Report. Canadian Cystic Fibrosis Foundation 1991.
11. Grimwood K, To M, Semple RA, Rabin HR, Sokol PA, Woods DE et al. Elevated exoenzyme expression by *Pseudomonas aeruginosa* is correlated with exacerbations of lung disease in cystic fibrosis. Pediatr Pulmonol 1993; 15: 135–139.
12. Corey M, McLaughlin FJ, Williams M, Levison H. A comparison of survival, growth, and pulmonary function in patients with cystic fibrosis in Boston and Toronto. J Clin Epidemiol 1988; 41: 583–591.
13. Boland MP, Stoski DS, MacDonald NE, Soucy P, Patrick J et al. Chronic jejunostomy feeding with a non elemental formula in undernourished patients with cystic fibrosis. Lancet 1986; I: 232–234.
14. Bertrand JM, Morin CL, Lasalle R, Patrick J, Coates AL et al. Short-term clinical, nutritional, and functional elements of continuous elemental enteral alimentation in children with cystic fibrosis. J Pediatr 1984; 104: 41–46.
15. Levy LD, Durie PR, Pencharz PB, Corey ML: Effects of longterm nutritional rehabilitation on body composition and clinical status in malnourished children and adolescents with cystic fibrosis. J Pediatr 1985; 107: 225–230.
16. Canadian Cystic Fibrosis Foundation: Report of the Canadian Patient Data Registry 1992; Toronto: Canadian Cystic Fibrosis Foundation 1993.
17. Fitzsimmons SC: The changing epidemiology of cystic fibrosis. J Pediatr 1993; 122: 1–9.
18. Corey M: Determinants of mortality in cystic fibrosis in Canada 1970–89. Ph.D. Thesis, University of Toronto 1992.
19. National Center for Health Statistics: Growth curves for children birth to 18 years. Washington DC: National Center for Health Statistics, 1977. (Vital and Health Statistics: Series 11, No. 165. United States Department of Health, Education and Welfare Publication, No 78-1650).

Cystic Fibrosis Pulmonary Infections:
Lessons from Around the World
ed. by A. Bauernfeind, M. I. Marks and B. Strandvik
© 1996 Birkhäuser Verlag Basel/Switzerland

CHAPTER 9
Cystic Fibrosis in Latin America

C. N. Macri[1], O. H. Pivetta[2], A. Gentile[1], E. G. Cafferata[2] and
M. C. Luna[2]

[1]Hospital de Ninos "Ricardo Gutierrez", 1425 Buenos Aires, Argentina
[2]Instituto Nacional de Genetica Medica, Las Heras 2670, 1425 Buenos Aires, Argentina

Historical Perspective

Fanconi first described fibrocystic disease of the pancreas in 1936. During the subsequent 25 years cystic fibrosis (CF) patients in Latin America were managed by individual doctors. In the 1960s a National Foundation was created in Argentina to improve care and promote medical-biochemical research in CF in this part of the world. This was a very important development for Latin American countries, where methods to diagnose and treat CF were often lacking, and most medical resources were focused on summer diarrhea, malnutrition and common respiratory and parasitic infections.

In 1974 the International Pediatric Congress in Buenos Aires, Argentina, hosted the first International Meeting on Cystic Fibrosis, bringing the clinical and research CF experts to Latin America from around the world. In 1977, a group of professionals and parents of CF patients created FIPAN, the Argentina Association to Fight Against Fibrocystic Disease of the Pancreas, a non profilt organization which gave a great thrust to the dissemination of the general knowledge of the disease. This institution collaborated in creating centers for medical and social assistance, by developing information services to "spread the word" regarding new research and treatment techniques. It also promoted ties with foreign entities, and sponsored participation at national and international meetings. These roots have grown in recent years to form the Latin American CF group, the Latin American CF Registry (REGLAFQ) and other associations to fight CF in these countries. These organizations are all affiliated with the International Cystic Fibrosis (Mucoviscidosis) Association, (ICF) and have helped sponsor studies on the incidence and pathology of CF in Latin America, as well as neonatal screening in Argentina [1].

In 1989 a genetic and molecular study of CF in Latin America was presented for the first time [2]. As a result, research aimed towards perinatal genetic studies increased and important discoveries were made on the frequency of the different mutations, especially the $\Delta F508$ mutation. In spite of the advances in the understanding of the disease and the interaction between Latin American countries and developed nations, less than 8% of the potentially affected CF population in Latin America are registered in CF Centers. This estimate is based on data from REGLAFQ [3], which registered 75% of the Latin American population (1223 CF patients are registered from an estimated total of 16 856). Likewise, the annual number of newly diagnosed cases is small. For example, in 1991, there were only 193 new cases reported from a theoretical 2177 affected births (83 had been born that year), indicating 97% of CF cases are underdiagnosed. Underdiagnosis and lack of regionalized care are reflected by a low life expectancy for CF patients in Latin America, far below that observed in developed countries.

Incidence of Fibrocystic Disease of the Pancreas in Latin America

The true incidence of CF in the continent is not yet known. Many Latin American countries are submerged in social and economic problems, have minimal technological advances and lack modern communication tools, making it difficult to both recognize and register new patients. A better estimate of the incidence of CF, might be achieved through regional neonatal screening programs (4), however this has not been possible due to the high cost involved.

In a previous observation, conducted in the City of Buenos Aires and its environs, the incidence of CF was determined for 9931 newborns from 11 maternity wards [1]. The detection of two affected children implies an incidence of one in 4966 live births. This is lower than the classic description of 1:2500 for predominantly Caucasian countries, but higher than the incidence of CF among the Black and Oriental races.

To address this a Latin American Registry, CF REGLAFQ, was created, with the purpose of improving our CF patient knowledge by documenting the incidence of CF in Latin American countries. If we had a more precise idea of the incidence in the region we could improve the treatment of this disease. For example, there are many pharmaceutical companies which do not distribute pancreatic enzymes in some areas because they are not aware of the real scope and geographic distribution of cystic fibrosis.

In order to better understand the real scope of CF in Latin America, the expected incidence, obtained from the latest population figures, was corrected for ethnic composition based on the anthropological study of the different Latin American populations [4]. The results are shown in Table 1. This table shows the racial composition of 11 Latin American

Table 1. Theoretical incidence of CF in Latin-American countries by race

Country Race	Argentina	Brazil	Cuba	Mexico	Colombia	Uruguay	Puerto Rico	Panama	Chile	Costa Rica	El Salvador	Totals
White	28 735 667	82 251 638	7 593 460	2 704 698	6 048 200	2 682 900	–	417 960	3 888 310	2 449 082	51 070	143 197 405
Incid.	241	941	53	34	60	27		4	30	86	1	1473
Mestiza	2 873 567	7 001 707		68 969 784	17 237 370	298 100	3 522 037	1 207 440	8 813 502	284 823	4 545 230	23 754 560
Incid.	8	27		241	60	0.7	10	4	68	10	89	577
Mulatto	19 157	43 071 557	1 560 300		4 233 740			116 100		53 600		49 054 454
Incid.	0	236	5		21			0.6		2		265
Indigenous	191 571	230 068		8 114 092	604 820			232 200	10 384	510 700	1 489 281	
Incid.	0.4	0.1		3	0.2			0	2	0.4	10	14.4
Black	9 578	141 306 079	1 248 240		2 116 870			348 300		53 600		17 912 667
Incid.	0	24	1		3			0.5		2		30
Total	31 829 540	14 671 049	1 040 200	81 140 922	30 241 000	2 981 000	3 522 037	2 322 000	12 961 032	2 851 085	5 107 000	325 501 665
Incid.	250	1 228	59	336	148	21	10	9	100	100.4	100	2 361 4

Table 2. Theoretical % of CF patient by race as suggested by REGLAFQ

Race	White	Mestizo	Mulatto	Indigenous	Black
Theoretical FQ	66	20	13	0.02	1
REGLAFQ	90	3	7	0.1	0.3

Table 3. Distribution of the 51 Latin-American CF centers

Country	
Argentina	12
Brazil	11
Chile	1
Costa Rica	1
Colombia	2
Cuba	10
El Salvador	1
Mexico	5
Panama	1
Paraguay	1
Uruguay	4
Venezuela	2

countries, representing more than 75% of the population of the continent. The theoretical incidence was corrected for race. With a total Latin American population of 325 501 665, one should expect, after consulting various embassies for birth rates, about 2361 affected births per year; a far cry from the 83 cases identified in 1991. Table 2 gives us an idea of the probable racial composition of CF patients in the continent. When compared to the numbers obtained from REGLAFQ the results indicate improved diagnosis and reporting among the Caucasian population, since 90% vs the theoretical 60% of the patients diagnosed belong to this sub-group. This is probably because the Caucasian population in Latin America, because of its socioeconomic status, has greater access to those health care facilities found only in large cities. Only 12 Latin American countries have CF centers (Table 3) [5–8]. Currently there is a plan in Argentina to educate health care professionals in rural areas about the diagnosis and management of CF.

Genetics

The gene responsible for the CF phenotype is located in the q31 position of the long arm of chromosome 7 [9]. This gene codes for a 1480 base pair glycoprotein associated with the cell membrane, known as CF transmembrane conductance regulator (CFTR). To date, there are more than 550 known allele variants, the most common being the deletion of 3 base pairs that encode for phenylalanine in the F508 position, known as ΔF508. The frequency of this mutation varies based on race and the population under study, but is most commonly seen in the Caucasian race and in the Northern European region where it reaches 88% in Denmark [10] and decreases toward southern Europe (e.g. Spain = 45%) [11].

In Latin America, 42% of the population is primarily of southern European background, while 58% are of very heterogenous origin (Table 4). With the use of RFLPs and PCR technology, it has been possible to determine the frequency of certain mutations in Latin America, including ΔF508, G542X, R553X and N1303K.

Because of the ethnic composition of the continent, one would expect the frequency of the ΔF508 mutation to be low since the majority of the Caucasian population is descended from areas where the incidence of the mutation is low (Table 5). Brazil has a frequency of the ΔF508 mutation of 47% [12], Argentina 64% [13] and Mexico 35% [14].

The values clearly show a lower than expected frequency in Mexico and a higher than expected frequency for Argentina. In the case of Mexico, Lorena Orozco [14] concludes that this may be due to: i) limited number of cases studied, ii) the predominantly Hispanic (40%) vs indigenous (50%) ethnic origin of the Mexican population (notably, the indigenous population of Mexico is different from the indigenous population of other Latin American countries) and iii) the possibility that, in developing countries, a large number of children afflicted with CF die without a diagnosis, including those homozygous ΔF508 mutation patients who present with severe pulmonary illness and pancreatic insufficiency.

In Argentina, a country with a larger proportion of Caucasians in the population, the possibility existed than a important ancestral contribu-

Table 4. Racial proportions in Latin-America

Race	Caucasian	Mestiza	Mulatto	Indigenous	Black
Percentage	42	33	16	3	6

Table 5. Percent mutations in three Latin-American countries

Country mutation	Argentina	Brazil	Mexico
DF508	64	42	35
G551D	—	1	—
G542X	3	5	1.5
R553X	—	1	3
N1303K	—	4	—

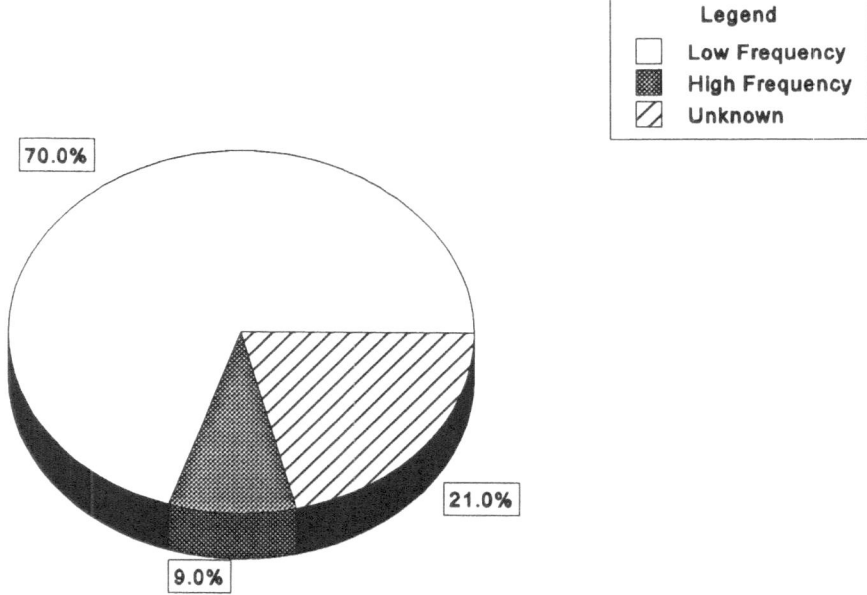

Figure 1. Distribution of country of origin among CF patients in Argentina.

tion from countries with a high incidence of the ΔF508 mutation might be found. A study completed in 1992 [15], which analyzed the European ancestry of the Argentina CF population showed that only 9% came from countries where the frequency of the ΔF508 mutation was greater than 50% (Figure 1).

The conclusions of this study probably overestimate disease severity due to a greater probability that those patients who are homozygous are diagnosed because they present with much earlier symptomatology.

The first studies of the relationship between genotype and phenotype were done in Argentina [15] and Brazil [2]. In Brazil, differences in the frequency of ΔF508 mutation were found among the different states studied; this may have been due to the different regional ethnic composition. Statistical differences were also noted for pancreatic insufficiency present in 93% of the homozygous ΔF508 mutation (28/30) vs 67% (28/42) without the mutation. There were no significant differences between pneumopathology and meconium ileus.

The Buenos Aires group studied 52 patients, 26 of whom were homozygous for ΔF508, 15 ΔF508/? and 11?/? (Figure 2). The results showed the presence of meconium ileus only in patients that had one or more ΔF508 alleles, although the differences were not significant. The ?/? group showed more severe pulmonary disease, no difference in gastrointestinal involvement, and a Shwachman score of less than 70 points.

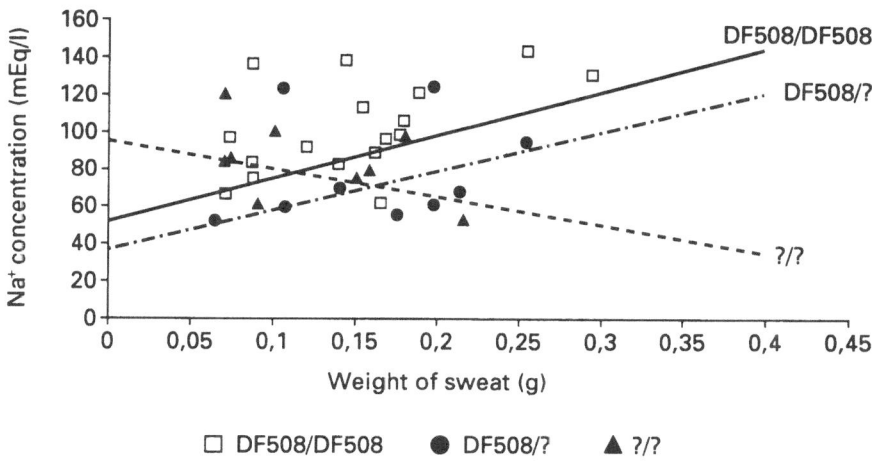

Figure 2. Na⁺ concentration vs weight of sweat in different genotypes. For further details, see text.

There was a statistically significant positive correlation between the sweat weight and Na concentration in the ΔF508/ΔF508 and ΔF508/? groups, but there was a negative correlation in the ?/? group.

In a more recent study [17], the ratio between $Cl^-:Na^+$ in the sweat of genotypically identified patients was greater than 1 in the homozygous ΔF508 group in 85.7% of the cases (6/7) and in only 26.8% for the heterozygous group (2/7) ($p = <0.025$). When the Na^+ concentration was plotted vs weight of sweat, the results were again duplicated (Proceedings of the V Latin American Congress on Cystic Fibrosis).

Currently, the possibility of utilizing the $Cl^-:Na^+$ ratio as a phenotypic marker for homozygous ΔF508 is being studied. A $Cl^-:Na^+$ ratio of >1, along with other phenotypical characteristics such as moderate or severe pancreatic insufficiency, meconium ileus and early onset of the illness, makes us suspect that we are confronted with a patient with the ΔF508 genotype. This is important in this area of the world where molecular studies are not always possible. This ratio may also be of great importance for the genetic assessment in cases where the homozygotic subject is not available.

Latin American Epidemiological Aspects

A retrospective study of CF care was conducted between 1960 and 1989 for the purpose of motivating and informing the Latin American medical community. All Latin American countries and centers were asked to participate. A preliminary list of 102 hospitals and pediatric centers that treated CF and other chronic respiratory diseases was developed. Each center was asked to collect information about their patient population.

Of the 102 centers contacted, 34 (36.7%) responded to the survey. A total of 1827 patients were identified from 10 countries: Argentina, Brazil, Colombia, Chile, El Salvador, Mexico, Paraguay, Puerto Rico, Dominican Republic and Uruguay. The results of this retrospective study conducted to start REGLAFQ at the end of 1990, showed the following: of 1827 patients followed from 1965–1989, 52.9% of the patients were male, 47.1% female. More than half of the patients were living and being followed (53.1%), 29% had died and 17.7% were lost to follow up.

Age at Diagnosis and Age at Admission/Entrance to Health Centers

In this retrospective study, the mean age at diagnosis was 3.7 years ± 5.22, and the mean age of entrance to clinics/health centers was 4.5 years ± 6.1 (Table 6). Analysis of the mean age at diagnosis, along with data from the retrospective register and the last REGLAFQ reports (1990, 1991) showed a delay in diagnosis with respect to the number of cases reported in developed countries [16, 18]. The values are consistent with those found at the Hospital de Niños Ricardo Gutierrez (HNRG), 3.28 ± 4.2 years [20]. This data is worrisome since clinicians and epidemiologists consider that early diagnosis improves the prognosis and increases survival in relation to the initiation of therapeutic modalities [21–28].

The mean age of entry into health centers was not very different from the age at diagnosis, suggesting that the majority of children were diagnosed at the start of their hospital care or shortly before that. A child's clinical progression varied considerably based on his or her clinical status at the time of admission.

Of these patients, 49.4% were severely clinically compromised upon admission (Shwachman Score) during the first decade of the study (1960–1969), while 45.6% and 18.4% were severely compromised during 1970–1979 and 1980–1989 respectively (Figure 3). This decrease was

Table 6. Age at diagnosis, start of study, and death of Latin-American children with CF

Age	Median	Standard deviation
At diagnosis	3.7	5.22
At start of study	4.51	6.1
Death	6.68	8.46

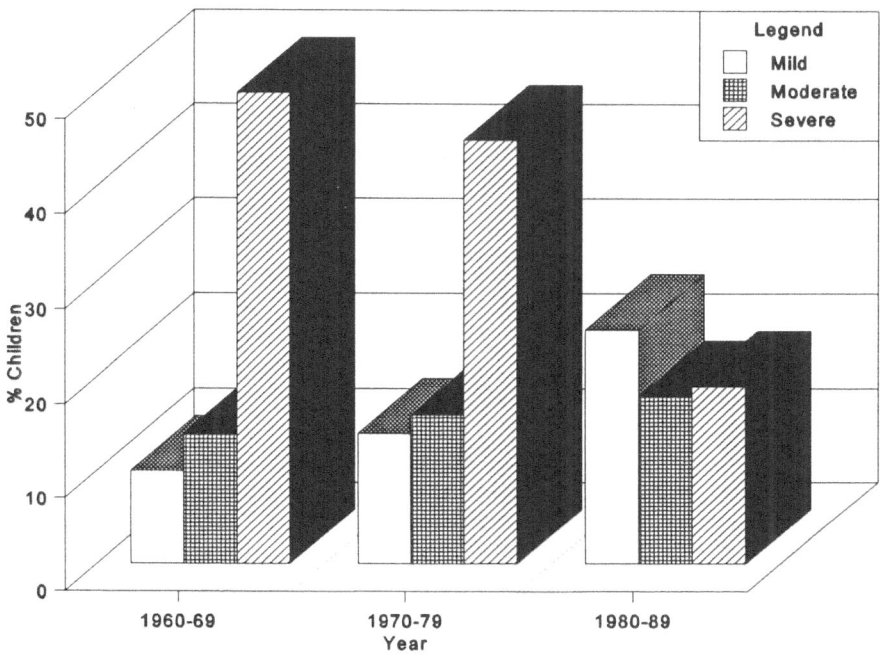

Figure 3. Clinical severity of CF upon admission to center.

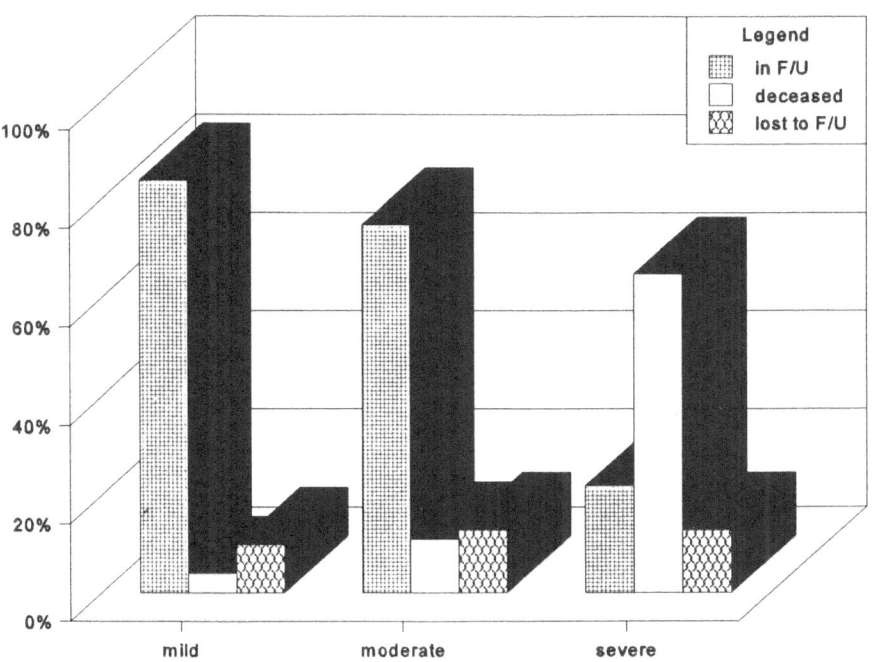

Figure 4. Outcome based on severity upon admission to CF center.

probably due to a greater understanding of the disease by the pediatricians during the last time period. Of those who were admitted with mild
disease, 83.4% were still living and in follow up in the last year, while
only 22.9% of those with severe disease were living (Figure 4).

Mortality Rate

In the retrospective Latin American study, the mortality rate was
determined to be 6.2% and 6.3% in each registry year (1990 and 1991),
with a mean age at death of 6.68 ± 6.4 and 6.14 ± 5.9 years, respectively. Only approximately 10% of the patients were above 18 years old.
The first study period (1960–1969) had GMR of 33.6%, vs 23.3%, the
second period (1970–1979) and 19.3% in the last period (1980–1989).
In the 29 years under study, there was an increment and then a
decrement in the mortality rates and a frank decreasing trend after 1984
(Figure 5), yet in 1989, the mortality rate was still 15.1%. This decrease
in the last few years could be related to more aggressive intravenous
chemotherapeutic regimens [27], to the commercialization of the enteric
coated lyophilized pancreatic enzymes in Latin America during the last
decade, and perhaps to a slight improvement in early diagnosis.

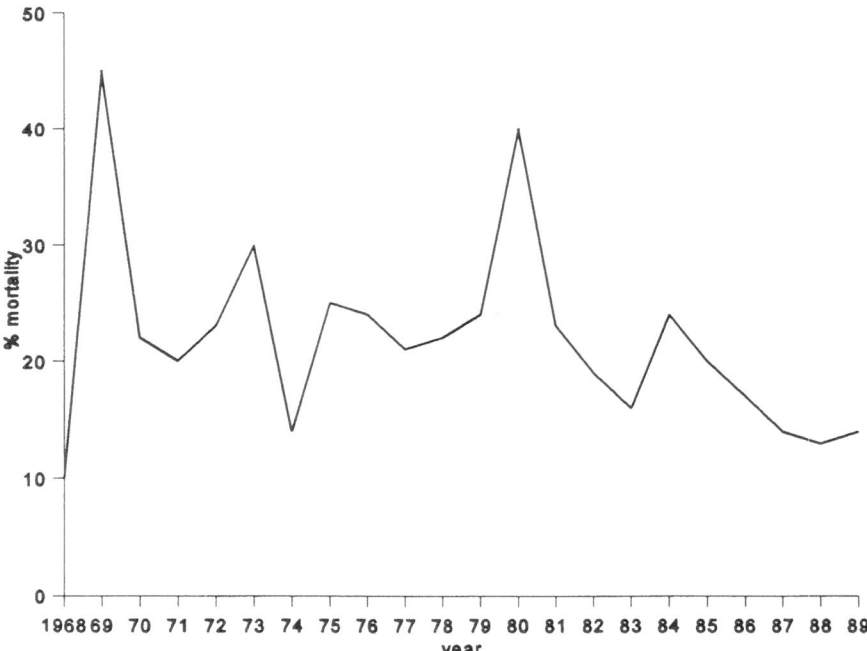

Figure 5. CF mortality: weighted rate.

Survival

The survival of CF patients has notably improved in the last few years in various parts of the world. In a recent report from the Canadian CF Registry [28], the mean age of survival was 31.8 years in the period between 1986–1990. Of those diagnosed in 1990, 67% had been born in the same year. The North American CF Registry for 1988 tracked 60.4% of patients diagnosed in the first year of life, whereas only 14 patients over 40 years old were registered [21]. With respect to total survival, as determined by the number of years since diagnosis or admission to a CF center, 50% of the children in the Latin American study were still living 6 years after admission to the center. This number decreased to 26.2% at 10 years and 10.7% at 15 years after admission to a CF center (Figure 6).

The appearance of new antibiotics and more potent medications to combat respiratory infections – the true pacemaker of this disease – have augured a better global survival. The patient's sex is not a prognostic factor in survival, a finding similar to that described in Australia [29]. Initially there was a slight difference favoring males: 50% of males had a survival of 6 years after admission, while 50% of females only survived 5.6 years. The differences between the sexes were equili-

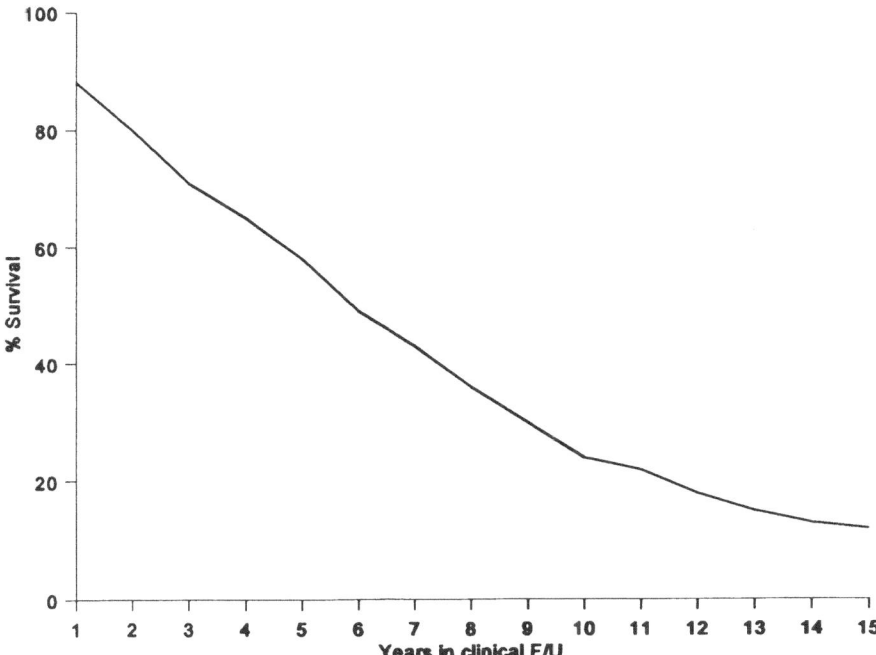

Figure 6. Total survival since admission to CF center.

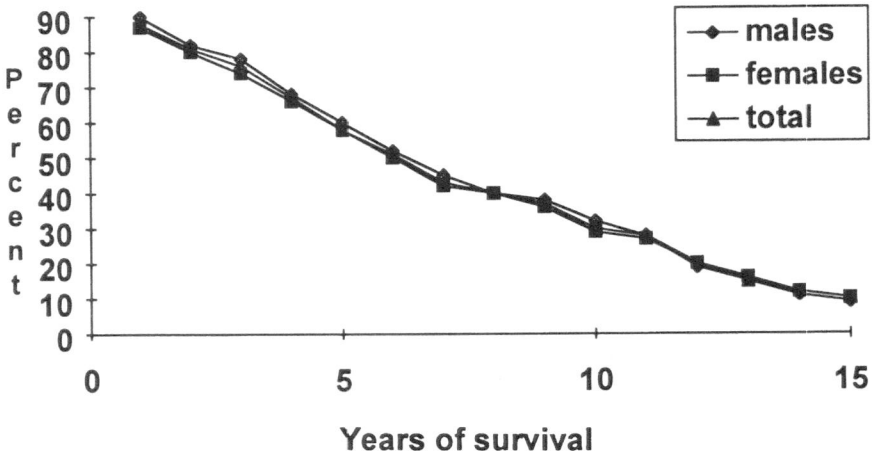

Figure 7. Years of survival by sex.

brated after 12 years of follow up. After 15 years of follow up in a CF center 9.3% of males vs 10.4% of females had survived (Figure 7).

The study of survival of patients based on the year of admission to a CF center for follow up demonstrated that in the years between 1960–1969, 50% of the patients had survived 8 years, while between 1970–1979 and 1980–1989 the years of survival were 6.7 and 6 years, respectively (Figure 8). The survival of patients during the first decade studied is striking. This may be attributed to the opening of the first

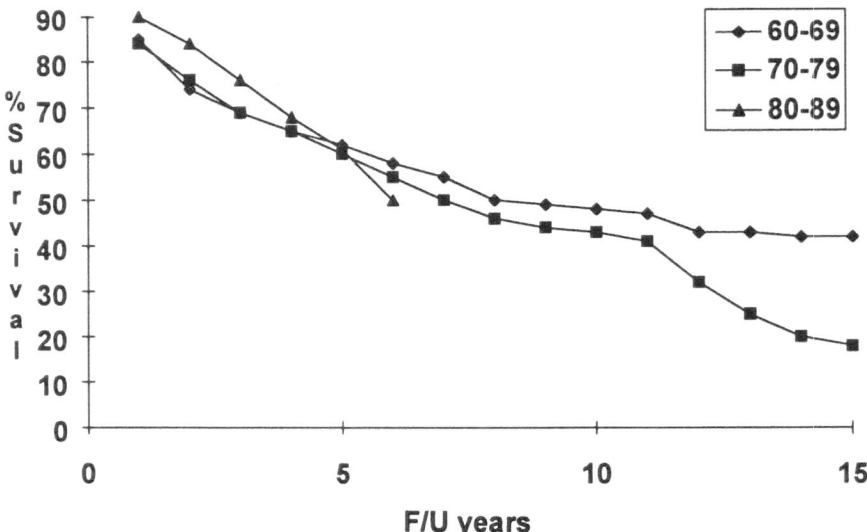

Figure 8. Survival based upon decade patient began F/U.

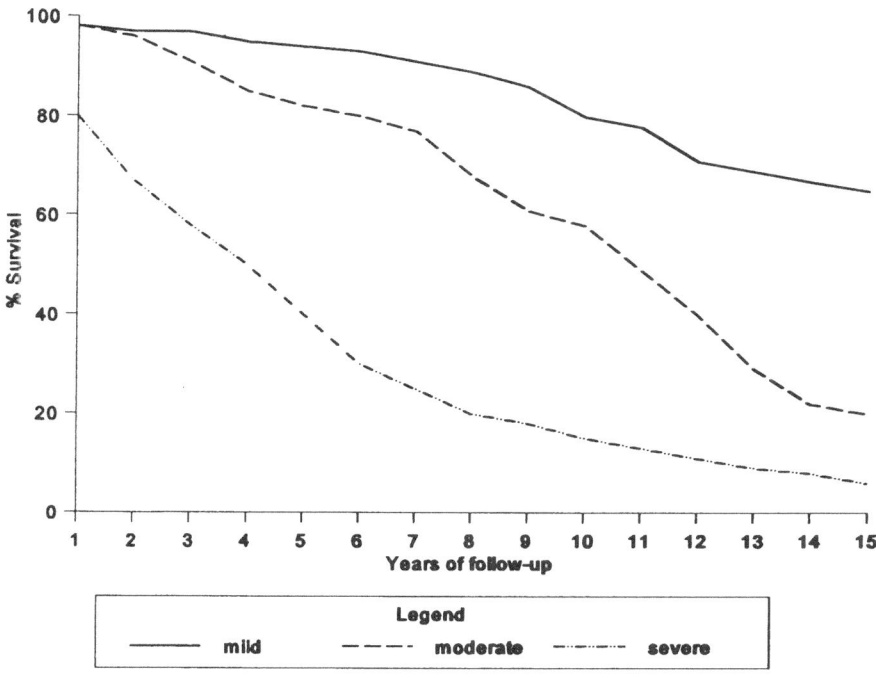

Figure 9. Survival of CF patients based on severity at start of follow-up.

centers capable of diagnosing and treating these types of patients. A better survival, 65.2% after 15 years of follow up, was seen with children who entered with less severe forms of the disease. Of the patients who entered with a more severe form of the disease, only 50% had survived 4 years, while 50% of those with moderate disease had survived 11 years (Figure 9). Younger children – less than 1 year of age – had lower survival than those children admitted at an older age (Figure 10). While 50% of children less than 1 year of age survived only 3–4 years, 50% of the older children survived 6–7 years.

When a child with CF has frank respiratory symptoms (cough, abundant secretions, signs of chronic obstructive bronchitis, and hypoxemia), malabsorption, and malnutrition etc., it is possible for the pediatrician to suspect CF and for a rapid diagnosis to be made. At this stage, however, the pulmonary deterioration is greater. This explains why children who were diagnosed and received early intervention survived less than older children who entered with less symptomatology, since in areas where many difficulties exist in the treatment and diagnosis of the disease, early detection of the illness implies a greater deterioration for the patient. Even as the therapeutic focus has improved in intensity and quality, increasing the survival for the patients remains a

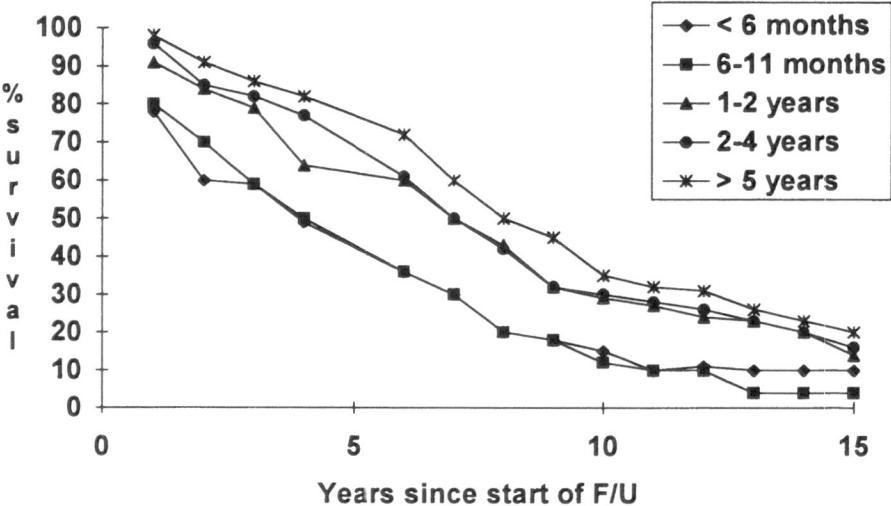

Figure 10. Outcome based on age at start of follow-up.

challenge. The introduction of more potent medications has allowed us to be more optimistic with respect to the improvement of global survival.

In summary, preliminary data of this study provide a global idea of CF in Latin America over a long period of time. Apparently in the first stages of the study the detection of CF patients were delayed, subsequently leading to the progression of their disease. The under-registration of these patients must have been important and in general these patients were severely compromised when they arrived at centers, leading to the increased mortality. This situation began to reverse itself in the 1980s and by 1985 the results were more encouraging. The next few years should prove whether the trend is favorable.

Clinical Aspects

We wish to emphasize some aspects, mainly nutritional and pulmonary, that are typical for the CF population in Latin America. The anthropometric parameters of some Latin American children with CF are certainly worrisome. In the period between 1990–1991, 52% of the registered patients were below the 3rd percentile for weight and yet, paradoxically, between 64% and 71% had received no nutritional support [30, 31]. These changes were already evident in the retrospective study conducted by HNRG in which CF had affected the anthropometric growth of these patients in direct relation to disease severity. Thus only 9.6% of the mild cases presented with low height for age, while almost half of the severely affected children were below the 3rd percentile for height and almost 80% were below the 3rd percentile for weight. Weight was more affected than height.

Pulmonary Function

Bronchial obstruction, common in children with CF, can easily be measured by volume-time curves (PFT) in children over age 6. In a previous study, important obstructive parameters were found that were directly related to clinical severity and Shwachman's Clinical Score [32, 33]. In 205 patients with CF studied by REGLAFQ, 40.4% of the children were noted to have Forced Expiratory Volume (FEV_1) values below 50% of normal. The values for Forced Vital Capacity (FVC) were also below 50% in 27.8% of the patients. In the second year of the REGLAFQ study, this parameter improved; 34.5% had FEV_1 below 50% and 20.0% of the patients' FVC values were below 50%. It is clear that the predominant element is severe obstruction of the mid and smaller airways, probably aggravated since we are dealing with children who lack proper treatment. Only 24.8% had normal FEV_1 values (above 80%). The deterioration of pulmonary function gains more importance given the young age of the patients studied. The study, although not longitudinal, allowed us to measure how pulmonary function logically deteriorates as age increases.

Bronchial obstruction can begin early in CF. In a recent study, 18 asymptomatic infants (12 males, 6 females) with a mean age of 20.3 years (range 1–3.1 years) were studied via thoracic–abdominal compression. An increase was shown in the relationship Peak Expiratory Flow/Tidal volume, along with important restrictive parameters in the flow volume curves [34]. Compliance was also diminished when compared to a group of asthmatic infants.

This early alteration in infant CF patients who are not severely affected could be related to an early alteration in the elastic recoil of the lungs in these patients. Also the caliber of the airway in this infant group was significantly less than found among asthmatic children. While patients in this study were evaluated in an apparently normal clinical status, with normal auscultatory findings and arterial oxygen saturation, pulmonary function findings showed significant alterations. The advantage of these methods of study are obvious since they are neither invasive, nor do they require general anesthesia. They allow us also to quantify the degree of change in the bronchial diameter after the administration of bronchodilators, and perhaps broaden our understanding of the normal pulmonary development in infancy. However, the majority of Latin American countries have no access to tools necessary for these types of studies.

Complications

By 1990 the majority of clinical complications were found among children less than 1 year of age and in malnourished patients: 64% of the complications were among children with weight less than the 10th percentile and of those, 50% were below the third percentile [30]. The situation was also similar in 1991. Given the low mean age of the study population, some of the complications more frequently seen in adulthood had a low incidence (e.g. pneumothorax).

The mean ambulatory visits were 4.88 and 5.46 for 1990 and 1991 respectively, which seems reasonable given the socio-economic situation in Latin America. The mean number of hospital days was 26.7 and 32.5 days, although for children diagnosed in this study year the mean was approximately 40 days. These results suggest a short hospital stay during this year. Malnutrition and infection are more than reason enough to hospitalize these children. The mean hospital days suggest that patients were hospitalized primarily to fulfill the diagnostic phase.

Microbiology and Antibiotics

In Latin America, the respiratory tracts of 80% of the CF patients, regardless of age, are colonized with pathogenic bacteria. Surprisingly, this is true even in patients less than one year of age. In HNRG, the most frequent pathogen is *Pseudomonas aeruginosa*, as seen by other authors [35–37], including 50% isolates with mucoid strains. The presence of the latter is usually associated with chronic colonization [38]. The viscosity of the mucoid variety is related to alginate, a polysaccharide (polymer of manuronic and gluconic acid) which may contribute to the pathogenesis of these strains by resistance to phagocytosis, and decrease permeability to antibiotics and antibodies. *Pseudomonas cepacia* is not a worrisome agent at this time since REGLAFQ detected only 2% during 1990–1991.

HNRG isolated *Staphylococcus aureus* in 46.2% of the specimens, a slightly different number from previous studies in the same hospital [39–43]. However, in the 1991 multicenter study, *S. aureus* was isolated in lower numbers (28.9% in 943 patients). The incidence of *Haemophilus influenzae* in HNRG and in REGLAFQ was only 3.8%, less than that reported by other authors [35]. Usuallly "no type B" was isolated and was associated with *S. Aureus* or *S. aureus* and *Pseudomonas*. There is a low incidence of other enteric bacteria – *Klebsiella, E. coli, Enterobacter* etc, associated with *S. aureus*. As far as antibiotic susceptibility in the HNRG sutdy, ceftazidime resistance was low (8.3%), perhaps related to the scarce utilization of this drug in our environment. It was striking to find low resistance to aminoglycosides.

Scientific Investigations

In 1974, work with animal models, using mice litters, was begun in Argentina. The most frequently used was DBA/2J cri which has an alteration at the electrolyte level in the parotid and sweat glands, as well as a cribiform degeneration of the central nervous system (41). Spermatozoan motility of this litter was studied in order to see ciliary movement in the presence of CF sera, healthy controls [45, 46].

Other studies include cleansing and clearance of pathogens [47–49], exocrine pancreatic secretion [50–55] and biliary secretion [56] of this litter in comparison to other litters. New mutations were seen in mice [57] and reproductive studies were conducted on other mice litters [58, 59]. Kallikrein–kinin system studies were conducted on mice colon and on sweat obtained from CF patients [60–62]. Currently, different Latin American countries are conducting basic and applied research studies ranging from casuality to non-conventional therapies.

Final Reflections

What is the real magnitude of CF in the context of health care in Latin America? This report indicates the magnitude of the problem is significant. It is true that inconveniences exist, such as the growing cost of health care, insufficient clinical research and lack of proper technology. These factors often compromise the efforts to improve diagnostic aspects and treatment of complex diseases and high operational cost, as seen with CF.

Based on these results it is necessary to organize, select and implement regional follow up programs for prevention and treatment of the disease, keeping in mind the social and economic aspects of each area. This would represent a step towards improved survival and a mechanism of feedback among centers that traditionally have had poor communication among themselves or have been involved only with the Northern Hemisphere [63].

Acknowledgement

We gratefully acknowledge the translation from Spanish to English by Ofelia Vargas-Shiraishi, Infectious Diseases, Children's Hospital of Orange County, California.

References

1. Pivetta OH, Macri CN. Newborn screening meconium BM test for cystic fibrosis. Proc. 1er Congreso Latinoam. de FQ. 1986. Bs. Aires.

2. Raskin S, Rozov T, Caldieri J, Abreu F, Marostica P, Giugliani R, Ficher E, Silveira T, Rosario N, Ludwig N, Phillips A, Pilloto RA. Fibrose cistica no Brasil: Análise de DNA e correlaço genotipo/cuadro clínico. Actas del IV Congreso Latinoamericano de Fibrosis Quística, Montevideo, Uruguay, 1991.
3. REGLAFQ: Macri CN, Gentile A, Manterola A, Maillie A, Castorina A, Tomezzoli S, et al. 1990.
4. Pivetta OH. Guiding Principles of the Formulation of National Programs for the Prevention and Control of Cystic Fibrosis in Developing Countries. WHO. 1989.
5. Comas Juan. Antropología de los Pueblos Iberoamericanos. Biblioteca Universitaria Labor, Barcelona, España. 1974.
6. Cystic Fibrosis International Directory 1993.
7. Annual Members Reports I.C.F.(M).A. 1992 y 1993.
8. Información personal del Grupo Latinoamericano.
9. Rommens JM, Iannuzzi MC, Kerem B, Drumm ML, Melmer G, Dean M, Rozmahel R, Cole JL, Kennedy D, Hidaka N, Zsiga M, Buchwald M, Riordan JR, Tsui LC, Collins FS. Identification of the cystic fibrosis gene: chromosome walking and jumping. Science 1989; 245: 1059–1065.
10. Kere J, Savilahti E, Norio R, Estivill X, de la Chapelle A. Cystic Fibrosis mutation ΔF508 in Finland: other mutations predominant. Human Genetics 1985(4): 413–415.
11. Chillón M, Nunes V, Casals T, Gimenez FJ, Fernandez E, Benítez J, Estivill X. Distribution of the ΔF508 mutation in 194 Spanish cystic fibrosis families. Human Genetics 1985(4): 396–397.
12. Raskin S, Phillips A, Kaplan G, McClure M, Dawson E, Cardieri JM, Marostica P, Abreu F, Giugliani R, Rosario N, Reis F, Ludwig N. and Diniz E. DNA data suggest the incidence of CF in Brazil may be tenfold more than observed. Annual Meeting at the American Society of Human Genetics, Oct, 1992.
13. Olek K, Pivetta OH, Döring G. Fibrosis Quística: Estudio de 25 familias argentinas con sondas ligadas de DNA. Actas del III Congreso Latinoamericano de Fibrosis Quística. Mexico DF. Mexico 1989.
14. Orozco L, Lezana JL, Chavez M, Valdez H, Moreno M, Carnevale A. Estudio Molecular de la Mutación ΔF508 y Análisis Genético de una Muestra de Pacientes con Fibrosis Quística. Bal Médico Hospital Infantil Mexico 1992.
15. Pivetta OH, Luna MC. Influencia del origen poblacional sobre la frecuencia de la mutación ΔF508 en la Argentina. Actas del V Congreso Brasileiro de Pneumonología Pediatrica – V Congreso Latinoamericano de Fibrosis Quística – V Jornada Brasileira de Fibrose Cistica. Recife, Brasil, 1993.
16. Pivetta OH, Olek K. Relación entre la deleción ΔF508 y la expresión clínica en pacientes Fibroquísticos. Actas del IV Congreso Latinoamericano de Fibrosis Quística, Montevideo, Uruguay, 1991.
17. Luna MC, Pivetta OH. Relación Cl^-/Na^+ en sudor. Marcador Fenotípico de la mutación ΔF508? Actas del V Congreso Brasileiro de Pneumonología Pediatrica – V Congreso Latinoamericano de Fibrosis Quística – V Jornada Brasileira de Fibrose Cistica. Recife, Brasil, 1993.
18. Davidson AG, Anderson CM. Diagnosis of cystic fibrosis. Br Med J 1971; 4: 362–364.
19. Macri CN, Gentile A, Manterola A, Maillie JA, Tomezzoli S. Estudio clínico epidemiológico Latino Americano de la fibrosis quistica. Archivos Argentinos de Pediatría, tomo 80, 1992.
20. Macri CN, Gentile A, Manterola A, Tomezzoli S y Galanterik L. Fibrosis quística: Veintiun años de seguimiento clínico. Rev. Hospital de niños Buenos Aires Vol XXXII N° 140/141 172–183 Oct–Dec 1990.
21. Cystic Fibrosis Foundation, CF Patient Registry Data 1988, Bolletin.
22. Barbero GJ. The diagnosis of Cystic Fibrosis: problems and new vistas. 1982; 1000 years of Cystic Fibrosis. Univ. Minnesota, Minneapolis.
23. Kelly HW, Lovato C. Antibiotic use in cystic fibrosis. Drug Intell Clin Pharm 1984; 18: 772–782.
24. Khaw K, Adeniyi-Jones S, Pena Cruz V et al. The effect of caloric supplementation on growth parameters in children with cystic fibrosis. CF Annual Club Abstr. 1978.
25. Shwachman H. Progress in the studies of mucoviscidosis. Pediatrics 1951; 7: 153.
26. Shwachman H. Therapy of cystic fibrosis of the pancreas. Pediatrics 1960; 25: 155.

27. Donati MA, Guenetti G, Auerbach H. Prospective controlled study of home and Hospital therapy of cystic fibrosis pulmonary disease. J Pediatr 1987; 111: 28–33.
28. Canadian Cystic Fibrosis Foundation. CF patient Registry Data 1988.
29. Shwachman H, Kulczicki LL. A long term study in 105 patients with cystic fibrosis. Am J Dis Child 1970; 270.
30. Informe Multicéntrico LA, REGLAFQ año 1990 (not published).
31. Informe Multicéntrico LA, REGLAFQ año 1991 (not published).
32. Macri CN, Alvarez AR. Enfermedad Fibroquística: Correlación clínico-Funcional. Arch Arg Ped 1971; LXIX: 173–182.
33. Macri CN, Alvarez AR. Enfermedad Fibroquística: Sintesis de nuestra Experencia. Rev Htal Niños Buenos Aires 1977; XLX 75: 135–144.
34. Kofman CN, Teper AM, Alducin J, Maffey AF, Macri CN. Evaluación de la Función Respiratoria en niños Fq. menores de tres años. I Jornadas Uruguayas de Neumonología Pediátrica. Libro de Publicación 82–83: Oct. 1992.
35. Hernandez C, Rubeglio E, Macri C. Incidencia de *Pseudomonas* en la enfermedad fibroquística. Abst I Congreso Latinoamericano de Fibrosis Quística. Buenos Aires, Mayo 1986.
36. Hernandez C, Galanternik L, Procopio A, Rubeglio E, Macri CN. Estudio microbiológico de la flora de vías repiratorias de pacientes con Enfermedad Fibroquística del Páncreas (FQ). I congreso Latinoamericano de Fibrosis Quística, Buenoa Aires, Mayo de 1986.
37. Hernandez C, Galanternik L, Macri CN. Bacteriologia de la flora respiratoria en pacientes con Enfermedad Fibroquistica. II Congreso Latinoamericano de Fibrose Cistica. Brasil, Agosto de 1987.
38. Galanternik L, Macri CN, Woloj M, Hernandez C. Incidencia Bacteriana en esputos de pacientes con Fibrosis Quistica en un periodod de dos años: comparación con experiencias previas. Actas del III Congreso Latinoamericano de Fibrosis Quística, México D.F. México, Julio 1989.
39. Galanternik L, Macri CN, Woloj M. *Pseudomonas cepacia*: su rol en pacientes fibroquísticos en el hospital de niños Ricardo Gutierrez. Actas del IV Congreso Latinoamericano de Fibrosis Quistica. Montevideo, Uruguay, 1991.
40. Garcia de Dávila MT, Marco I, Macri CN. Enfermedad Fibroquística: revisión y análisis clínico anatómico de autopsias durante 20 años. Actas del I Congreso Latinoamericano de Fibrosis Quística, Buenos Aires, Argentina, Mayo 1986.
41. Hernandez C, Rubeglio E, Macri CN. Incidencia de *Pseudomonas* en la enfermedad fibroquística. Actas del I Congreso Latinoamericano de Fibrosis Quística, Buenos Aires, Argentina, 1986.
42. Hernandez C, Galanternik L, Procopio A, Rubeglio E, Macri CN. Estudio microbiológico de la flora de vías respiratorias de pacientes con Enfermedad Fibroquística del Páncreas (FQ). I Congreso Latinoamericano de Fibrosis Quistica, Buenos Aires, Argentina, 1986.
43. Hernandez C, Galanternik L, Macri CN. Bacteriología de la flora respiratoria en pacientes con Enfermedad Fibroquística. II Congreso Latinoamericano de Fibrose Cística. Brasil, 1987.
44. Kaiser D, Pivetta OH, Rennet O. Autosomal recessively inhered electrolite excretory defect in parotid of cribiform degeneration mouse mutant: Possible analogy of cystic fibrosis. Life Sci 1974; 15(4): 803–810.
45. Pivetta OH, Labal ML, Sordelli DO. Serum cilitoxic activity in mutant mice with some hereditary alterations resembling cystic fibrosis. Pediat Res 1977; 13: 1133–1136.
46. Pivetta OH, Macri CN, Sordelli DO, Tuozzo SN, Determinación de actividad sérica de lecitinas en individuos homocigotas y heterocigotas para la enfermedad fibroquística. XV Jornadas Htal de Niños Buenos Aires. dic. 1980.
47. Sordelli DO, Cassino RJJ, Macri CN, Kohan M, Dillon MA, Pivett OH. Effect of cystic fibrosis (CF) serum on the kinetics of phagocytosis of pulmonary alveolar macrophages (PAM). Pediat Res, vol 15 n°2. Actas del 17mo Congreso Latinoamericano de Investigación Pediátrica. 1981.
48. Sordelli DO, Cerquetti MC, Cassino RJJ, Pivetta OH. Lung unspecific microbicidal defenses in a possible animal model for cystic fibrosis. Pediat. Res, vol 15 n°2. Actas del 17mo Congreso Latinoamericano de Investigación Pediátrica. 1981.
49. Sordelli DO, Cassino RJJ, Labal M, Pivetta OH. Depuración bacteriana pulmonar disminuida en ratones con degeneración cribiforme. Medicina 1980; 39: 457.

50. Basabe JC, Bruno L, Pivetta OH, Canales L, Cresto JC. Somatostatin as a hormone of the endocrine pancreas: Somatostatin secretion. Pediat Res, vol 15 n°2. Actas del 17mo Congreso Latinoamericano de Investigación Pediátrica. 1981.
51. Cassino RJJ, Sordelli DO, Cerquetti MC, Pivetta OH. Pulmonary defenses against *Pseudomonas aeruginosa* as a function of age in a possible animal model for cystic fibrosis (CF). Pediat Res, vol 15 n°2. Actas del 17mo Congreso Latinoamericano de Investigación Pediátrica. 1981.
52. Basabe JC, Pivetta OH, Bruno L. Karabatas L, Aparicio N. Somatostatin as a hormone of the endocrine pancreas: β cell sensitivity to its inhibitory action. Pediat Res, vol 15 n°2. Actas del 17mo Congreso Latinoamericano de Investigación Pediátrica. 1981.
53. Calvo EL, Vaccaro MI, Maille AJ, Pivetta OH. An experimental model to perform dynamic studies of exocrine pancreatic secretion in mice. Acta Physiol Latinoam 1984; XXXIV, n° 1: 9–13.
54. Calvo EL, Vaccaro MI, Maille JA, Emiliani R, Pivetta OH. Estudio *"in vivo"* de la secreción de calcio por el páncreas exócrino del ratón. Relación con la secreción enzimática. Acta Physiol Latinoam 1986; 36, n°1: 10–13.
55. Vaccaro MI, Pivetta OH, Maille AJ, de Caboteau L, Calvo E, Función pancreática exócrina en ratones endocriados. Determinación de actividad enzimática en secreción obtenida por microcanulación coledociana retrógrada. Rev Soc Argent Biol 1979; 54–55: 151–152.
56. De Matos D, Buzzalino ND, Pivetta OH. A new mutant mouse. Nutrition and pancreatic studies. Communicaciones Biológicas, 1984; 3, N°2: 249–260.
57. De Matos D, Buzzalino ND, Pivetta OH. In *"In vitro"* capacitation of spermatozoa in different strains of mice: The acrosome reaction. Medicina 1987; 47: 500–504.
58. Zucollo A, Martiarena J, Luna MC, Pivetta OH, Villagra A, Catanzaro OL. Actas del Congreso "Kinin 91" Munich, Alemania, 1991.
59. Catanzaro OL, Vaccaro MI, Vila SB, Martinez Seeber AL, Pivetta OH. Kallikrein and amylase contents in tissues from a mutant mouse model for human cystic fibrosis. Life Sci 1982; 32: 825–831.
60. Catanzaro OL, Vila SB, Pivetta OH. Comparative studies on kinin and kininase activity of pulmonary lavage fluid from mutant mouse model for CF and reserpinized mouse. II Congreso Latinoamericano de Fibrose Cistica. Belo Horizonte, Brasil, 1987.
61. Zucollo A, Martiarena J, Luna MC, Pivetta OH, Villagra A, Catanzaro OL. The Kallikrein-Kinin system of sweat in normal and CF subjects. Agents and Actions 1992; 38, N°3: 493–498.
62. Maille JA, Calvo E, Vaccaro MI, de Cabouteau L, Pivetta OH. An experimental model to study bile and exocrine pancreatic secretion from mice. Laboratory Animal Science, 1981; 31, N°6.
63. Macri CN. Perspectives of Cystic Fibrosis in Latin America. Abstract 3rd Latin American CF Congress. 1989. México.

CHAPTER 10
Pulmonary Infections in Venezuelan Patients with Cystic Fibrosis

Sonia Alvarez de Garcia Tuñon and Heberto Reyes

Department of Pediatrics, University School of Medicine, Central University of Venezuela, Venezuela

Introduction

Cystic fibrosis is considered an important health problem in different decades of life. It causes high morbidity and mortality as a consequence of chronic and recurrent pulmonary infections [1, 2]. In addition, it is responsible for a large variety of manifestations, i.e. pancreatic insufficiency, nasal polyposis, pulmonary disease, sinusitis, rectal prolapse, hyperglycemia, short stature, etc. Therefore, it is considered a complex disease which calls for management by a multidisciplinary team, including pneumonologists, infectologists, pediatricians, gastroenterologists, cardiologists, nutritionists, therapists, etc. [3]. This strategy, together with early diagnosis and timely initiation of treatment, greatly improve patient survival. The approximate annual cost of treatment in Venezuela is US$10 000 per patient, making it very difficult to provide adequate therapy to low income patients without financial assistance from public and private institutions.

The disease is known to be inherited in an autosomal recessive manner. The CF mutated gene was discovered to be located on chromosome 7 [4]. The CF gene product was named the cystic fibrosis transmembrane conductance regulator (CFTR) [5]. The basic gene defect in cystic fibrosis consists of the deletion of the three basic pairs causing the loss of the phenylalanine aminoacid sequence in position 508 of the protein (CFTR protein) [5].

The $\Delta F508$ mutation is present in 70% of cystic fibrosis chromosomes, never in normal chromosomes. There exists a large variety of mutations in cystic fibrosis; more than 200 CF alleles have been identified in the CFTR gene [6], considered geographically heterogeneous. Certain mutations may be common to a specific ethnic group. The determination of the mutation present in the cystic fibrosis patient (genotype–phenotype correlation) is helpful in management and prognosis [5].

The incidence of CF is variable, based on the ethnic distribution of specific regions. It is known that there is a high incidence of the disease in Caucasian populations, reported to be 1 in every 2000 live births [5].

In Venezuela, some regions have a higher disease incidence. For instance, the Andean-Coastal region in the northern part of the country, including Caracas, the capital, and the main seaport of Venezuela, La Guaira, which was the main landing site of our colonizers.

It is important to note that our ancestors and colonizers were Europeans and that the Venezuelan population is made up of a mixture of races: whites, mixed blood, native Indians, and Blacks. Most of our population is of mixed blood.

Cystic Fibrosis Patients in Venezuela

The following is a review of 55 children selected from a sample population of 200 patients with cystic fibrosis. The diagnostic age, current age, sex, race, current nutritional status, significant personal history, significant family history, clinical manifestations, diagnostic procedures, complications, treatment and mortality are reported (Tables 1-10).

Table 1 exhibits a high frequency of diagnosis between 0 and 2 years (18:55).

A General Registry of CF patients in Venezuela was first developed in 1991. Currently, there are 200 patients registered, with only 13 over the age of 12 years (range 13-28 years, median 16 years). It is difficult to estimate the true census of patients with CF in Venezuela at this time.

Management of these older patients follow the same guidelines as for patients under age 12. Hence, antibiotic, nutritional, and respiratory therapies are standard and are administered and supervised by multidiscisplinary care teams.

Monitoring of disease course and results of therapy include radiographic, microbiologic, and pulmonary function assessments.

Pseudomonas aeruginosa predominates as the respiratory pathogen isolated from the sputum from these older CF patients; *Staphylococcus aureus* and *Klebsiella* sp. are also common. Mycobacteria have not been found.

Table 1. Cystic fibrosis in Venezuelan children. Relation of diagnostic age/number of subjects

Diagnostic age	Number of subjects
0-11 months	10
12-23 months	8
2-6 years	25
7-12 years	7
over 12 years	5

Pulmonary function tests indicate a severely restrictive impairment in approximately 25% of the CF patients over 12 years and moderate restriction in the remainder.

Almost one-half of the older patients (over 12 years of age) have gastroesophageal reflux, and one-quarter have hiatal hernias. Approximately one-half have moderate to severe nutritional deficiencies, and we have one older patient with pancreatitis and another with hepatic cirrhosis. Other complications in the older CF patients in Venezuela include some evidence of bronchiectasis demonstrated by computerized tomography scars in all 13 patients and chest deformity in 50%.

Sinusitis is also a frequent complication in older CF patients in Venezuela. Among the 13 patients in our registry over 12 years of age, five have had surgery for multiple polyps and most have clinical or CT scan evidence of sinus inflammation.

In a study carried out by Macri et al. [7] on the epidemiology of CF in Latin America, the average age at diagnosis was after the third year of life. In Table 2, the sample demonstrates a slight increase of females over males (30/55) representing 55%. Other authors report an increase of males.

Table 3 exhibits a slightly higher prevalence of the disease among our white patients representing approximately 40% of the sample (22/55). For the most part, the white race in this country is made up of descendants of the Spaniards who came during the Conquest, and followed much later by migratory flows from European countries.

The mixed blood patients make up 36% (20/55) of our study population. They are products of Spanish and Indian blood (our first inhabitants), the third place being occupied by mulattos with 24% (13/55), and these are the product of whites mixing with blacks (from the African continent).

Most of our patients presented with a high degree of malnutrition, 71% (39/55) were below the 50th percentile per weight. It is important

Table 2. Gender of 55 Venezuelan cystic fibrosis patients

Gender	Patients
Female	30/55
Male	25/55

Table 3. Race of Venezuelan patients with cystic fibrosis

Race	Patients
White	22/55
Mixed blood	20/55
Mulatto	13/55

to note that the sample was taken in a public hospital which receives patients from the lower income groups. To the problems of CF are added nutritional deficits of essential nutrients (Table 4).

At this time, of the total of 55 patients, 51 are under control and four have died. The nutritional status of the children included in the sample has greatly improved as is denoted in Table 5, once they were submitted to the treatment plan. At this time, 61% (31/51) are at the 50th percentile and only 14% (7/51) are at the 3rd percentile. The clinical and family histories of Venezuelan cystic fibrosis patients are listed in Tables 6 and 7, respectively. Fifty-five percent of 51 patients had been immunized with the BCG vaccine during the first month of life.

The most common respiratory features are set out in Table 8 and include pneumonia, pansinusitis, chronic cough, and asthma. It is a well

Table 4. Nutritional status at time of diagnosis of cystic fibrosis

P3	39/55
P10	12/55
P50	4/55

P = percentile.

Table 5. Current nutritional status in the same 55 Venezuelan patients with cystic fibrosis

P50	31/55
P10	13/55
P3	7/55
Mortality	4/55

P = percentile.

Table 6. Clinical history of Venezuelan CF patients (reported by parents)

Clinical features	Patients	Percentage
Lung infection	42/55	76%
Chronic cough	37/55	67%
Respiratory allergy	36/55	65%
Chronic diarrhea	36/55	65%
Upper airway obstruction	25/55	45%
Anemia	16/55	29%
Neonatal jaundice	13/55	24%
Rectal prolapse	12/55	22%
Short stature	7/55	13%
Edematous syndrome	6/55	11%
Intestinal obstruction	4/55	7%
Meconium ileus	4/55	7%
Heat shock	4/55	7%
Hydrocele	1/55	2%

Table 7. Family history of Venezuelan cystic fibrosis patients

Clinical features	Family	Percentage
Respiratory allergies	38/55	69%
Diabetes mellitus	6/55	11%
Previous offspring who died with CF	6/55	11%
Parents were smokers	4/55	7%
Fat intolerance	1/55	2%

Table 8. Respiratory manifestations in Venezuelan CF patients

Clinical diagnosis	Respiratory symptoms	Percentage
Pneumonia	(46/55)	87%
Pansinusitis	(41/55)	75%
Chronic cough	(40/55)	73%
Asthma	(38/55)	69%
High airway obstruction	(23/55)	42%
Adenoid hypertrophy	(18/55)	31%
Turbinate hypertrophy	(6/55)	11%
Otitis	(3/55)	5%

known fact that CF causes a high prevalence of respiratory manifestations resulting from the airway changes which cause alterations of the mucus secretions (increased production and quality deficit) affecting clearance and other functions [7].

The main gastrointestinal symptoms were gastroesophageal reflux, steatorrhea and chronic diarrhea (Table 9). These gastric manifestations in CF patients are a direct consequence of the genetic alteration or secondary to pancreatic insufficiency [8]. The chloride impermeability of the intestinal epithelial membrane affects the quality of the secretion in

Table 9. Gastrointestinal manifestations in Venezuelan CF patients

Gastroesophageal reflux	(39/55)	71%
Steatorrhea	(27/55)	50%
Chronic diarrhea	(23/55)	41%
Esophagitis	(15/55)	27%
Rectal prolapse	(9/55)	16%
Hiatal hernia	(5/55)	9%
Duodenitis	(3/55)	5%
Duodenogastric reflux	(3/55)	5%
Abdominal pain	(3/55)	5%
Intestinal malabsorption	(1/55)	2%
Pancreatitis	(1/55)	2%
Milk protein intolerance	(1/55)	2%

the intraluminal space as thicker mucus invades the secretory and exocrine intraductal spaces leading to obstruction, inflammation and fibrosis of the ducts, in addition to causing dysfunction of proximal tissue. An increased sodium reabsorption has also been shown, apparently related to the abnormal apical transmembrane conductance of this element [9, 10].

Laboratory Diagnostic Work Up

The following studies are included in the diagnostic work up for CF in Venezuela:

a) Sweat Electrolytes
b) PCR (polymerase chain reaction)
c) Enzymatic Studies
d) Ultrasound
e) Fat Determinations

a) **Sweat Electrolytes:** patients exhibit increased levels of Na^+ and Cl^- in sweat. The study is carried out three times with the pilocarpine method (>50 mg of sweat), with silver electrodes. The same specially trained staff are used in every case.

b) **PCR (polymerase chain reaction):** using DNA probes (direct technique). This procedure is used to establish the existing mutation. The test costs approximately US$20 in this country. It is carried out on our patients, their parents and siblings, in order to look for carriers, mild and asymptomatic forms. Among the 55 patients detailed above, 20 were found to be infrequent mutation heterozygotics, representing 36%. It is probable that these results could explain the low mortality rate in this group of patients.

c) **Enzymatic Studies:** using duodenal intubation and pancreazymin and secretin. This study serves to evaluate pancreatic enzymes and bicarbonate production.

d) **Ultrasound:** is used to determine the pancreatic structure.

e) **Stool Fat Determination (Van de Kramer method):** stools are collected for three days, on admission and thereafter to control results of therapy. There is a considerable increase in every case.

Lung Disease Diagnosis: Radiologic studies are done in every patient at the time of initial diagnosis, quarterly for one year and every six months thereafter. Radiographic diagnosis is also used as needed for the diagnosis and management of acute pulmonary exacerbations.

Etiological Diagnosis: Bacteria determinations are fundamental in lung disease. Systematic cultures are done every 3 months on every patient, and with every case of pneumonia. Bronchoscopy is used for infants and for the rest, a sputum test.

An example of the microbiologic status of our patients is provided by a review of the 55 patients reported above. A total of 99 potentially pathogenic strains were isolated. *Staphylococcus aureus* was most prevalent (37 strains or 37% of the total strains identified), *Pseudomonas aureus* 35 strains (35% of the strains isolated), followed by *Haemophilus influenzae* (19% of strains isolated), *Pseudomonas cepacia* [11] (3%), and *Klebsiella pneumoniae* and *Aspergillus fumigatus* in one case each. No mycobacteria were isolated in any of these patients.

Many had mixed pulmonary infections. The most frequent association observed was *Staphylococcus aureus*, *Pseudomonas aeruginosa*, and *Haemophilus influenzae* in 20% of cultures.

Lung Function Tests

Another important test in lung infections and CF in order to complete patient evaluation is lung function. The information it provides is very useful to follow the disease, to assess respiratory therapy and as an exploratory method to observe the degree of pulmonary alteration in asymptomatic patients. The earliest defect observed is an increase of residual volume and airway resistance. Initially, obstruction of peripheral airways is observed, trapping of air and a deterioration of ventilation–perfusion.

The airway obstruction is measured with the Flow-Volume curve. In the above cohort the pattern observed was severely restrictive in five (9%), and was moderately restrictive in 3 of 55 patients (5%).

Additional Studies

The prevalence of positive findings is illustrated by a review of the 55 Venezuelan patients we have detailed. Forty had pansinusitis as revealed by a CT scan of the paranasal sinuses (75%); 18% had slight hypoxemia; 5% had hypoxemia with hypercapnea; and 4% had moderate hypoxemia. The 24-hour pH and endoscopy and biopsy studies demonstrated gastroesophageal reflux in 71%.

Again, using the 55 patient cohort as a sample, the most frequent complication was bronchiectasis caused by recurrent and chronic infections, mechanical processes and also due to the presence of gastroesophageal reflux, the latter being the most frequent GI manifestation in CF (Table 10). Contrary to what is reported by other authors, cor pulmonale, atelectasis, and respiratory failure were seen in a low percentage of our cases. Two patients among the 55 were found to have a pulmonary abscess.

Table 10. Complication of CF in Venezuelan Patients

Bronchiectasis	(16/55)	29%
Cor pulmonale	(3/55)	5%
Chest deformity	(3/55)	5%
Atelectasis	(2/55)	4%
Lung abscess	(2/55)	4%
Heart failure	(1/55)	2%
Respiratory failure	(1/55)	2%
Lung fibrosis	(1/55)	2%
Esophageal varix	(1/55)	2%
Liver cirrhosis	(1/55)	2%

Treatment

Treatment is individualized according to age at diagnosis, genophenotypical alterations, number of complications and sequelae. It is comprehensive as it includes pulmonary anti-infection therapy, gastrointestinal therapy geared to correct the pancreatic deficit and measures to improve the nutritional status of patients.

The anti-infectious therapy is designed to clear lung infection and to minimize or delay the inflammatory reaction and the progressive pulmonary lesions [4].

The most frequent reason for hospitalization in our patient population is recurrent pulmonary infections. Hospitalizations have declined as a result of the quarterly bacteriological screening practiced on all CF patients. When a culture is positive and the patient is asymptomatic, ambulatory treatment is initiated according to bacterial sensitivity. It can be in the form of a nebulizer for three, four, and up to six months along, or associated with oral antibiotics.

Hospitalization depends on several factors including age, the patient's condition, or associated manifestations and radiological findings. I.V. antimicrobial treatment is initiated with a combination of antimicrobials in order to cover the spectrum including the main pathogens which cause pulmonary infection. It is varied according to the clinical results, the culture, and the sensitivity tests.

In addition to anti-infectious treatment, patients also receive beta-adrenergics (nebulizations), terbutaline, fenoterol, fenoterol with bromuro of ipatropio or salbutamol (ventolin). In Venezuela, we use ventolin with good results. Lung function tests are performed before and after treatment. Other medications used are inhaled corticosteroids for high airway obstruction caused by endonasal polyposis. All CF patients are included in a physical therapy program to improve their respiratory function.

Gastrointestinal therapy is mostly geared to the correction of the different Gl tract pathologies (gastroesophageal reflux, duodenogastric reflux, intestinal dysmotility, etc.) which worsen the pulmonary disease, interfere with nutrient absorption and affect adequate utilization of pancreatic enzymes.

The **pancreatic deficit** is treated with enzymes (lipase) or pancreatic extracts.

The nutritional status of patients is improved with an increase of 130% over their basal requirements of all nutrients, vitamins and minerals [4]. Where there is infection, requirements are increased by 150%.

Final comments

Chronic and recurrent pulmonary infections continue to be the main cause of morbidity-mortality in Venezuelan patients with CF. The low mortality rate observed in our patient population is probably due to the infrequent heterozygotic mutations found in our genetic studies.

At this time there is great hope that genetic therapy will provide the means to correct the genetic defect of CF. Recent efforts are also directed to the search for a safe and immunogenic conjugated *Pseudomonas aeruginosa* vaccine for CF [12].

In Caracas, Venezuela there is a Cystic Fibrosis Association integrated by the community of parents of affected children. It provides counselling by a multidisciplinary team of physicians and specialized staff. The contributions of private enterprises are used for the acquisition of medication, instruments and research requirements in order to provide care for patients from the lower income groups.

Acknowledgement

The authors wish to acknowledge the collaboration of Dr Ana Navas, The Children's Hospital JM de los Rios and the University Hospital of Caracas. We greatly appreciate the editorial supervision provided by Dr Melvin I. Marks and Joyce Bagan, Memorial Miller Children's Hospital, Long Beach, California.

References

1. Neils H. Cystic fibrosis infection. Schweiz med Wachr 1991; 121: 105–109.
2. Cahen P, Le Bourgeois M, Delacourt C, et al. Prueba de la actividad bactericida del suero como indicador pronostico en las exacerbaciones pulmonares agudas de la fibrosis quistica. Francia. Pediatr 1993; 35(2): 78–83.
3. Castro EH, Suarez C. Diagnostico y tratamiento de la fibrosis quistica. Sistema Nacional de Salud 1992; 15(3): 66–67.

4. Patterson JM, Budd J, Goetz D, Warwick WJ. Family correlates of a 10-year pulmonary health in CF. Pediatric 1993; 91(2): 383–389.
5. Beaudet AL. Genetic testing for cystic fibrosis. Pediatric Clinics of North America 1992; 39(2): 213–227.
6. Kubesch P, Dork T, Wulbrand U, et al. Genetic determinants of airways' colonization with *Pseudomonas aeruginosa* in cystic fibrosis. Lancet 1993; 341: 189–193.
7. Macri C, et al. Cystic fibrosis in Latinoamerican. IV Congress Lationamerican Cystic Fibrosis, Montevideo, 1991.
8. Navas-Ramirez A. Fibrosis quistica. Ediciones Interamericana 1993;50–60.
9. Goldstein JL, Nash T. Rectum has abnormal ion transport but normal C amp binding protein in cystic fibrosis. Am J Physiol 1988; 254: 719–724.
10. Elborn JS. Fourth Annual North American and 1990 International Cystic Fibrosis Conference. Thorax 1991; 46: 72–73.
11. Saijan SU, Fostner JF. Identification of the mucin binding adhesive of *Pseudomonas cepacia* isolated from patients with cystic fibrosis. J Clin Invest 1992; 89: 657–665.
12. Lang S, Ruedeberg WJ. Safety and immunogenicity of *Pseudomonas aeruginosa* conjugate: a vaccine in cystic fibrosis. Lancet 1991; 338: 1236–1237.

Cystic Fibrosis Pulmonary Infections:
Lessons from Around the World
ed. by A. Bauernfeind, M. I. Marks and B. Strandvik
© 1996 Birkhäuser Verlag Basel/Switzerland

CHAPTER 11
Pulmonary Infection in Cystic Fibrosis:
The Australian Approach

Peter D. Phelan

Department of Pediatrics, University of Melbourne, Parkville 3052, Victoria, Australia

Introduction

Death in patients with cystic fibrosis is almost always the result of failure to control the progressive lung infection so characteristic of the disease. Consequently this aspect of management has received predominant attention in CF centres in Australia but the importance of maintenance of optimal nutrition, control of gastrointestinal symptoms, prevention of salt depletion and psychosocial support of patients and families are integral aspects of optimal management.

Organisation of Cystic Fibrosis Care in Australia

Australia is a country of 7 682 000 km² with a population of 18 million of which about 95% is Caucasian in origin. It is a federation comprising seven sovereign states which are primarily responsible for the administration of health care. Most of Australia's population is along the eastern and south-eastern seaboard and three cities, Sydney, Melbourne and Brisbane, account for almost 50% of the population.

In New South Wales, the largest state (population about 5 million), there are four CF centres providing care for children and one for adults. In Queensland, there are two centres for children and one for adults. In each of Victoria, South Australia and Western Australia there is one paediatric and one adult centre. The Victoria Centre provides consultative support to paediatricians in Tasmania who look after patients with cystic fibrosis. The population of the Northern Territory is far too small to justify a centre.

This review is based on the practices of the CF Centre in Melbourne, the capital city of Victoria (area 227 000 km²), which has an integrated paediatric centre at the Royal Children's Hospital and an adult centre at the Alfred Hospital. It is the oldest centre in Australia (established

1953) with 420 patients under the age of 21 and an adult component of approximately 120 patients up to the age of 60. Patients normally transfer from the paediatric service to the adult service soon after completing formal secondary education but the time is flexible depending on the patient's needs and wishes. However, there is a strong view that once the patient has achieved social and economic independence he/she should shift to adult care.

The Melbourne Centre looks after virtually all patients with cystic fibrosis from a population of 4.5 million. Its treatment practices are similar to those in the other centres in Australia and the heads of approximately half those centres trained in Melbourne. This article reflects the general approach to CF management throughout Australia.

The Melbourne Clinic

As already mentioned, the Melbourne Clinic currently manages virtually every patient with CF in Victoria and the southern part of New South Wales. Newborn screening was introduced in 1989. The screening service is run by the Murdoch Institute based at the Royal Children's Hospital, and works in close collaboration with the hospital's Department of Thoracic Medicine which is responsible for the CF Clinic. When parents are notified that their child has been identified by the screening programme as having CF either because of DNA mapping or an elevated sodium and chloride in sweat, an appointment is made within 24–48 hours to meet the personnel of the clinic.

Prior to the introduction of newborn screening, 42% of patients (other than those with meconium ileus and those diagnosed by routine testing because of a family history) were diagnosed prior to the age of 6 months and a further 19% between 6–12 months, and similar percentages between 1–2 years and 2–5 years. Fewer than 2% of patients were diagnosed over the age of 5. Twenty percent of patients presented with meconium ileus and 12% were diagnosed because of a family history.

Four paediatric thoracic physicians are involved in the clinic and each is primarily responsible for approximately 100 patients. There is a very close working relationship with three paediatric gastroenterologists, infectious disease physicians and paediatric surgeons. There are two physiotherapists, a social worker/clinic coordinator and dietitian attached to the clinic.

At the time of diagnosis patients are almost always admitted to hospital and more recently to the hospital's care-by-parent unit. During this time there is an intensive education programme for parents, baseline investigations (including a 3-day fat balance) are performed, a therapeutic regime established and if there is lung disease present, it is treated. If there is no lung disease, the period in hospital is usually about five days. During the first 12 months patients are normally seen every 6–8 weeks but once progress is satisfactory, routine reviews are normally every three months. Some patients will have a return journey of 500 km for a clinic visit.

Comprehensive care is provided to patients living in the metropolitan area of Melbourne and the adjacent region (approximately 75% of patients). Those living in the rural area of the state will normally also see the regional paediatricians who work in very close association with the clinic. Regional clinics are held with regional paediatricians in three non-metropolitan centres on a 6-monthly basis. These are the only centres with sufficient numbers of patients to justify regional clinics.

At a clinic visit patients will normally be seen by the same thoracic physician whom they will regard as "their doctor". Those over 6 years of age have their lung function measured. From the age of 12–13 patients are seen on their own without their parents. Generally the patients are also seen by the physiotherapist, dietician and clinic coordinator/social worker.

The adult service is based in a general hospital about 5 km from the Royal Children's Hospital. It is staffed by two adult thoracic physicians who have a major commitment to cystic fibrosis. Two additional thoracic physicians who are involved in the hospital's heart/lung and lung transplantation service also participate in the clinic. In addition there are physiotherapist, dietitian, social worker and occupational therapist.

Management of Lung Disease

The two principles in the management of lung disease are the removal of excess tracheo–bronchial secretion and the treatment of any bacterial infection present. Of course, the maintenance of good nutrition is important and the adoption of a very positive attitude by patient, parents and caregivers is crucial to achieving an optimal outcome.

Removal of Excess Tracheo–Bronchial Secretion

Physical exercise and physiotherapy, preferably in combination, are used to remove excess tracheo–bronchial secretion. Effective coughing is the cornerstone and plays the major role in both physical exercise and physiotherapy. Patients are taught how to cough effectively and actively discouraged from suppressing their cough.

Exercise
The importance of physical activity is stressed from the time of diagnosis. Families are counselled to adopt the lifestyle which includes regular

physical activity. Once children commence school, they are encouraged to join all available sporting activities and to continue these throughout their school years. Participation with peers in sports that are enjoyed is the best way of maintaining an active lifestyle. It certainly is the impression of the clinic staff that those patients who are physically active and engage in regular sport are the fittest but whether this is the cause or effect is impossible to determine.

Social pressures are often against girls, as they enter the teenage years, maintaining active participation in regular sport. To what extent this withdrawal from regular physical activity plays a part in the progression of lung disease, still regrettably seen in some adolescent females, is impossible to determine. Towards the end of secondary schooling when studies become so important and at the time of leaving school it may be increasingly difficult for both men and women to maintain regular sport. Much counselling and support is essential to ensure that the regular lifestyle of early school years is maintained into adult life. The particular physical activities that adults will maintain are those that they enjoy and can do with their friends.

As well as helping to clear tracheo–bronchial secretions, regular sporting activities seem to maintain good general health, stimulate appetite and are important for self-esteem. To see patients with cystic fibrosis achieve excellence in sporting activities provides a very powerful incentive.

Physiotherapy

Formal physiotherapy probably has an important role to play in the management of the lung disease of cystic fibrosis but again there has been little scientific evaluation. In our clinic all families are taught how to do physiotherapy at the time of diagnosis. This is basically postural drainage and stimulated coughing. From the age of 5 or 6 patients are taught how to cough effectively and directed coughing becomes a major component of treatment. The use of PEP masks also seem to be useful particularly in those with large amounts of sputum.

We have become increasingly concerned about postural drainage and its possible contribution to gastroesophageal reflux and therefore to further lung damage. This is currently a matter of active evaluation [1].

In the early years of life, if the child is cough-free, parents are encouraged to do physiotherapy once most days. If after the age of 4 or 5 the child is cough-free and physically very active, then regular physiotherapy is suspended as long as the child remains well and engages in regular sport. For exacerbations of cough, physiotherapy is resumed twice daily. For children with a minor chronic cough, once daily physiotherapy is recommended and for those with moderate to large amounts of sputum twice daily treatment is encouraged. Whenever possible physiotherapy is undertaken after a period of physical activity.

The patients are encouraged to become independent of other caregivers with their physiotherapy from about the age of 9 or 10. Active cycle of breathing, forced expiration, directed coughing and PEP masks seem to be very helpful in achieving this degree of independence.

It is recognised that compliance with regular physiotherapy is far from satisfactory, particularly among teenagers. We try to have a very honest approach with our patients and develop alternate strategies if they are unwilling to do regular physiotherapy. For some chronic sputum producers, regular physical activity has to be accepted as a substitute with the patient agreeing to resume physiotherapy during exacerbations. This honest approach and negotiation of an appropriate therapeutic regime with the patient does seem to improve overall compliance. Authoritarian approaches to treatment will almost invariably be counterproductive.

Treatment of Bacterial Infection

It seems logical to treat bacterial lower respiratory infection with antibiotics that are effective against the particular pathogen. This presents two difficulties in patients with cystic fibrosis. The first is how to diagnose the presence of bacterial infection and secondly how to establish what is the pathogen.

Diagnosing Bacterial Infection

It has been a principle in the clinic for many years that if a child has a loose cough, it can be assumed that bacterial infection of the lower respiratory tract is present. It is only recently that bronchoalveolar lavage is being used to determine the accuracy of this principle.

Our recent studies using bronchoalveolar lavage at the time of diagnosis have indicated that *Staphylococcus aureus* may be present without symptoms but if *Pseudomonas aeruginosa* is present in the first 1–2 years of life, almost invariably there will be a loose cough. We have had infants who have had a loose cough associated with respiratory syncytial virus infection but without bacterial pathogens in the lower respiratory tract.

There are as yet no studies in older children to correlate the presence of a loose cough with bacterial pathogens in the lower respiratory tract. However, it seems reasonable to assume that if purulent sputum is produced, then there is almost certainly infection in the lower respiratory tract.

The presence of other physical signs in the chest, deteriorating general health, anorexia, weight loss and fever, indicates more serious infection and treatment is not deferred until they appear.

Microbiological Diagnosis

If there is difficulty in diagnosing the presence of bacterial infection, the determination of the responsible pathogen provides no less a daunting task. Our own studies have indicated a poor correlation between findings on throat swabs and on bronchoalveolar lavage in infants, particularly for the presence of *S. aureus* [2]. *P. aeruginosa* in a throat swab does not necessarily indicate its presence in the lower respiratory tract. Others have also reported the limitations of oropharyngeal swabs in identifying lower respiratory pathogens [3]. Studies have yet to be done in older children and adults correlating sputum microbiology and that obtained from bronchoalveolar lavage not contaminated by upper respiratory secretion.

Approximately 80% of our patients who produce sputum culture *P. aeruginosa* from it. We have adopted the principle that if *P. aeruginosa* is cultured once from a patient, it can be assumed that it will then be present permanently. *Burkholderia cepacia* has not been a problem in our clinic. We have suspected that we do not culture adequately *S. aureus*, particularly in the presence of a heavy growth of *P. aeruginosa*. Our recent studies using bronchoalveolar lavage in infants at the time of diagnosis would seem to reinforce the earlier view that *S. aureus* is the primary bacterial pathogen [2] and we have always tried to cover for this in our antibiotic therapy even if we have not been able to demonstrate it on microbiological culture.

We do not do routine throat swabs or culture sputum from our patients who are sputum-producers. As already implied, the reliability of these investigations as an indicator of lower respiratory tract pathogens remains to be confirmed. When patients are admitted to hospital for treatment of an exacerbation, sputum is collected by the physiotherapist and cultured. This is done particularly to determine sensitivities of the *P. aeruginosa* so that if there is not improvement after 5–7 days of initial therapy, there may be antibiotic sensitivities to guide changes.

Antibiotic Therapy in Ambulatory Patients

If a child is cough-free, has normal or near normal pulmonary function, normal or near normal chest x-ray and is growing well, regular antibiotic therapy is not used. If such a child develops a loose cough, antibiotics effective against *S. aureus* and *Haemophilus influenzae* are commenced promptly. Most parents will have an appropriate antibiotic at home or at least a prescription for one and will commence this without reference to the clinic. However, if they are uncertain whether to commence antibiotics or not, they are encouraged to discuss this with their thoracic physician. If the cough is trivial, trimethoprim sulphamethaxozole may be used but more commonly amoxycillin with clavulanic acid is the initial therapy. This is normally continued until the cough has cleared completely for about 7–10 days. If after 2–3 weeks therapy the cough is not improving, the parents are asked to contact their thoracic physician and further therapy is discussed. Generally this would result in the addition of ciprofloxacin to their regime on the assumption *P. aeruginosa* is likely to be present but occasionally oral chloramphenicol is used particularly if the patient has cultured only *S. aureus* or *H. influenzae*. Inhaled antibiotics, colistin 1 million units twice daily, gentamicin or tobramycin, 80 mgs twice daily may be added, particularly if it is thought important to avoid hospitalisation.

If after a further 2 weeks the cough has not cleared and particularly if there has been failure of return to normal lung function, admission to hospital will be arranged for more intensive treatment.

Children with a persistent loose cough or who are chronic sputum producers, those with impaired lung function (FEV_1 less than 75% predicted normal) or an abnormal chest x-ray or whose growth is suboptimal despite an adequate caloric intake, will generally be on long term oral antibiotics. In a few patients with minor chronic lung disease this will be trimethoprim sulphamethoxazole but for the majority of patients it will be amoxycillin with clavulanic acid. A few patients have intolerable gastrointestinal symptoms with this combination but most of these seem to be able to tolerate a combination of flucloxacillin and amoxycillin. Exacerbation of lung disease in this group, manifested by increasing cough and sputum, deterioration in lung function or impaired general health are treated by the addition of ciprofloxacin and perhaps also an inhaled aminoglycoside. Failure of improvement after 2–3 weeks of this additional therapy again is likely to lead to a hospital admission.

The small group of patients with severe lung disease are treated more intensively on an ambulatory basis. These are patients who produce moderate to large amounts of sputum every day, have an FEV_1 usually of less than 60% normal, whose growth is impaired or as adults have difficulty in maintaining weight and have limited exercise tolerance. They are normally kept on long term amoxycillin with clavulanic acid with the addition on a 2-weekly alternating basis of oral ciprofloxacin and an inhaled aminoglycoside.

Oral chloramphenicol is still occasionally used to treat exacerbations of lung disease in those on long term antibiotics and occasional patients with severe lung disease find alternating chloramphenicol and amoxycillin with clavulanic acid on a monthly basis helpful.

A few adolescents and adult patients who chronically produce small amounts of sputum find they are not helped by regular oral antibiotics. They prefer to limit the use of these to periods of exacerbation. These are usually very active patients who maintain excellent general health.

Inpatient Use of Antibiotics
A few patients admitted with a minor exacerbation of lung disease will be treated with oral flucloxacillin and intravenous aminoglycoside.

However, the vast majority of those admitted are started on intravenous ticarcillin with clavulanic acid plus aminoglycoside, usually gentamicin. This is irrespective of sputum microbiology and bacterial sensitivity. The only exception is if a patient has been in hospital in the previous 2–3 months and has failed to respond to this combination but had improved with a different combination, then this latter will be used. Most patients improve after 7–10 days and are discharged once their sputum has cleared or returned to normal volume, their lung function has returned to baseline, weight has been regained and there has been restoration to normal health. If after 7–10 days these have not been achieved, then antibiotic therapy is reviewed on the basis of sputum microbiology and sensitivity. Therapy may be changed to ceftazidime, imipenem, or aztreonam with a different aminoglycoside. If after a further 1–2 weeks, the previous baseline is not achieved, then it is assumed that some deterioration is permanent. We have found that periods of hospitalisation in excess of 3 weeks rarely are beneficial.

Home intravenous therapy has not been used in the child and adolescent patients. In Australia there has been no financial imperative to drive the introduction of this form of therapy. Much is achieved in hospital in the way of patient counselling, effective physiotherapy and family relief. However, in adult patients the situation is different and home therapy has been used to allow continuation of education and work. Generally the patient is an inpatient for 3–4 days initially and once stabilised, therepy is continued at home with nursing support. However, the impression is that home therapy is not as effective as inpatient treatment.

We do not routinely admit patients to hospital – their admission is based on symptoms and what objective measurements of deterioration are available. Further, we have never instituted treatment for a particular pathogen grown in sputum simply on its presence and consequently we have not followed the practice of some clinics of treating intensively *P. aeruginosa*.

The principles of treatment outlined, antibiotic therapy, physiotherapy and physical activity, have never been properly evaluated on a controlled double-blind basis. The antibiotic regime in particular is based on clinical experience and some scientific rationale. The three important lower respiratory pathogens in cystic fibrosis are *S. aureus*, *H. influenzae* and *P. aeruginosa*. Our antibiotic regimes have been developed to treat those. It is recognised that much of the oral antibiotic therapy will not treat *P. aeruginosa* but the role that organism plays at least in less serious lung disease remains far from clear. Regrettably there are few valid double-blind controlled trials of antibiotic therapy in cystic fibrosis and there are daunting tasks in undertaking them. Until they do become available, antibiotic therapy will continue to be based on impression and hope rather than strong science.

All that is available is looking at the overall outcome of the management of cystic fibrosis. Clearly the outcome has improved dramatically in the last 30 years. The various factors that have contributed to this are a matter of much debate. Probably the most important has been the development of centralised care in major clinics by staff who are committed to cystic fibrosis and who have managed to project a positive approach to patient and family as well as to themselves.

The Outcome

The median age of survival in all patients managed in the Melbourne Clinic since 1974, the time from which the clinic managed almost all patients in the state with cystic fibrosis, is 26.1 years. Based on the experience of patients managed over the last 10 years, the predicted 80% survival is to 18 years and 50% to 30 years. Measurement of quality of life is much more difficult but most surviving late adolescents and young adults are in full time education or full time employment [4]. About 6% of patients under 20 have severe lung disease and this is the only group whose lifestyle is seriously compromised.

In Figure 1 the mean and 95% confidence limits for FEV_1 based on the best annual measurement in all patients over the age of 6 since 1974 is given. Data for patients beyond the age of 25 are relatively small and

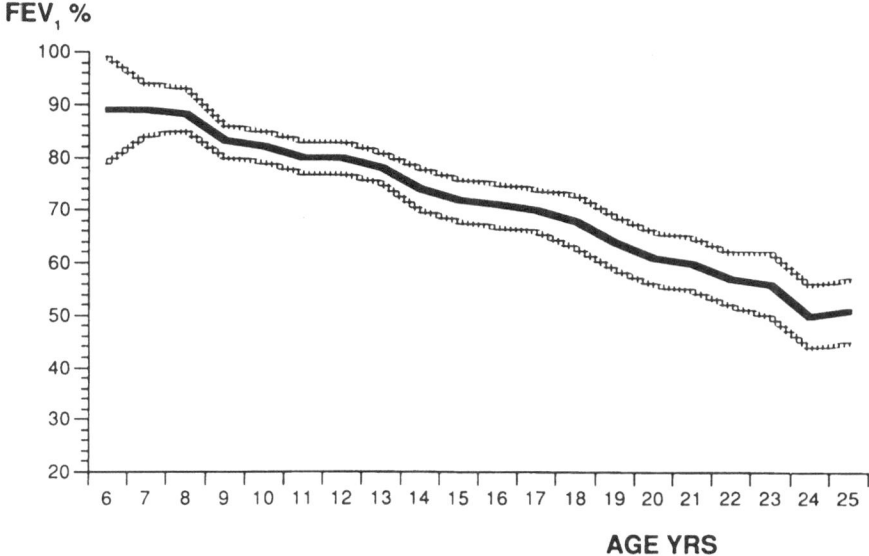

Figure 1. Mean and 95% confidence limits of FEV_1 measured annually in patients from 6–25 years managed at the Royal Children's Hospital – Alfred Hospital, Melbourne CF Clinics from 1974–1993. Bold = mean. Hatched = 95% confidence limits.

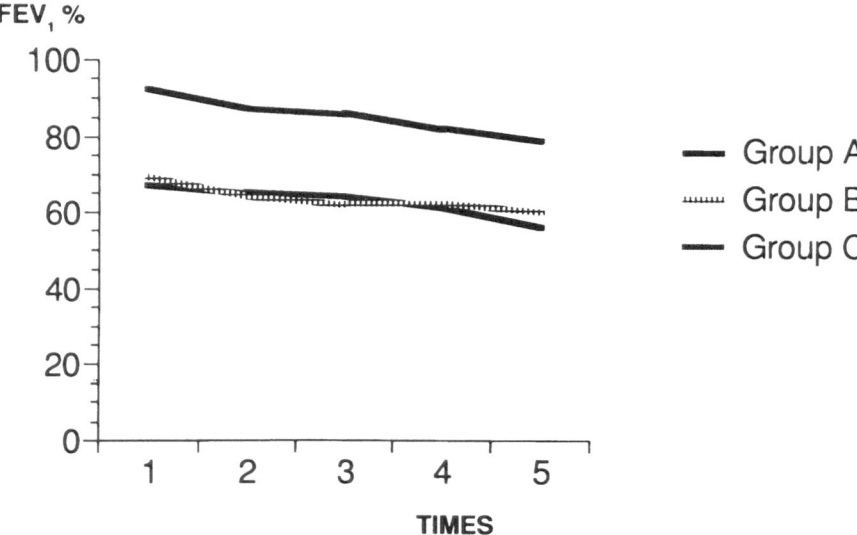

Figure 2. Mean FEV$_1$ measured annually in patients with CF according to culture from sputum of *P. aeruginosa*. Group A (66 patients) were free of *P. aeruginosa* on 5 occasions 4 years apart. Group B (61 patients) cultured *P. aeruginosa* first at time 3 after being free of it for at least 2 years previously. Group C patients (160 patients) had *P. aeruginosa* on all 5 occasions.

there is considerable variation. There is approximately a 2% annual loss in predicted FEV$_1$ between 6 and 25 years.

In Figure 2, the relationship of culture of *P. aeruginosa* to FEV$_1$ is given. Group A were patients free of *P. aeruginosa* over a 4 year period, Group B were patients who cultured *P. aeruginosa* after 2 years of freedom (Time 3) and then had it cultured for 2 subsequent years. Group C had *P. aeruginosa* in their sputum in 5 successive years. Patients in Group A were significantly younger at the commencement of the study (6.3 ± 0.6) than Group B (11.7 ± 0.7) and Group C (12.1 ± 0.5). The rate of decline in FEV$_1$ is similar in the 3 groups taking into account the younger age at entry of Group A. There was no increase in the rate of decline in FEV$_1$ (Group B) after the first culture of *P. aeruginosa*, a finding also reported from the Toronto Clinic [5]. However, the lack of reliability of sputum cultures in detecting lower respiratory tract colonisation of *P. aeruginosa* must be recognised in interpreting these data.

Our approach of prompt admission to hospital for treatment of exacerbations of lung infection does put substantial demands on patients, families and health care services. During each year over the last 10 years an average of 156 paediatric patients have been admitted (approximately 40% of the paediatric clinic), with about 50% of these being admitted on one occasion, 21% on two occasions, 11% on three occasions and 18% more than three occasions. This means an average of 350 CF admissions to the Royal Children's Hospital per year with a mean length of stay of about 12.5 days. About 25 of these are for newly diagnosed patients.

Summary

Optimal management of cystic fibrosis is still a matter of controversy despite the dramatic advances that have occurred in the last 30 years. This paper reviews the approach to management of lung disease in one major clinic but it is readily acknowledged that there is little scientific evidence to justify the approach adopted. How much validation of the current therapies can be achieved is uncertain and probably therapy will continue to be used on the basis of clinical experience rather than scientific proof. A number of new forms of therapy are currently being proposed and it is to be hoped that they will be properly evaluated before they are introduced so that the current unscientific approach will not continue with these new, potentially very expensive therapies. In their evaluation, it probably will be important not only to look at improvements they achieve but to do a true cost benefit analysis. Perhaps there may be more effective use of the monies that these new therapies cost, in improving other aspects of CF care. A small gain in lung function for the expenditure of $10 000 per year may be less beneficial than spending a similar amount of money on more participation in regular sporting activities or better nutrition.

References

1. Button BM, Heine RG, Catto-Smith AG, Phelan PD, Olinsky A. Effect of postural draining chest physiotherapy on gastro-oesophageal reflux in infants with cystic fibrosis. Am J Respir Crit Care Med 1995; 151: A738.
2. Armstrong DS, Grimwood K, Carzino R, Carlin J, Olinsky A, Phelan PD. Bacterial colonisation of the lungs in infants with cystic fibrosis diagnosed by newborn screening. Am Rev Respir Dis 1993; 147: A463.
3. Ramsey BW, Wentz KR, Smith AL, Richardson M, Williams-Warren J, Hedges DL et al. Predictive value of oropharyngeal cultures for identifying lower airway bacteria in cystic fibrosis populations. Am Rev Respir Dis 1991; 144: 331-7.
4. Allan JA, Phelan PD. Cystic fibrosis. The ability to survive disability. Med J Aust 1980; 1: 600-2.
5. Kerem E, Corey M, Gold R, Levison H. Pulmonary function and clinical course in patients with cystic fibrosis after pulmonary colonisation with *Pseudomonas aeruginosa*. J Pediatr 1990; 116: 714-9.

CHAPTER 12
Cystic Fibrosis in Japan

Y. Yamashiro, T. Shimizu, S. Oguchi, T. Shioya, S. Nagata and
Y. Ohtsuka

Department of Pediatrics, Juntendo University School of Medicine, Tokyo, Japan 113

Summary. We collected 104 CF cases among pure Japanese patients from the literature covering a period of 42 years from 1951 to 1993. A simple calculation based on the numbers of reported cases and live births in the period suggests that the estimated incidence of CF might be about one in 680 000 in the Japanese population. Twenty-eight percent of the total cases presented symptoms of meconium ileus, which is a higher frequency than that seen in the Caucasian population. This might probably reflect a genetic difference between CF of Northern Europe and Japan.

Cystic fibrosis (CF) is the most frequently seen lethal and autosomal recessive disease in the Caucasian population, affecting approximately 1 in 2000 births [1]. It is believed that the incidence of CF among Asian races including the Japanese is very rare [2]. We attempted to identify neonatal CF by using dried blood spots for measurement of trypsinogen concentration, but no case was detected in 32 000 samples in Tokyo [3]. We have therefore investigated CF in Japan epidemiologically in a study based on the literature.

Reevaluation of Diagnosis

All pure Japanese CF cases, recorded in either Japanese [4] or English [5, 6] journals were collected and the diagnosis reconfirmed by the following criteria:

1) positive sweat test (in cases reported after 1961)
2) exocrine pancreatic insufficiency (impaired function test(s) and/or maldigestion and malabsorption)
3) symptoms of lung disease (chronic or recurrent infections)
4) meconium ileus and/or a family history of CF.

More than two of the three criteria, except for positive sweat test, have to be fulfilled in the cases reported before 1960, because sweat test

Correspondence address: Y. Yamashiro, Department of Pediatrics, Juntendo University School of Medicine, 2-1-1 Hongo, Bunkyo-ku, Tokyo, Japan 113.

was first reported in the Japanese literature as a diagnostic tool for CF in 1960 [7]. More than three of the four criteria have to be fulfilled in the cases reported after 1969.

The first Japanese case of CF was reported in 1951 [8] and another 103 cases have been reported to the end of 1993. Although we found 124 cases to be reported as CF, only 104 out of 124 cases met our diagnostic criteria as described above. Consanguinity among the parents was found in 27 cases (26%) and a family history of CF was found in 27%. Thirty of the 104 cases (29%) were diagnosed in the neonatal period, 34 cases (33%) in the period from 1–12 months of age and 15 cases (14%) from 1–3 years of age. Altogether 62% of the cases were diagnosed by 12 months of age and 76% at 3 years of age. The diagnosis was not made until 16 years of age or even later in 8 cases (8%) (Table 1).

Sweat test was performed in 75 out of 96 cases (79%) after 1960 and 58 out of 65 cases (89%) after 1988. The method of sweat test used in the majority of cases (55 out of 58, 95%) after 1980 was pilocarpine iontophoresis.

Symptoms in Japanese Cystic Fibrosis Patients

All the neonatal cases except for one (29/30 97%, or 28% of the total number of cases), presented with symptoms of meconium ileus. The majority of cases which were diagnosed as toddlers had respiratory symptoms and those symptoms developed in 78% of the total cases. Exocrine pancreatic dysfunction was proved in 80% of the patients and manifested as diarrhoea or steatorrhoea resulting in nutritional disturbances (body weight ≤ 2SD). There was a 14-year old patient in whom symptoms of diabetes mellitus was the presenting ones for the diagnosis of CF [9]. Those patients, who were not able to be diagnosed until school age or adolescence might have had milder symptoms compared with those who were diagnosed at earlier ages (Table 2).

Nearly 78% of the cases who were diagnosed as toddlers showed respiratory symptoms presenting as persistent cough, wheezy breathing,

Table 1. Age at diagnosis of patients with CF in Japan

Age	No. of cases	%	Cumulative %
Neonate	30	28.8	28.8
1–12 mo	34	32.7	61.5
1–3 yr	15	14.4	75.9
4–7 yr	8	7.4	83.6
8–15 yr	8	8.7	92.3
16 yr ≤	8	7.7	100
Total	104	100	

Table 2. Major symptoms of 104 patients (M:57, F:47) with CF in Japan collected from the literature

	Percentage
Family history	28
Exocrine pancreatic dysfunction	80
Respiratory symptoms	78
Meconium ileus	28

and harsh and paroxysmal cough. Subsequently, almost all the cases who survived longer and those diagnosed later developed respiratory symptoms as frequent coughing with purulent sputum, dyspnoea, and recurrent and persistent bronchitis with barrel chest and finger clubbing. These symptoms were progressive and related to severe obstructive airway disease with emphysema, resulting in respiratory insufficiency and cor pulmonale.

Cultures made from sputum, cough and throat swabs of the patients most commonly yielded *Staphylococcus aureus* and occasionally *Haemophilus influenzae* was found. *Pseudomonas aeruginosa*, particularly the "mucoid" form was more common in those with progressive chest involvement. Once *P. aeruginosa* was isolated from the sputum of the CF patient, it was persistently found.

Treatment of Pulmonary Symptoms

The treatment of *P. aeruginosa* infection was carried out by intravenous administration of a combination of antibiotics: an aminoglycoside with either ureidopenicillin or one of the third generation of cephalosporins, i.e., ceftazidime. Continuous therapy, however, with an anti-staphylococcus agent from the time of diagnosis throughout life, plus intermittent therapy for *P. aeruginosa* were not routinely performed. Furthermore, chest physiotherapy which is very important as a preventive as well as therapeutic measure for chronic lung infection was not carried out routinely. Therefore, two important factors of treatment in the control of infection, the administration of antibiotics, and the removal of thickened bronchial secretion by chest physiotherapy, were not routinely performed in the past in Japan.

Twenty-eight (61%) out of 46 cases were deceased at the time of the national survey of CF in Japan in 1983. Thirty-two percent of the deaths occurred in the neonatal period, 58% by 6 months of age and 82% by 3 years of age. At least 4 CF patients older than 10 years survived in this country in 1994. Recently, the survival rate appears to be improving, but lack of management of the respiratory disease make it inferior to that in European countries and the US.

Approximation of Cystic Fibrosis Incidence

The incidence of CF in the non-Caucasian population is very low. A genetic study on CF carried out in Hawaii in 1967 indicated that the estimated incidence of CF in the Asian population including Japanese, Chinese and Koreans was about 1 in 90 000 live births [2]. We collected 104 pure Japanese cases of CF, which were accumulated from the literature during 42 years, which is the time since the first case report was published in Japan [8]. There were 71 216 272 live births in the last 42 years in Japan. A simple calculation from 104 CF cases and live births in the period suggests that the estimated incidence of CF in the Japanese population is at least one in 682 772 live births, or approximately one in 680 000.

This figure is consistent with the finding of no positive case in our measurement of trypsinogen in dried blood spots performed on 32 000 neonates in Tokyo, and the estimated incidence from the study in Hawaii. If the incidence of one in 90 000 was correct, we should have had 791 CF cases in Japan during the last 42 years, but we found only 104 cases. The authors do not suppose that the remaining 687 cases were lost without a definite diagnosis, although it is a possibility we can not deny. Because the findings of this study show that the majority of cases of CF (76%) were found by 3 years of age, this indicates that Japanese pediatricians and pediatric surgeons would have sufficient knowledge to make a diagnosis of CF. We consider that the real incidence is closer to our figure of one in 680 000 rather than one in 90 000.

An interesting finding in our study is that 28% of the total cases diagnosed in the neonatal period showed symptoms of meconium ileus (Table 2). This is in contrast to the fact that 5–10% of Caucasian CF cases presented with meconium ileus [10]. Whether the high incidence of meconium ileus in the Japanese CF patients relates to a clinically severe form of CF is not known. Probably this may reflect a genetic difference to CF in Northern Europe out of which 60–80% of all cases have a ΔF508 mutation [11]. Indeed, there are reports that genetic analysis of four Japanese CF patients demonstrated no ΔF508 mutation [12–14], a finding we have also confirmed recently in other CF patients in Japan (Kohsaka, Igarashi and Yamada, personal communication).

Although a rare disease in our population, we will try to further characterize CF in Japan.

References

1. Wood RE, Boat TF, Doershuk CF. State of the art of cystic fibrosis. Am Rev Respir Dis 1976; 113: 833–878.
2. Wright SW, Morton NE. Genetic studies on cystic fibrosis in Hawaii. J Hum Genet 1968; 20: 157–169.

3. A joint WHO/ICF(M)A meeting on the feasibility study on hereditary disease community control programmes (cystic fibrosis), June 1989, London.

4. Takita S, Chikaoka H, Suzuki M, Okuyama K. Survey of the incidence of cystic fibrosis in Japan and the typical case of cystic fibrosis experienced in our hospital. Tan-to-Sui, 1983; 4: 447-454.

5. Komi N, Seki Y. An analysis of 46 autopsy cases of Japanese children showing fibrocystic changes of the pancreas and one case of fibrocystic disease of the pancreas. Bull Tokyo Med Dent 1967; 14: 407-414.

6. Katayama H, Tanaka T, Kunihara G, Kuwabara N. Cystic fibrosis of the pancreas: Report of a Japanese autopsy case. Radiat Med 1985; 3: 137-143.

7. Tokuda S, Yanagisawa M. A case of probable cystic fibrosis. Shonika-Rinsho 1960; 13: 997-998.

8. Masuno S. Meconium ileus. Rinsho-igaku 1951; 36: 635-636.

9. Otani T, Seki T, Oishi T, Joh K and Kouda N. A case of a 14-year-old boy with cystic fibrosis complicated with diabetes mellitus. J Jpn Pediatr Soc 1992; 96: 1288-1293.

10. Goodchild MC and Dodge J. Cystic fibrosis, manual of diagnosis and management. 2nd ed, London: Balliere Tindall, 1985.

11. Super M, Schwartz MJ. Mutation of the cystic fibrosis gene locus within the population of the northwest of England. Eur J Pediatr 1992; 151: 108-111.

12. Komi N, Takahara H, Kunitomo K, Sasaki K. Cystic fibrosis – nationwide survey and genetic analysis of CF in Japan. Tan-to-Sui 1994; 15: 539-546.

13. Hanashiro E, Satoh Y, Ohtake A, Takayanagi M, Ohshima H, Suzuki H et al. Genetic analysis of cystic fibrosis. J Jpn Pediatr Soc 1993; 7: 2279-2283.

14. Shimizu T, Yamashiro Y, Yabuta K, Bartholomew D, Hubbard VS. Epidemiological and genetic study of cystic fibrosis in Japan. 4th Pan Pacific Congress of Paediatric Gastroenterology and Nutrition. September 1994, Tokyo, Japan.

Cystic Fibrosis Pulmonary Infections:
Lessons from Around the World
ed. by A. Bauernfeind, M. I. Marks and B. Strandvik
© 1996 Birkhauser Verlag Basel/Switzerland

CHAPTER 13
The General Approach to Cystic Fibrosis Pulmonary Infection in Russia

Tatiana E. Guembitskaia[1], Ludmila A. Vishnyakova[1],
Ludmila A. Zhelenina[1] and Nikolai J. Kapranov[2]

[1]*Cystic Fibrosis Centre, State Research Centre for Pulmonology, St. Petersburg 197089,*
[2]*Institute for Medical Genetics, Moscow 117573, Russia*

Summary. Cystic fibrosis (CF) is a disease with high mortality and morbidity among children and young people. The problem of aid to CF patients and their families started to attract attention of medical authorities in Russia only in recent years. According to the data of the National Russian Cystic Fibrosis (Mucoviscidosis) Association about 2000 CF patients were registered in the country (the population of Russia is 180 million people). The CF Centre in St. Petersburg has examined 231 CF patients aged from 0 to 49 during ten years. All the patients were repeatedly treated at the hospital and were under continuous dispensary observation. The mean life expectancy was 13.5 years. The main reason for the progression of the disease and death was chronic pulmonary infection, chronic *Pseudomonas aeruginosa* infection being noted in 39% ill children and in 24% adults. The organization of treatment to CF patients under the conditions of specialized centre, up-to-date antibacterial treatment and respiratory physiotherapy considerably improve the quality of life of patients.

Introduction

Cystic fibrosis (CF) is the most common inherited disease of the Caucasian population. Respiratory disease is the major cause of mortality and morbidity. The problem of organizing the aid to CF patients began to attract attention of medical authorities and public health institutions towards the end of 1980s. The first two CF Centres were organized by the end of 1989 in St Petersburg, later in Moscow. The tasks and the system of organization of aid to CF patients follow the European centres. Doctors working at the centres have been trained abroad (Denmark, Germany, England). It is difficult to give the real number of CF patients in Russia since there is no registration except in the central regions. Pediatricians do not diagnose all the CF cases. Screening of new-born infants was conducted only in a few maternity homes in Moscow and St Petersburg.

The birth rate of CF patients in Moscow is calculated to be 1:2500 newborns; annually 750 CF patients [12] are born in Russia. From 1989 genetic diagnosis of CF was developed, and molecular screening of all relatives of proband carriers for ΔF508 has been conducted. Prenatal diagnosis of pregnant women who already had a CF child and wanted family planning were carried out.

The most frequent mutation in Russia is ΔF508; the frequency of ΔF508 among Russian population is 55% of all CF⁺ chromosomes [1, 9]. Mutation 3732 del A is encountered rather frequently. Four different, previously unknown, mutations of the CF gene have been described – 1677 del TA (exon 10), E504Q (exon 10), S1196X (exon 19) and W1282R (exon 20) [10]. All of them are included in International Cystic Fibrosis Genetic Analysis Consortium. The major ΔF508 and the other mutations of CFTR gene are identified in 60% of all CF⁺ chromosomes at present in Russia. The severity of CF and its outcome in individual patients are to a large extent defined by the chronic infectious pulmonary process. The aim of the present study is to analyse the specificity of the infectious process in lungs of CF patients in Russia and present the main results of treatment.

Materials and Methods

We have during 10 years observed 231 CF patients, 181 children and 50 adults, 118 males (99 children and 19 adults), and 113 females (82 children and 31 adults). The age of the patients varied from one month to 49 years, the mean age of children being 7.6 ± 0.5 and of adults 27.7 ± 2.4 years. More than 70% of the children were aged from 3 to 14 years and only 25% were up to three years of age.

CF diagnosis was based on the clinical picture of the disease and positive sweat test, $Cl^- > 50$ mmol/L. Blood samples were sent to the Centre of Prenatal Diagnostics (headed by Prof. V. Baranov) for genotype examinations. Pulmonary X-ray examination, study of respiratory function, biochemical studies, bronchoscopy, examination of pancreatic function and ultrasonic examination were done. The complex of clinical data was evaluated by the Shwachman scoring system. Sputum or bronchial content was subjected to quantitative microbiological test once during 1–3 months. Quantitative bacteriological analysis of sputum specimens isolated pathogenic bacteria. The level of antibodies in blood samples was examined in the indirect hemagglutination test and by immunofluorescence. An antibiogram was made for each bacteriological analysis. Antibacterial treatment was prescribed according to sensitivity of isolated agents in the period of exacerbations and also at increase of titres in sputum against pathogenic agents, such as *Haemophilus influenzae*, *Staphylococcus aureus*, and *Pseudomonas aeruginosa*. Antibiotics were administered orally, intramuscularly and intravenously. The most frequently used were cephalosporins, aminoglycosides, polymyxines, beta-lactams, quinolones and imipenem. Antibacterial therapy was given both in hospitals and at home. All the patients received adequate nutrition and hydration, pancreatic enzymes (in tablets and microspheres), vitamins, respiratory physiotherapy including PEP-mask and inhalations with mucolytics.

Data were processed by methods of variation, statistics on IBM.

Results

Based on clinical data and the results of the sweat test the CF diagnosis was established in 22% of patients during the first year of life. In more than half of patients (54%) CF was confirmed during the first 5 years and in 38% at 5–10 years. Only in 4% was the disease revealed at a later period. The major mutation ΔF508 was encountered in 34% CF^+ chromosomes of children; in homozygous state in only 19 patients and heterozygous in 79. Other mutations, as 1677 del TA (2 patients), 3732 del A (2 patients) and W1282R (1 patient), were revealed in single cases. We failed to identify the genetic defect in a considerable number of patients (39%). In adults ΔF508 was discovered only in a compound state and in a frequency of 27%, 2 cases had the genotype ΔF508/ R334W (0.14).

The data obtained differ from others in Europe and probably reflect the genetic specificity in subjects of Slavonian origin who made up the main group of our patients, 90%; representatives of Asians and Jews made up 7% and 4% of patients, respectively. The marriage of relatives was found in only three families (Armenian, Jewish–Ashkenasi and Tartarian). Seventy-one percent of the patients had symptoms from the respiratory tract and insufficiency of pancreatic function. The pancreatic insufficiency was encountered in all patients homozygous ΔF508, in 86% of the heterozygous and considerably less (45%, $p < 0.02$) in patients with non identified genetic defect. The mutations 3732 del A, 1677 del TA, W1282R, were connected with severe insufficiency of pancreatic function. No lesion of pancreas was found in patients with genotype ΔF508/R334W.

Meconium ileus was observed in only 25% of cases and intestinal obstruction was diagnosed in two patients aged more than 5 years. Rectal prolapse, which was a frequent complication in previous years, was encountered very rarely (5%), probably reflecting a more adequate pancreatic enzyme therapy. Among CF patients with only malabsorption syndrome, biliary hepatocirrhosis was found in 8.5% of the patients. Diabetes mellitus was diagnosed in one girl of 6 years old, which is a considerably lower frequency than reported in the literature and might be related to the early death of our patients.

Different respiratory symptoms, from episodes of recurrent bronchitis to pronounced obstruction and formation of bronchiectasis, were clinically defined in all the patients. Along with genetically specified disorders of mucociliary clearance, an infectious inflammatory process in the lungs plays an important role in pathogenesis of respiratory tract lesions. The infectious inflammatory process in CF is polyetiological both in appearance, severity and in number of exacerbations. The most frequent agents of pulmonary infection are *Streptococcus pneumoniae. Haemophilus influenzae, Staphylococcus aureus* and *Pseudomonas aeruginosa* [8] but the role of these bacteria is different in children and adults and changes in the course of the CF diseases. Absence of pathogenic bacteria was seen in 9 patients (6.1%), mainly in those children not observed regularly at our Centre.

Both in the beginning of lung disease in CF and during the subsequent progress of the disease, *S. pneumoniae* and *H. influenzae* – the usual agents of acute respiratory tract infections in children (ARI) – play an important role. Pneumococcal infection was revealed in 75% of the children and 86% of adult patients. A high level of local immunity-IgA_1 and strict return dynamics of system immunity showed the prevalence of different acute forms of pneumococcal infections in children. Adults revealed a very high and stable level of antipneumococcal antibodies in serum, mean geometrical antibody titers (MGT) was 1:2085. High frequency of *S. pneumoniae* isolation from bronchial content support the suggestion of their role in the chronic infection of CF [15]. However, CF patients more frequently reveal pneumococcal antibodies than positive bacterial culture. This is certainly due to intensive antibacterial therapy. Beta lactamase activity of the main bacterial species promotes the impact of pneumococcus in the infectious process.

H. influenzae untyped strains was found in 52–65% of children and adults, both temporarily and more chronically. In spite of a high level of *H. influenzae* circulation among children, the appearance and the course of haemophilus infection are promoted by a low level of humoral immunity, established in 30% of patients only. However, a high level of system immunity was observed in adult patients, 50% of whom had antibody titers of 1:1280–1:2560, and MGT of 1:1640. The role of these bacterial in CF pathogenesis has been studied sufficiently. These bacteria play a triggering role in the onset of infection and in its aggravation. Besides, they have pathogenetic factors such as the ability to stimulate mucin formation, destroy the ciliary mechanism of respiratory airways mucous membrane, synthesize histamine, and also have elastase and cytolytic activity [14]. These and other factors of pathogenicity in combination with destructive action of polymorphonuclear leukocytes promote the progress of disease. *H. influenzae* and *S. pneumoniae* are involved in pulmonary infection during the whole life of CF patients but their role as the only pathogens is reduced with age of patients, since the bacteria were revealed in 22% of children and only in 3% of adults. This five fold difference is the result of the further course of the infectious process in CF patients and the subsequent contamination of the bronchial tree with *S. aureus.*

S. aureus was discovered in 43.5% of children and 65% of adults, mainly in children 7–9 years old (45–60%). Staphylococcus infection is more often associated with *H. influenzae* and Gram-negative bacteria (GNB). *S. aureus* causes mostly acute processes, more rare the chronic ones. The leading role of *S. aureus* in etiology of pulmonary infection was established in 18% of children and 31% of adult patients. Severe staphylococcal infection was the reason for death of 6 children (23%).

GNB are involved in infectious bronchial lesion of approximately 25% of children and 44% of adults and mostly in association with other bacteria. Clinical and microbiological comparisons and rather high level of antibodies with clear seroconversion give the possibility to evaluate the course of acute infection. But sometimes, the dissemination of bronchial tree with GNB is of colonization character. The development of chronic inflammatory process with this etiology was observed in some of the patients.

Prolonged examination of CF patients gave the possibility to observe the contamination of bronchial tree with non-mucoid strains of *P. aeruginosa* in patients with current *Staphylococcus* and/or *Haemophilus* infections. On the whole *P. aeruginosa* was found in 67 children (46%) and 17 adults (57%). First, the contamination cause colonization and/or development of acute infection. Similar primary transitory contamination was discovered only in 13% of children and considerably more often in adults (41%). *P. aeruginosa* very quickly acquires the chronic nature. Especially severe course is observed in *P. aeruginosa* during the first years of life. When studying the age specificity of etiology of the infectious process in children the maximum occurrence of *P. aeruginosa* (42–50%) falls in the 3rd–5th year of life. *P. aeruginosa* was the cause of death of 19 children (73%).

The primary contamination as well as further aggravation of the disease were mostly caused by non-mucoid strains of *P. aeruginosa*. Mucoid strains were isolated in severe courses of CF and usually in association with non-mucoid ones.

Burkholderia cepacia was isolated only in 4 children and one adult (2%). A very low occurrence of this type of bacteriae is the specificity of the CF course in our patients [13].

We found a lower score in the majority of patients infected with *P. aeruginosa* (average Shwachman score 53). None of these patients showed normal lung function: average of FVC was 50% of predicted value, and in 42% of the patients in this index was considerably lower. FEV_1 in patients with *P. aeruginosa* in the lungs also significantly differed both from the norm ($p < 0.001$) and the index in patients with non-*P. aeruginosa* infection ($p < 0.01$) and in more than half of the cases (58%) it was lower than 45% of predicted value.

In recent years the problem of therapy of the infection in CF has been actively studied (4–7). If treatment of pneumococcal and haemophilus infection and in some cases the staphylococcal infection requires 1–3 courses of antibacterial therapy, then *P. aeruginosa* infection requires considerably more efforts. During the last 3 years the strategy of separate hospitalization of patients with and without *P. aeruginosa* infection was introduced at our centre which considerably reduced cross-infection.

For treatment of *P. aeruginosa* infection we use 3–4 courses of intravenous antibacterial therapy during a year. The duration of each course is 2–3 weeks. We use the combinations of such antibiotics as cephalosporins, aminoglycosides, polymyxines, quinolones, imipenem, and other β-lactames. As a result we succeeded in achieving elimination of *Pseudomonas* from all children infected for the first time in 1991–1992. Such therapy permitted to achieve considerable improvement in the course of chronic *Pseudomonas* infection (duration of exacerbation reduced from 25 days to 16).

The most severe group of patients were children with multiresistant *Pseudomonas*. In these cases we used 4–6 courses of intravenous anti-*Pseudomonas* therapy during a year; as a rule we used a combination of 2–3 antibiotics. Such therapy permitted to obtain a positive result in the majority of cases. It was established that the earlier *P. aeruginosa* appeared in patients the more severe and prognostically more unfavourable was the disease. All the diseased children (mean age 7.5 years) were infected with *Pseudomonas* at an early age.

Discussion

We have succeeded in isolation of ΔF508 in 34% of CF children and 27% of CF adults. The obtained data differ considerably from the results of studies conducted in the USA and Western European countries [1] and, probably, are related to the genetic specificity of CF in subject of Slavonian origin. Besides, the analysis of the clinical material allowed to distinguish two types of courses in CF. Some children revealed late appearance of the infectious process with prevalence of *S. pneumoniae* and *H. influenzae* – usual agents of ARI – and prolonged remissions and subsequent addition of staphylococcal infections. In another group of children, *P. aeruginosa* developed during the first 2–5 years of age and quickly acquired a chronic colonization. It was the cause of death in 19 patients, i.e. in 75% of all diseased patients. Probably this severe CF course is defined genetically, since in 75% of these patients the mutation ΔF508 was observed. Most probably, the infectious lesions of the bronchial tree in CF pathogeneses is specified by a great number of different factors including the factors distributed by polymorphonuclear leukocytes [3, 4, 15]. Treatment of *P. aeruginosa* in CF is one of the main tasks of the clinicians. Prolonged observation of patients permits effective use of preventive therapy and obtaining positive results.

Acknowledgements

We are indebted to our colleagues from the Laboratory of Microbiology headed by Prof. L. Vishniakova, and from the Centre of Prenatal Diagnostics headed by Prof. V. Baranov who have contributed to the preparation of this chapter.

References

1. Baranov VS, Ivaschenko TE, Gorbunova VN, Livshitz LA, Venozinskis MT, Gembovskaya SA *et al.* Frequency of the F508 deletion in cystic fibrosis patients from the European part of the USSR. Hum Genet 1991; 87: 61–64.
2. Bogdanova AV, Gelenina LA, Blinova T, Mustafaev I, Kovaleva L, Perley V. La mucoviscidose au Centre de Saint-Pétersbourg. Etude clinique, génétique et thérapeutique. Pédiatre 1991; 27: 103–106.
3. Döring G, Maier M, Müller E, Bibi Z, Tümmler B, Kharazmi A. Virulence factors of *Pseudomonas aeruginosa*. Antibiot Chemother 1987; 39: 136–148.
4. Döring G. Chronic *Pseudomonas aeruginosa* lung infection in cystic fibrosis. In: M. Campa, M. Bendinelli, H. Friedman (eds.), *Pseudomonas aeruginosa* as an opportunistic pathogen. Plenum Press, New York 1993, pp. 245–273.
5. Feigelson J, Pecau Y, Gaultier L, Boule M. Cures intensives d'antibiotiques dans les mucoviscidoses évoluées. Nouv Presse Méd 1981; 10: 955–958.
6. Guembitskaia TE. Cystic fibrosis. Sov Krasny Krest 1991; 10: 16.
7. Guembitskaia TE. Organization of patient care, achievements and perspectives. IACFA Newsletter USA 1991; 31: 23–24.
8. Høiby N. Cystic fibrosis: Infection. Schweiz med Wschr. 1991; 121: 105–109.
9. Ivaschenko TE, White MB, Dean M, Baranov VS. A deletion of nucleotides in exon 10 of the CFTR gene in a Soviet family with cystic fibrosis causing early infant death. Genomics 1991; 10: 298–299.
10. Ivaschenko TE, Baranov US, Dean M. Two new mutations detected by single-stained conformation polymorphism analysis in cystic fibrosis from Russia. Hum Genet 1993; 91: 63–65.
11. Jensen T, Pedersen SS, Høiby N, Koch C, Flensborg EW. Use of antibiotics in cystic fibrosis. The Danish approach. Antibiot Chemother 1989; 42: 237–246.
12. Kapranov NJ, Kashirskaya NYu, Moin DM, Petrova NV, Simakova OJ, Khafizova ZA, Shabalova IA. A problem of mucoviscidosis: current advances and presentday issues. Vestnik AMN SSSR 1992; 4: 34–39.
13. Laraya-Caussay LR, Lipstein M, Huang N. *Pseudomonas cepacia* in the respiratory flora of patients with cystic fibrosis. Pediat Res 1977; 11: 502–504.
14. Vishnyakova LA. The role of different microorganisms and infectious processes in the origin and course of bronchial asthma. Sov Arch Internal Med 1990; 62: 59–69.
15. Vishnyakova LA. Pathogenesis of chronical bronchitis: new ideas. Sov Arch Internal Med 1993; 3: 8.

Cystic Fibrosis Pulmonary Infections:
Lessons from Around the World
ed. by A. Bauernfeind, M. I. Marks and B. Strandvik
© 1996 Birkhäuser Verlag Basel/Switzerland

CHAPTER 14
Cystic Fibrosis in Israel: Clinical and Microbiological Aspects

Eitan Kerem[1], Joseph Rivlin[2], Yaacov Yahav[3], Asher Tal[4], Amir Szeinberg[3] and Itamar Shalit[5]

[1]*Cystic Fibrosis Centers of Shaare Zedek Medical Center, Jerusalem 91031;* [2]*Carmel Medical Center, Haifa 34362;* [3]*Sheba Medical Center, Tel Hashomer 52621;* [4]*Soroka Medical Center, Ben-Gurion University, Beer Sheva 84101 and* [5]*Infectious Disease Unit, Tel-Aviv Medical Center, Tel-Aviv 64239, Israel*

Introduction

Cystic fibrosis (CF) is an inherited genetic disease characterized by progressive lung disease, pancreatic dysfunction, impaired growth, elevated sweat electrolytes, and other less common clinical findings including meconium ileus, nasal polyposis, and hepatobiliary disease [1]. Patients are diagnosed at different ages with various modes of presentation, and there is considerable variability in the severity or rate of disease progression of involved organs. Certain clinical characteristics of disease expression have been delineated to provide some explanation for the heterogeneity in the clinical course and survival amongst patients with this devastating genetic illness. For example, the patients with sufficient residual exocrine pancreatic function to permit normal digestion without the need for enzyme supplements – pancreatic sufficiency [2, 3] are generally diagnosed at a later age, with lower mean sweat chloride levels, milder respiratory abnormalities, normal growth into adulthood and a better overall prognosis than those with pancreatic insufficiency [3, 4]. Subsequently it was suggested that the extreme variability in disease severity in patients with cystic fibrosis is not a consequence of relative preservation of pancreatic function but is a result of different CF gene mutants, which confer mild or severe phenotypes [5]. In this regard, ΔF_{508} and W1282X were mutations associated with severe phenotypic expression [5, 6] and R117H and 3849 + 10 kb were mutations associated with less severe phenotype [7, 8]. Severe mutations are characterized by early age at diagnosis, presence of meconium ileus, higher levels of sweat chloride, pancreatic

Correspondence address: Eitan Kerem M.D., Department of Pediatrics, Pulmonary and Cystic Fibrosis Clinic, Shaare Zedek Medical Center, Bait Vagan St., Jerusalem 91031, Israel.

insufficiency, lower nutritional status, and worse survival. However, similar variability in pulmonary function was observed among patients with severe and less severe mutations [5–7]. Thus, severity of pulmonary disease could not be attributed to type of genetic mutation only. It was therefore suggested that other factors, genetic or environmental, are responsible for the variability found in severity of lung disease among patients with identical genotype. In this regard comparison of CF patient status and treatment between different countries, with different genetic background, climate, standards and way of living, may contribute to the understanding of the variability in disease presentation in cystic fibrosis.

The Population in Israel

The population of the state of Israel comprises approximately 5 million inhabitants of whom 79% are Jews and 21% Arabs. Of the Jewish population, 39% are of Ashkenazi Jewish origin and 39% of a non-Ashkenazi (Sephardi) origin. In 22% the ethnic origin could not be determined (The Israeli Annual Statistics Bulletin – 1993). The term Ashkenazi Jews designates Jews who settled in North-West Europe since the 6th century. It is used in contradistinction to the Sephardi Jews; Jews who originated in Spain and now include all non-Ashkenazi Jews. There were waves of emigration of Ashkenazi Jews to Eastern Europe in the 15th–16th centuries, and to North America, Israel and several other countries in the 18th–20th centuries. The non-Ashkenazi Jews originate from countries along the Mediterranean Sea, Near East, Asia and Africa. Since Jews tended to live in relatively closed isolated communities, one would expect to find among them a limited number of CF mutations.

In a recent survey we found that there is a high variability in the incidence of CF among different ethnic origins in Israel. The incidence of CF among Ashkenazi Jews is 1:2500 live births, with five mutations responsible for 95% of the genetic defects, whereas the incidence of CF among Jews immigrated from Iraq and Iran is 1:32 000 and 1:39 000 live births respectively. Overall the incidence of CF in Israel among Jews and Arabs is about 1:5000 live births.

Methods

A questionnaire was sent to four different CF centers in Israel: Carmel Medical Center, Haifa; Sheba Medical Center, Tel Hashomer; Soroka Medical Center, Beer Sheva; and Shaare Zedek Medical Center, Jerusalem. These centers are located in different parts of the country.

The questionnaires focused mainly on the nature of pulmonary infections in cystic fibrosis, including questions relating to ethnic background, age at diagnosis, mode of presentation, previous complications,
present pulmonary function, bacterial cultures, type of treatment and
development of resistance to antimicrobial agents.

Sputum, if obtainable, or deep pharyngeal auger suction was taken in
each clinic visit every 3–6 months, or during respiratory exacerbations.
Culture material was processed on standard agar media (blood, Mac-
Conkey's, chocolate, and salt mannitol agar). Organisms were identified
by standard methods and results were usually given semiquantitatively.
Antimicrobial susceptibility was determined by the Kirby–Bauer
method.

The Student t-test was used to compare group means (± standard
deviation) for continuous variables. Proportions were compared by
chi-square analysis.

Results and Discussion

Clinical Characteristics of the Israeli CF Population

A total of 124 questionnaires were returned. This number represents
about half of the total Israeli CF patient population. There were 100
families of whom 80 had 1 child with CF, 16 had 2 children with CF,
and 4 had 3 children with CF. Of the 124 patients (57% males) 79%
were Jews and 21% Arabs. Of the Jews, 60% were of Ashkenazi Jewish
origin. The mean age of all patients was 10.98 ± 7.57 years (median 9.9,
range 0.2–35 years), this being considerably lower than that of patients
from Boston or Toronto [9]. As shown in Figure 1, 2.4% of the patients
were less than 1 year of age, 27% were less than 5 years of age and 51%
less than 10 years of age. At present, there are no data regarding
survival of CF patients in Israel.

Cystic Fibrosis Presentation in Israel

Overall the median age at diagnosis was 0.23 years (mean 1.81 ± 3.94
years, range 0–20 years); lower than that found in Boston or Toronto
[9]. Of these 74% were diagnosed before 1 year of age, 13.5% between
1–5 years of age, and 7.4% were diagnosed after the age of 10 years.

In 80% of the patients the diagnosis of CF was made within the first
year of appearance of symptoms. When we excluded patients who were
diagnosed at birth (cases of meconium ileus, or known sibling with CF),
CF diagnosis was made more than 1 year after the appearance of
symptoms in 25% of patients, and more than 5 years in 9% of patients

CUMULATIVE %

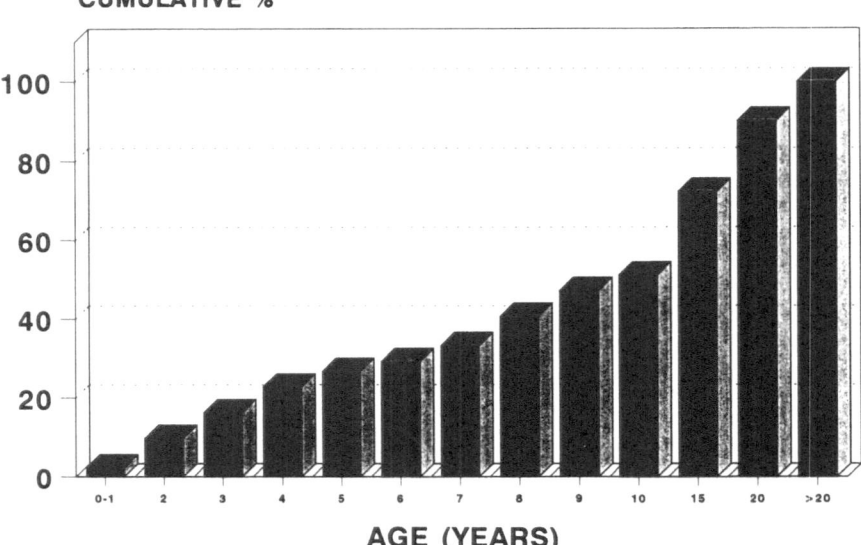

AGE (YEARS)

Figure 1.   Cumulative percentage of current age of Israeli CF patients, 1993 (n = 124).

(Figure 2). The relatively older age of diagnosis and longer interval from appearance of symptoms to diagnosis can be attributed, at least partially, to the presence of a mild mutation $3849 + 10$ kb in about 10% of the Ashkenazi Jewish population. This mutation is associated with pancreatic sufficiency and normal sweat electrolyte values, thereby leading to a delay in diagnosis [7].

The most common mode of presentation was gastrointestinal symptoms (failure to thrive, fat and vitamins malabsorption), being present in 81% of patients (Table 1). In 12% of patients these were the only symptoms. Fifty-one percent of the patients presented with respiratory symptoms (recurrent respiratory infections, asthma) while only 8% had

Table 1. Mode of CF presentation among Israeli patients

Symptom	n	%
Failure to thrive	70	56
Recurrent pneumonia	44	35
Fat malabsorption	33	27
Asthma	30	24
Meconium ileus	26	21
Relative with CF	21	17
Vitamin deficiency	6	5
Salt deficiency syndrome	2	1.6

Some of the patients had more than 1 symptom at diagnosis.

CUMULATIVE %

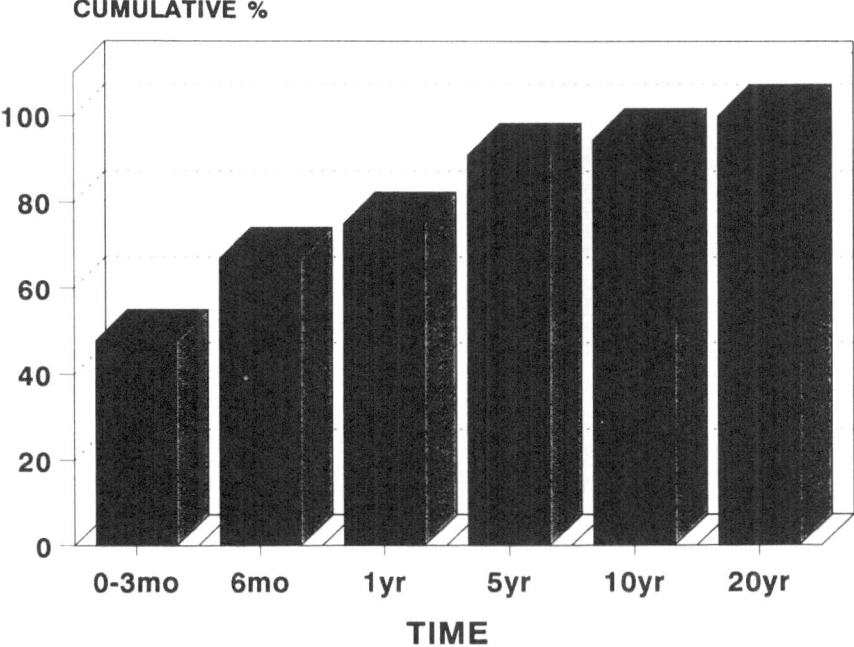

Figure 2. Cumulative percentage of time from appearance of first symptoms to diagnosis in Israeli CF patients (n = 124). Time shown excludes patients diagnosed at birth.

respiratory symptoms as a single manifestation. The rate of meconium ileus in our population was 21%, higher than 10–15% previously reported in other populations from Canada and USA [10, 11].

It is interesting to note that although 24 of our patients had an older sibling with CF, the diagnosis was made in only 6 before the appearance of symptoms. In the remaining cases parents tended to wait until symptoms had appeared before requesting sweat electrolytes tests.

Current Clinical Status

The mean FEV_1 of our patients (mean age 10.98 ± 7.57 years) was $67.6 \pm 22.8\%$ predicted (median 68% predicted), mean FVC $78.1 \pm 19.2\%$ predicted (median 81% predicted), and mean FEF_{25-75} was $55.1 \pm 32.1\%$ predicted (median 48.5% predicted). Figure 3 shows the distribution of pulmonary function values in our patient population. Of these, 55% had normal FVC, 40% had normal FEV_1 (above 80% predicted), and 42% had normal FEF_{25-75} (above 70% predicted).

The mean percentile for weight of our patient population was 26.0 ± 24.5 (median 15), and for height was 28.0 ± 25.8 (median 25).

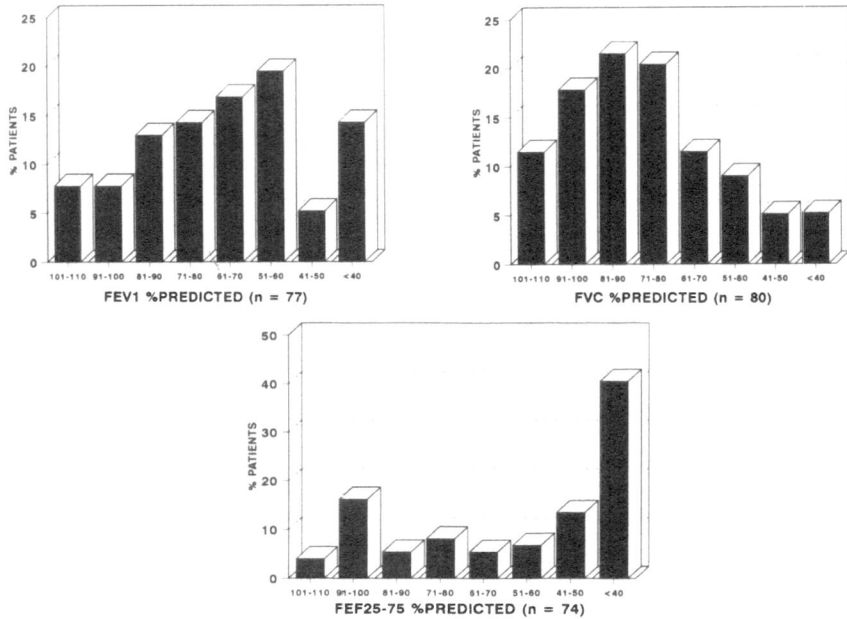

Figure 3. Distribution of pulmonary function tests among Israeli CF patients in 1993. Mean age 10.98 ± 7.57 years.

Figure 4 shows the distribution of weight and height percentiles in our patient population. Forty-six percent of the patients were under the 10th percentile for either weight or height. This indicates the relatively poor nutritional status of our patients. The rate of pancreatic sufficiency was 9%, lower than the 15% which was reported from Toronto [3, 4].

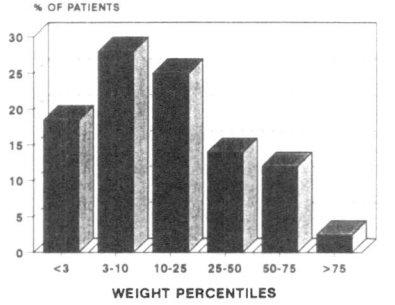
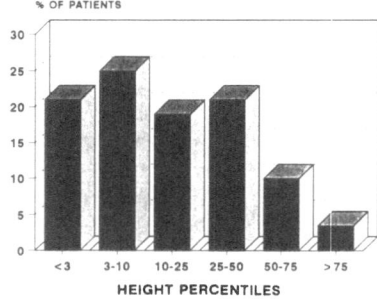

Figure 4. Current percentiles for weight and height of Israeli CF patients in 1993. Mean age 10.98 ± 7.57 years (n = 124).

Table 2. Complications among Israeli CF patients (n = 124)

Complication	n	%
Nasal polyps	19	15
DIOS*	16	13
Raised serum liver enzymes	14	11
Diabetes	9	7
Rectal prolapse	9	7
Hemoptysis	9	7
Liver cirrhosis	6	5
Hypoelectrolytemia	6	5
Pneumothorax	0	0

*DIOS – distal intestinal obstruction syndrome.

The most common complications were nasal polyps, distal intestinal obstruction syndrome and impaired liver function tests (Table 2). It is interesting to note that none of the patients in this study had a pneumothorax.

Steroids (oral or inhaled) were administered to 23% of the patients for a mean period of 16.5 ± 13.4 weeks.

Bacteriological Data

In 66% of the patients bacteria were isolated from sputum cultures. The most common microorganism cultured in our patient population was *P. aeruginosa* (50% of patients), followed by *Staphylococcus aureus* (23.4%), *Haemophilus influenzae* (18.5%), and *Streptococcus pneumoniae* (5%) (Figure 5). In many cases more than one microorganism was cultured either concomitantly or on different occasions. Different proportions were reported from Canada [12]; in their study *P. aeruginosa* accounted for 70% of isolates, *Staphylococcus aureus* for 10–15%, *Klebsiella* and *Escherichia coli* for 20%, *Haemophilus influenzae* for 10%, and *Pseudomonas cepacia* for 20%. *Pseudomonas cepacia* was not isolated in any sputum culture from our patients. Furthermore, this microorganism has never been isolated from sputum cultures obtained from the Israeli CF patient population (unpublished data). We have no explanation for the absence of *Pseudomonas cepacia* in our patient population, in contrast to the reports from North America and Europe which indicate an increase in its isolation rate. However, selective media for growth of *Pseudomonas cepacia* are not used routinely in Israel for processing sputum from CF patients.

There has been a gradual and constant change in the respiratory bacterial flora over the years. Mearns *et al.* [13] who followed CF patients between the years 1950–1971 showed that the isolation of *Staphylococcus aureus* fell from 45% to 12%. Its isolation rate in infants

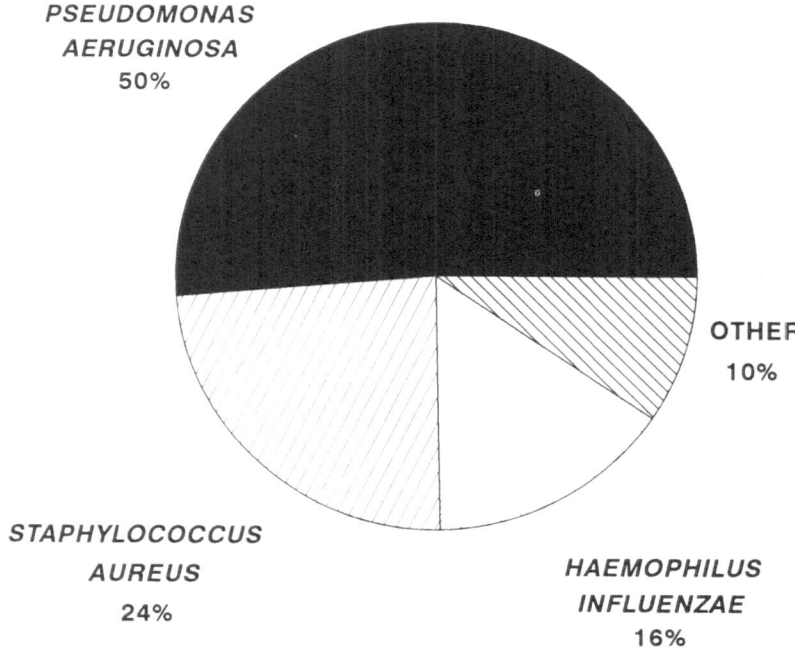

Figure 5. Percentages of bacteria isolated from sputum cultures in Israeli CF patients during the year 1993. *P. cepacia* was not isolated. More than 1 isolate recovered in some of the cases (*n* = 124).

under 1 year of age fell from 86% to 30%. The isolation rate of *P. aeruginosa* increased from less than 1% in 1956 to 30% in 1972. In Toronto, the prevalence of *P. aeruginosa* increased from 60% in 1970 [12] to 82% in 1988. It is possible that this change is a reflection of the increase in survival of patients with cystic fibrosis, an increase in the use of broad spectrum antibiotics, or a change in the virulence of these microorganisms.

At the time of infection, patients colonized by *P. aeruginosa* had similar pulmonary function values and weight and height percentiles to those colonized by *Staphylococcus aureus* and *Haemophilus influenzae* (Table 3). Although mean pulmonary function values were close to normal, nutritional status was poor in most of the patients at the time of any bacterial colonization. This may reflect the general finding of poor nutritional status among our patients (Figure 4). There seems to be a tendency towards a later age of first colonization with *Staphylococcus aureus* and *P. aeruginosa* as compared to *Haemophilus influenzae* and *Streptococcus pneumoniae* (Table 3). However, the variability of the age of colonization was very high for all the bacteria isolated. It has been previously shown that the prevalence of *P. aeruginosa* colonization in the respiratory flora of CF patients increases with age [14, 15], while

Table 3. Clinical characteristics of CF patients at the time of colonization

Type of bacteria	n	Age of colonization (years)	% tile Wt	FEV_1	FVC	$FEF_{25\ 75}$
P. aeruginosa	62	7.3 ± 6.4 (6.0)	17.0 ± 20.1 (10)	68.9 ± 21.2 (72)	64.6 ± 22.6 (78)	57.2 ± 27.0 (46)
Haemophilus influenzae	35	6.3 ± 5.0 (4.0)	17.8 ± 21.1 (10)	70.2 ± 18.8 (66)	78.2 ± 21.3 (64)	64.1 ± 27.9 (59)
Staphylococcus aureus	34	7.1 ± 5.6 (6.3)	14.7 ± 18.9 (9.5)	64.7 ± 22.9 (65)	74.9 ± 24.5 (78)	56.1 ± 30.1 (45)
Streptococcus pneumoniae	10	6.3 ± 5.0 (4.2)	15.8 ± 17.5 (3)	No data	No data	No data

Values are given as mean ± SD. in brackets are median values. Pulmonary function variables are presented as % of predicted values.

Staphylococcus aureus is more prevalent in infants and young children [13]. We have no explanation for the tendency for *Staphylococcus aureus* colonization to occur in our CF patients at an older age. This could be due to earlier treatment with anti-staphylococcal agents, a shift towards more selective antipseudomonal agents, or a change in the virulence of the bacteria.

Generally, the appearance of a microorganism in the sputum was not associated directly with respiratory exacerbation. Only two patients demonstrated a change in sputum cultures during respiratory exacerbation.

Pseudomonas aeruginosa

Almost every patient with CF will have *P. aeruginosa* colonization of the respiratory tract at some point during the course of the disease [16–19]. This colonization continues [16–19] for years, usually until the patient's death. However, it is still not clear when, where and why this occurs. *P. aeruginosa* is ubiquitous in the environment, yet the source of the *P. aeruginosa* colonizing CF patients is unknown. It has been suggested that patients with CF acquire *P. aeruginosa* from other patients already colonized by this microorganism, or from a common environmental source [16, 20–22].

As shown in Table 3 the age of colonization by *P. aeruginosa* in Israeli CF patients varies considerably. The rate of colonization increased with age (Figure 6A): 7.2% of patients under 1 year, 17.6% of patients under 5 years and 31% of patients under 10 years of age. However, in those colonized, most *P. aeruginosa* colonizations occurred at a relatively young age, similar to the findings reported from Toronto [15]. Of the patients colonized by *P. aeruginosa* (n = 62), 17.6% were

A

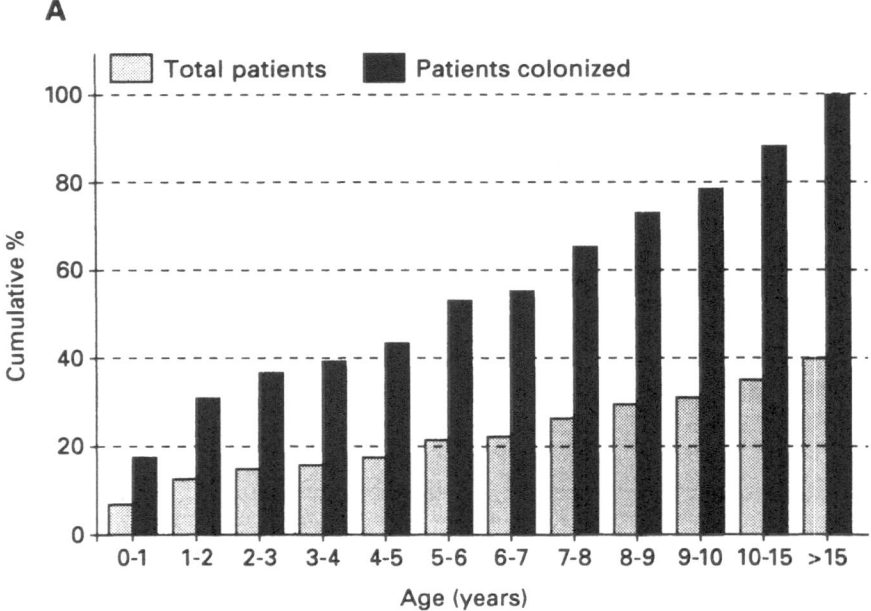

B

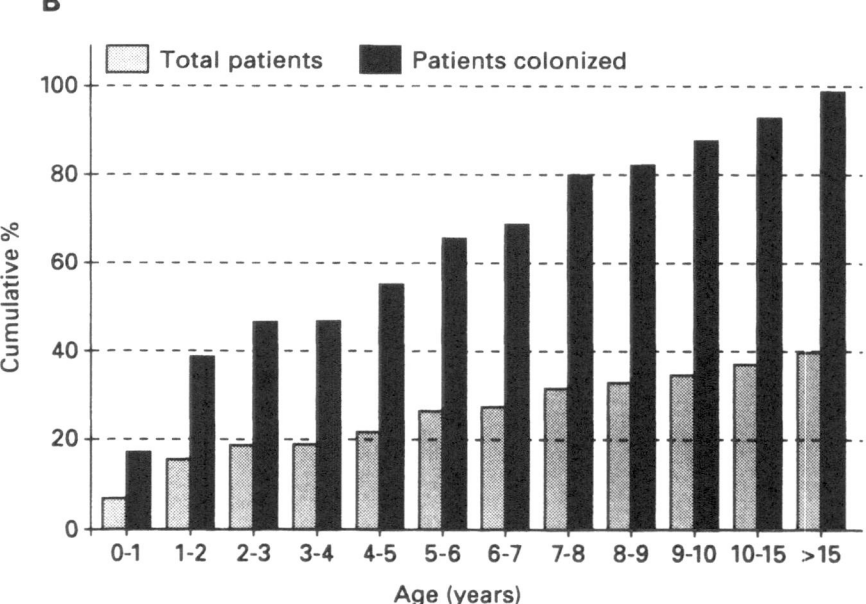

Figure 6. (A) Cumulative percentage of *P. aeruginosa* colonization by age for all CF patients (n = 124). (B) Cumulative percentages of *P. aeruginosa* colonization by age for CF patients diagnosed before 1 year of age (n = 91).

Table 4. Comparison of clinical characteristics between patients colonized and not colonized by *P. aeruginosa*

	Colonized	Not colonized	p
n	62	62	
Age at diagnosis. y	2.3 ± 4.4	2.3 ± 3.3	NS
	(0.23)	(0.23)	
Current age. y	14.4 ± 8.2	7.5 ± 4.8	<0.001
	(13.5)	(7.5)	
Diagnosed after 1 year			
of age. %	34	16	0.022
Pancreatic sufficiency. %	11	6	NS
Meconium ileus. %	10	24	0.031

Values are given as mean ± SD. in brackets are median values.

colonized before 1 year of age. 43% before 5 years of age, and 78% before 10 years of age (Figure 6A). These rates of colonization are considerably lower than those reported from Canada [15], England [13], or Denmark [23]. When patients colonized by *P. aeruginosa* were compared to non colonized patients (Table 4), the colonized patients were older, had a higher percentage of diagnosis after 1 year of age, a higher percentage of pancreatic sufficient patients, and a lower incidence of meconium ileus. These differences were likely to reflect the older age of patients with *P. aeruginosa* or the difficulty in obtaining sputum from the younger patients, rather than true risk factors for *Pseudomonas* colonization.

In order to investigate the rate of acquisition of *P. aeruginosa* more accurately, we studied a subgroup of patients who were diagnosed under 1 year of age and being followed at our clinics (n = 91). *P. aeruginosa* was cultured in 36 patients (40%) at a mean age of 5.4 ± 5.2 years (median 4.75). As shown in Figure 6B these patients tended to be colonized by *P. aeruginosa* at an earlier age compared to those diagnosed after 1 year of age. Again, most of the colonizations occurred at a relatively young age. Of the patients diagnosed before 1 year of age and colonized by *P. aeruginosa*, 56% were colonized before 5 years of age, and 89% before 10 years of age (Figure 6B).

Antimicrobial Therapy

There was no standard mode of therapy for pulmonary disease in CF patients in the 4 Israeli centers. Some physicians prescribed antimicrobial treatment for continuous use, while others recommended treatment only during respiratory exacerbations. The most common antimicrobial preparations used for oral treatment of pulmonary exacerbations were amoxicillin-clavulanate, first-generation cephalosporins, cloxacillin, ciprofloxacin and trimethoprim-sulphamethoxazole. The extent of antimicrobial therapy may reflect CF severity. Of our patient population, 75% received at least one course of oral antimicrobial therapy for 14–21 days during the last year (1993), 55% received two or more courses, and 14%, four or more courses.

The parenteral antimicrobial agents most commonly used to treat pulmonary exacerbation in CF patients were a combination of aminoglycosides with either ceftazidime, imipenem, or occasionally unreidopenicillins. Intravenous antimicrobial treatment was required by 32% of the patients during the last year, 14% on more than one occasion.

Daily antimicrobial therapy was administered orally to 40% of patients, and as inhalations of aminoglycosides or colistin to 30.7%. Six percent of patients were treated intravenously every 3–4 months according to the protocol of Pederson *et al.* [20].

Oral ciprofloxacin was given to 23%, including children under 12 years of age, in most of the cases for up to three weeks. In 36% of these patients, emergence of resistance to ciprofloxacin was documented. Susceptibility to ciprofloxacin was regained in some of the patients after discontinuation of the drug.

Of the 62 patients in whom *P. aeruginosa* was isolated from sputum cultures, 21 developed resistance to antimicrobial agents: 16 developed resistance to aminoglycosides, five to ciprofloxacin and one to ceftazidime. The latter patient had *P. aeruginosa* strain with multiple resistance to ciprofloxacin, aminoglycosides and ceftazidime, after being treated with these drugs.

Of the 29 patients in whom *Staphylococcus aureus* was isolated from sputum, 12 developed resistances: six to aminoglycosides, five to ciprofloxacin, and one to methicillin. In most of the patients, prior to the development of resistance, an agent to which *Staphylococcus aureus* developed resistance had been used.

Summary

There was no standard way of treating pulmonary disease amongst the different Israeli CF centers. The patient population in this study from four CF centers, representing 50% of the Israeli CF patient population, was younger than the CF patient population in the major CF centers in North America. Our patients were diagnosed at a younger age with most of the patients being under the age of 6 months. Overall, the nutritional status of our patients was poor, considering the relatively young age of our patient population. In 66%, bacteria were isolated from sputum cultures, with *P. aeruginosa* cultured in 50% of them. The rate of colonization by *P. aeruginosa* increased with age, but was lower than that reported from other centers in North America and Europe.

The colonization tended to occur at a relatively young age, with 43% of colonizations occurring before age 5 years. So far, *Pseudomonas cepacia* has not been isolated from any of our patients. *Staphylococcus aureus*, cultured in about 25% of our patients, tended to be cultured at a later age than was previously reported. Most of our patients received two or more courses of oral antimicrobial therapy, with 40% receiving it on a daily basis. In one third of the patients receiving ciprofloxacin emergence of resistance to ciprofloxacin was documented.

Acknowledgement

We would like to thank Yael Vila MsC, Tel-Aviv Medical Center, for help with statistical analysis.

References

1. Boat TF, Welsh MJ, Beaudet AL. Cystic fibrosis. In: CR Scriver, AL Beaudet, WS Sly and D Valle, editors: The metabolic basis of inherited disease. 6th ed. New York: McGraw-Hill, 1989; 2649–80.
2. Gaskin KJ, Durie PR, Lee L, Hill R, Forstner GG. Colipase and lipase secretion in childhood-onset pancreatic insufficiency: delineation of patients with steatorrhoea secondary to relative colipase deficiency. Gastroenterology 1984; 86: 1–7.
3. Gaskin K, Gurwitz D, Durie P, Corey M, Levison H, Forstner GG. Improved respiratory prognosis in patients with cystic fibrosis with normal fat absorption. J Pediatr 1982; 100: 857–62.
4. Corey M, Gaskin K, Durie P, Levison H, Forstner G. Improved prognosis in CF patients with normal fat absorption. J Pediatr Gastroenterol Nutr 1984; 3: Suppl 1: S99–S105.
5. Kerem E, Corey M, Kerem B, Rommens J, Levison H, Tsui LC, et al. The relationship between genotype and phenotype in cystic fibrosis, analysis of the most common mutation (ΔF508). N Engl J Med 1990; 323: 1517–22.
6. Shoshani T, Berkun Y, Yahav Y, Bashan N, Yahav Y, Rivlin Y, et al. A new mutation in the CFTR gene, composed of 2 adjacent DNA alterations, is a common cause of cystic fibrosis among Georgian Jews. Genomics 1993; 15: 236–7.
7. Augarten A, Kerem B, Yahav Y, Noiman S, Rivlin J, Tal A, et al. Mild cystic fibrosis and normal or borderline sweat in patients with 3849 + 10 kb C → T mutation. Lancet 1993; 342: 25–7.
8. Dean M, White MB, Amos J, et al. Multiple mutations in highly conserved residues are found in mildly affected cystic fibrosis patients. Cell 1990; 16: 863–70.
9. Corey M, McLaughlin FJ, Williams M, Levison H. A comparison of survival, growth, and pulmonary function in patients with cystic fibrosis in Boston and Toronto. J Clin Epidermiol 1988; 41: 583–91.
10. Kerem E, Corey M, Kerem B, Durie P, Tsui LC, Levison H: Clinical and genetic comparisons of patients with cystic fibrosis, with or without meconium ileus. J Pediatr 1989; 114: 767–73.
11. Del Pin CA, Czyrko C, Ziegler MM, Scanlin TF, Bishop HG. Management and survival of meconium ileus. A 30-year review. Ann Surg 1992; 215: 179–85.
12. Corey M, Allison L, Prober C, Levison H. Sputum bacteriology in patients with cystic fibrosis in a Toronto hospital during 1970–1981. J Infect Dis 1984; 149: 18.
13. Mearns MB, Hunt GH, Ruthworth R. Bacterial flora of respiratory tracts in patients with cystic fibrosis, 1950–1971. Arch Dis Child 1972; 47: 902–7.
14. Kerem E, Corey M, Gold R, Levison H. Pulmonary function and clinical course in patients with cystic fibrosis after pulmonary colonization with *Pseudomonas aeruginosa*. J Pediatr 1990; 116: 714–9.

15. Kerem E, Corey M, Stein R, Gold R, Levison H. Risk factors for *Pseudomonas aeruginosa* colonization in cystic fibrosis patients. Pediatr Infect Dis 1990; 9: 494–8.
16. Hoiby N. Microbiology of lung infections in cystic fibrosis patients. Acta Pediatr Scand (Suppl) 1982; 301: 33–54.
17. Laraya-Cuasay LR, Cundy KR, Haung NN. Pseudomonas carrier rates of patients with cystic fibrosis and members of their families. J Pediatr 1976; 89: 23–6.
18. Hoiby N. Prevalence of mucoid strains of *Pseudomonas aeruginosa* in bacteriological specimens from patients with cystic fibrosis and patients with other diseases. Acta Pathol Microbiol Scand (Suppl) 1975; 83: 549–52.
19. Kulczycki LL, Murphy TM, Bellanti JA. Pseudomonas colonization in cystic fibrosis. A study of 160 patients. JAMA 1978; 240: 30–4.
20. Pedersen SS, Jensen T, Hoiby N, Koch C, Flensbory EW. Management of *Pseudomonas aeruginosa* lung infection in Danish cystic fibrosis patients. Acta Pediatr Scan 1987; 76: 955–61.
21. Hoiby N, Pedersen SS. Estimated risk of cross-infection with *Pseudomonas aeruginosa* in Danish cystic fibrosis patients. Acta Pediatr Scand 1989; 78: 395–404.
22. Zimakoff J, Hoiby N, Rosendal K, Guilbert JP. Epidemiology of *Pseudomonas aeruginosa* infection and the role of contamination of the environment in cystic fibrosis clinic. J Hosp Infect 1983; 4: 31–40.
23. Hoiby N. Microbiology of lung infections in cystic fibrosis patients. Acta Pediatr Scand (suppl) 1982; 301: 33–54.

Cystic Fibrosis Pulmonary Infections:
Lessons from Around the World
ed. by A. Bauernfeind, M. I. Marks and B. Strandvik
© 1996 Birkhäuser Verlag Basel/Switzerland

CHAPTER 15
The State of Cystic Fibrosis in Turkey

M. Demirkol[1], Z. Erturan[2], G. Hüner[1], T. Baykal[1], G. Kurdoğlu[1]
and Ö. Ang[2]

[1]University of Istanbul, Istanbul Faculty of Medicine, Department of Pediatrics,
Division of Nutrition and Metabolism, 34390 Çapa, Istanbul, Turkey
[2]University of Istanbul, Istanbul Faculty of Medicine, Department of Microbiology, 34390 Çapa,
Istanbul, Turkey

Summary. Cystic fibrosis (CF) represents a major health problem in developed countries. Although its distribution is worldwide, there is little awareness of its prevalance in most developing countries.

In Turkey the infant mortality rate is still very high (59/1000). Respiratory infections and diarrhea are important causes of infant mortality (13% and 9%, respectively) (1). There are no reliable statistical data available for the incidence of CF in our country. Probably some infant deaths which are listed under respiratory and gastrointestinal problems are due to CF, because of lack of diagnosis.

There is a specific aspect to be considered in Turkey. Consanguineous marriages are very common (21%) (2). Therefore we see a large number of inherited metabolic diseases, for instance phenylketonuria (PKU). The mean incidence of PKU is 1:10 000 all over the world, whereas its incidence in Turkey is 1:6 000 according to our studies (3). CF leads to mortality, but PKU to a sequal, mental retardation. We believe that because of the lack of diagnosis we cannot reach patients with CF in our country, but patients with PKU who survive with mental retardation are more easily diagnosed since newborn screening is not organized nationwide as yet.

Diagnosis of CF is being made primarily in hospitals or specialized centers that can provide subsequent health care. There are no special CF clinics in Turkey. CF patients are followed in a few number of children's hospitals of medical schools in the metropolitan areas where there are special out- and inpatients departments for CF as in our center. The total number of the CF patients who are followed in these centers does not exceed 250 to our knowledge. It will be necessary to develop new approaches in developing countries, where tertiary care facilities are limited, and to give more emphasis to early treatment in a primary care setting to reach the level of care of the developed countries.

From January 1985 to July 1994, among 5342 patients with sweat test indication (4), we detected chloride values greater than 60 mEq/L in 81 patients (1.5%) by Gibson's pilocarpine iontophoresis method (5). 68 patients of those with high chloride values were then referred by their doctors to our CF polyclinics for differential diagnosis.

The diagnosis of CF was based on a positive quantitative sweat test in the presence of one or more of the following clinical features: typical pulmonary problems, documented exocrine pancreatic insufficiency or a positive family history.

In 61 patients, 30 males and 31 females, who had high sweat test values, the diagnosis of CF was established with suggestive clinical features. In seven patients the diagnosis of CF was ruled out (two celiac disease, one glycogen storage disease type I, one congenital adrenal hyperplasia, one Addison disease and two protein–energy malnutrition) and they were excluded from the CF group.

Family History

In our CF families the percentage of consanguineous marriages is very high (39%). Half of our patients had siblings with clinical findings suggestive of CF (48%) who were not diagnosed while they were alive.

Age of Diagnosis

The age of diagnosis of CF patients (n = 61) was between one month and 10.8 years (median: 6 months). Table 1 shows the distribution of CF patients according to their age at initial diagnosis. In 72% of the cases the diagnosis was established during the first year of life, from which 50.8% was during the first six months. If we compare these results with the literature, in our study group we have a higher frequency of CF diagnosis in the infancy period. Approximate figures taken from various sources for age at diagnosis are 50% during infancy and 30% during the first six months (6). This high frequency is probably due to the fact that patients with less severe clinical symptoms at an older age are undiagnosed.

Initial Clinical Presentation

In our study there is an increased number of CF patients with respiratory and intestinal problems compared to the literature (Table 2) (6).These patients had a severe clinical picture at initial diagnosis and were therefore quickly referred to our center.

Table 1. Distribution of CF patients according to their age at initial diagnosis

Age at initial diagnosis	CF patients n (%)
0–3 months	21 (34.4)
4–6 months	10 (16.4)
7–12 months	13 (21.3)
1–2 years	5 (8.2)
3–4 years	5 (8.2)
5–10 years	7 (11.5)

Table 2. Clinical findings of CF patients at the time of initial diagnosis, compared with approximate figures taken from various sources (6)

Presenting features	Study group (% of CF patients)	Literature (% of CF patients)
Meconium ileus	6.6	15.0
Persistent or acute respiratory problems	31.3	25.0
Respiratory + intestinal problems	44.2	15.0
Intestinal problems	14.8	30.0
Family history	0	10.0
Others	3.2	5.0

Assessment

Pancreatic Function

For the assessment of exocrine pancreatic function the measurement of fat balance with a three day stool collection and quantitation of chymotrypsin activity in a fresh stool sample are the main applications. In our study group 87% of CF patients showed pancreatic insufficiency.

For the endocrine pancreatic dysfunction blood and urine glucose levels are checked and glycosylated hemoglobin levels are monitored yearly after the age of ten. We have only one patient with diabetes mellitus.

Nutritional State

Growth is the best guide of nutritional adequacy [7]. Anthropometric measurements such as body weight, length, triceps skinfold thickness, midarm circumference and biochemical evaluation as albumin, prealbumin, transferrin, retinol binding protein, carotene, iron, iron binding capacity, ferritin, lymphocyte count and creatinine height index are routinely performed [8].

Malnutrition was one of our major clinical findings of CF at initial diagnosis. Approximately 70.5 and 57.4% of patients with CF were less than the 10th percentile for body weight and height for their age-sex group, respectively. Weight for height at initial diagnosis was 82.9 ± 14.1%. The weight for height of 62.5% of the patients were below 90%.

Pulmonary Function

We could only recently start pulmonary function studies in patients above six years of age.

Microbiology

Sputum cultures are obtained at each control or on any sign of infection. From young patients who are not capable of excreting sputum, nasopharyngeal aspirates or throat swabs are taken.

During our follow up 33 patients (54%) had positive sputum for one or more microorganisms. 19 patients (31%) had at least one positive sputum culture for *Pseudomonas aeruginosa*. Most of these (n = 15) were transient infections which responded to antipseudomonal therapy whereas the remaining four patients had persistent colonization [7].

Sputum cultures were positive for *Staphylococcus aureus* in 17 patients (28%), *Klebsiella pneumoniae* in 16 patients (26%), *Haemophilus influenzae* in 3 patients (5%), *Candida albicans* in 7 patients (11.5%) and *Aspergillus fumigatus* in 3 patients (5%), Other microorganisms diagnosed were *Escherichia coli*, *Streptococcus pneumoniae* and *Enterobacter* spp. The age of colonization with *Pseudomonas aeruginosa* was between 2 and 21 years (median; 10.5 years).

In 1994, a new protocol was started for the microbiological sputum evaluation of CF patients in the department of microbiology. The sputa were liquefied with sputolysin and then diluted [9]. To follow the success of the treatment colony counting was performed. The selective media used were antibiotic-free Tryptic Soy agar (TSA), McConkey agar, sheep blood agar, chocolate agar with a bacitracin disk and TSA with imipenem or polymyxin B.

The strains with a green pigment were identified as *P. aeruginosa*. The antibiotic susceptibility of the strains was determined by the Kirby-Bauer method [10].

In the department of microbiology procedures like minimum inhibitory concentration (MIC), pyocin typing and API system are not routine yet. There are some technical difficulties in managing routine materials. The strains are freeze-dried to perform MICs, pyocin typing and API in the future according to the procedures of Bauernfeind *et al.* [11]. The differentiation between bacteria of the same species is now made by their different colony morphology, pigmentation and antibiotic susceptibility.

Since March 1994, 34 sputa and one throat swab from 17 different CF patients (7 females and 10 males) were examined with the new protocol. The youngest patient was 3.5 months old and the oldest was 21 years old. The isolate numbers and the colony count ranges are shown in Table 3, the susceptibility to antimicrobial agents in Tables 4 and 5.

The methicillin-susceptible *Staphylococcus aureus* (MSSA) were susceptible to a broad range of antibiotics. The majority of the *K. pneumoniae* strains was widely susceptible except for 5 isolates from the same patient which were multiresistant and susceptible only to imipenem.

Table 3. Bacterial isolate and colony counts

Microorganism	No. of patients	No. of strains	Colony count range
Nonmucoid *Pseudomonas* spp. (other than *P. cepacia*)	7	17 (13 with green pigment)	$10^1 - 10^8$
Mucoid	2	5	$10^1 - 10^7$
MRSA	5	10	$10^2 - 10^7$
MSSA	6	7	$10^2 - 10^9$
K. pneumoniae	9	15	$10^2 - 10^8$
S. maltophilia	2	4	10^4
B. cepacia	0	no isolate	0
E. coli	3	4	$10^2 - 10^7$
Enterobacter spp.	2	2	10^7
Morganella morganii	1	1	10^2
H. influenzae type b	1	1	$> 10^8$
Non group a beta hemolytic *Streptococcus*	1	1	10^1
Enterococcus spp.	1	1	10^1
Candida spp.	11	21	$10^2 - 10^4$
Aspergillus spp.	5	9	$10^1 - 10^3$

Table 4. Antibiotic susceptibility of 10 methicillin resistant *S. aureus* strains

*Antimicrobial agents	Susceptible	Intermediate-moderately susceptible
Vancomycin	10	0
Chloramphenicol	8	2
Netilmicin	8	1
Ciprofloxacin	4	4
Ofloxacin	5	3
Amikacin	0	1
Tetracycline	0	1

*Clindamycin, fusidic acid, teicoplanin, rifampicin, fosfomycin were not tested.

Table 5. Antibiotic susceptibility of 18 *Pseudomonas* spp. strains

Antimicrobial agents	Susceptible	Intermediate-moderately susceptible
Tobramycin	16	2
Imipenem	16	1
Amikacin	8	3
Ciprofloxacin	7	8
Netilmicin	5	5
Ofloxacin	5	3
Cefoperazone + Sulbactam	4	7
Gentamicin	4	1
Ceftazidime	4	—
Aztreonam	3	2

The most frequently used agent for antistaphylococcal prophylaxis was cotrimoxazole. Three strains of *S. aureus* were resistant and two intermediately susceptible to this drug.

The results from these 17 patients are not enough to give us a general overview of the microbiology of CF in Turkey. But this new study is going on and we hope to give better results in the near future.

Molecular Study

DNA analyses were performed for 24 CF families for the mutations ΔF508, 1677delTA, Δ1507, G551D and R553X. Of the 48 alleles of the CF patients only 9 (18%) were positively for ΔF508, and 3 (6%) for 1677delTA.

Management

General Approach of Care

In our center the CF patients are followed at a special outpatient clinic by our medical attendants, a dietitian and a pediatrician. The good collaboration with the Department of Microbiology of the same Faculty supports the medical therapy of CF patients. We are in need of a physiotherapist who is specialized for CF which is an important part of the therapy (8). The pediatricians try to give this knowledge to the parents with the manuscripts and video films which were obtained from the German CF Foundation, and try to practice it on the patients.

Follow Up

In our center our program for CF therapy is to normalize growth and nutritional status as early as possible after diagnosis and prolong infection free periods (12). To attain these we follow the patients younger than one year of age every month, and older patients every other month and on any sign of infection noticed by the family. The families are informed about the symptoms, treatment and genetic aspects of CF by our team in family meetings, which are arranged every month. Nutritional management, physiotherapy and early intervention for infections are our main applications. Our goal is to establish good nutrition as it will prevent pulmonary infection (13).

Hospitalization

The patients are hospitalized at initial diagnosis for accurate diagnosis, baseline assessment, nutritional rehabilitation, treatment of pulmonary infections, teaching physiotherapy, education and afterwards if there are complications. The median duration for hospitalization is 26 days/per year (range: 7–84 days).

Prophylaxis

Immunization against whooping cough, measles, tuberculosis, H. influenzae, influenza and hepatitis B infections are given to CF patients.

Nutritional Therapy

The achievement and maintenance of energy balance in CF is one of the central aims of clinical management, based on the recognition of malnutrition as a major prognostic factor adversely affecting survival [14].

The CF diet is prescribed to compensate for the increased energy, protein, vitamin and mineral requirements as minimum 120–150% of RDA. A normal fat diet in large amounts has demonstrated that energy intake could be enhanced and weight gain sustained [14]. The diet of our CF patients contains the normal percentage of fat but for the patients with oxygenation problems we increase the fat percentage of the diet. The protein requirements of CF patients have ranged from 2.5–4 g/kg body weight per day.

There is no single, optimal nutritional supplement for use in CF patients. Dietary counselling advice is tailored to the individual, suitable products selected according to the child's age, individual needs and taste with supplement being added as necessary.

Elemental diets are widely used in the management of CF [15]. They tend to be unpalatable and expensive. CF infants on human milk or standard formulae with enzyme supplements who had failure to thrive are started semielementary diet containing medium-chain triglycerides (MCT).

The desired aim of nutritional management is to achieve equilibrium by non-invasive intervention and with methods which are compatible with normal life style [14]. Supplemental feeding with elemental diet during periods of hospital treatment for respiratory infections will enhance weight gain, but the increased weight is not maintained when the patients return home. Therefore we educate parents for tube feeding at home. When such children are maintained on nocturnal tube feedings at home, weight and height velocity can be sustained at an increased rate over several months but the gains cease when the tube feeding is discontinued [15]. For the older patients we use enteral nutrition naso-gastrically. Now we are planning to apply gastrostomy for some CF patients [16]. Total parenteral nutrition is seldom indicated for those CF patients with severe malnutrition who need short term nutritional treatment.

Vitamin and Mineral Supplementation

To avoid vitamin deficiency we begin with 150% of the RDA recom-mendations of fat-soluble vitamins and mostly we increase the dosage as following the serum vitamin levels in our laboratory. And if there is still a need of vitamin support, we use water-soluble forms of these vitamins instead of fat-soluble form.

Pancreatic Insufficiency

To improve the impairment of fat absorption we use enteric coated microspheres in pancreatic insufficient patients (8). Creon (Kali-Chemie Pharma) is now the only preparation for this purpose in Turkey. The dosage is adjusted according to the frequency and the fat content of the stools and to the weight gain of the patient.

Pulmonary Therapy

Inhalation Therapy

Aerosol therapy is used before postural drainage and for the delivery of medication.

Physiotherapy

At initial diagnosis respiratory problems were in 74% of our CF patients. We experienced severe pulmonary infections especially at the admission during the infancy period. Some of these children were lost (n = 14, 73.7%). During the follow up of the CF patients the rate of pulmonary problems increased to nearly 100%.

We recommend physiotherapy three or four times a day for about 20 minutes after the administration of physiologic saline with a nebulizer.

Bronchodilators are not used on routine physiotherapy but prescribed if there are indications such as prolonged expiration time or wheezing. Oral mucolytics are used continuously. Inhaled N-acetylcysteine is prescribed for a short period of 3 or 5 days when there is difficulty in the drainage of the mucus. Oral N-acetylcysteine is used more frequently.

Antibiotic Therapy

Prophylactically we had given continuous TMP-SMX to our CF patients. Our results were not statistically significant when compared to the patients not receiving prophylaxy and therefore we ceased this prophylactic therapy.

On any acute exacerbation which may be characterized by loss of appetite, weight loss, deteriorating lung function, X-ray changes, fever, increased cough and sputum or increased CRP, ESR or leucocytosis broad spectrum antibiotic treatment is started immediately (8). One of our problems for antibiotic therapy is that there are no oral narrow spectrum antistaphylococcal antibiotics on the market.

For antipseudomonal therapy drugs such as ceftazidime plus aminoglycoside or oral ciprofloxacin depending on the age of the patient are used in two different groups comparing the effects of therapies. The duration of the infection free period will be evaluated between the transient pseudomonas infections.

For persistent *P. aeruginosa* colonization the policy is to admit patients on a regular basis every three months for a course of antipseudomonal therapy regardless of symptoms and to begin inhalation therapy with aminolgycosides, and if necessary with colistin in patients with persistent colonization and pathologic findings of the lungs.

If the clinical findings and laboratory assessments show infection and there is no response to medication after a week or ten days the therapy is changed according to the resistance patterns. The antibiotic mostly chosen for such occasions is imipenem.

Therapy of Complications

Meconium ileus

The incidence of meconium ileus (6.6%) is low in our group if we compare this with the literature (10–20%) [6]. It could be explained by the lack of CF diagnosis in the surgery departments where we also try to bring the CF knowledge.

Meconium ileus equivalent

Our older patients complained from abdominal pain at times and we try to adjust the dosage of pancreatic supplementation according to their needs. Only three of our patients had "Meconium ileus equivalent". Medical and conservative treatments such as N-acetylcysteine were sufficient.

Salt Depletion

Out country has hot and dry summers and the salt loss becomes a real life threatening problem. Severe electrolyte imbalance is experienced in a few patients especially during infancy and early childhood. We supply or patients with extra salt during summer or any occasion causing increased perspiration such as high fever.

Hypoalbuminemia

In our CF patients mean serum albumin level at initial diagnosis was 3.29 ± 0.8 g/dl. 32% of our patients had hypoalbuminemia defined as serum albumin levels below 3.2 g/dl.

Liver Disease

Hepatic fibrosis is a common finding in older CF patients. With improved survival, we expect that its incidence will increase. We don't have any patients with cirrhosis or its complications. One of our patients who was given ursodeoxycholic acid [17] now eight years old has persistent elevation in serum transaminase levels with cholestasis.

Hyperglycemia

Diabetes mellitus is a complication of CF at the 2nd decade. We have only one patient, who is 21 years old with diabetes mellitus. The rare incidence of diabetes mellitus in our CF group could be explained with the small number of our adolescent patients.

Psychosocial and Financial Problems

After the diagnosis the family is informed on CF, its clinical findings, treatment and genetic aspects. A demanding regimen of treatment is expected from them and they have to face many problems during follow up. We also try to discuss and share these problems in family meetings.

At the beginning the families experience shock, denial and depression. They are advised by our team.

The crowded families, the low level of the parent's education and the long distance to the therapy center are the main social problems.

The low rate of health insurance leads to main financial problem in the therapy. Parents who are not insured are faced with a new problem of finding a new job with insurance that requires a minimum waiting period of four months.

Survival

During follow-up 19 patients (8 females and 10 males) died between two months and 9 4/12 years (median: 4 months). Overall mortality rate was 31.3%. Most of them died shortly after diagnosis with a median of 30 days after referral (range: 9 days – 1 1/12 years). In 14 patients (73%) severe pulmonary infections leading to acute respiratory failure were the main cause of mortality during infancy.

The clinical syndrome of protein energy malnutrition in CF patients remain a significant source of morbidity and mortality within 6 months of life (15). All the patients (100%) who died with CF had malnutrition. These children had relative weight; $69.3 \pm 7.5\%$ (range: 53–80%). The relation between mortality and age of the patients is shown on Table 6. Our mortality rate is decreasing with respect to time by the use of assisted ventilation, better monitoring and therapeutic means.

Now 42 CF patients are being followed in our center. The average age of the group $5\ 6/12 \pm 4\ 8/12$ years (range: 6 months – 21 4/12 years) is still very low. We had two patients one girl and one boy surviving to adolescence who are in full-time education and employment.

Table 6. The relation between mortality and age of CF patients

Age (months)	CF patients who died n (%)
0–3	9 (47.4)
4–6	4 (21.0)
7–12	3 (15.8)
13–24	2 (10.5)
25–48	0 (0)
49–120	1 (5.3)

Conclusion

The improvement in survival of CF patients in developed countries over the past two decades have increased mean life expectancy. Many adult patients with CF at present are fully integrated into society and have an acceptable lifestyle. In our CF group the average age is still very young with only two surviving adolescents [18].

In developed countries CF causes progressive lung disease, chronic pancreatic insufficiency and cirrhosis of the liver. We are dealing with acute respiratory infections and malnutrition due to intestinal problems because CF patients don't live long enough to develop the diseases stated. The situation prior to 1930s when affected children died from maldigestion and malabsorption or from pulmonary infection still exists in parts of the world where CF is fequently not recognized as in our country. High infant mortality from common causes like respiratory and gastrointestinal disorders in developing countries may in fact be masking CF [12]. Recent reports indicate that, when appropriate diagnostic facilities exist, CF is often found.

Our first aim is to bring the knowledge of CF to medical staff for better diagnosis and especially for an early diagnosis. Secondly we are trying to approach the parents by spreading information through the mass media.

International collaboration is required to provide internationally useful guidelines for treatment, to promote initiatives in public health, and to assist in the dissemination of educational material. These will be most valuable steps for developing countries, where underdiagnosis of CF is widespread. We are aiming to educate the general public, as well as medical personnel and other health professionals about the disease. There is still a great deal of organizational work to be done.

References

1. Government of Turkey – UNICEF programme of cooperation. The situational analysis of mothers and children in Turkey. Ankara: UNICEF Turkey Office, Yeniçağ Press, 1991.
2. Tunçbilek E, Ulusoy M. Consanguineous marriages in Turkey. Journal of Population Science, 1989; 11: 37.
3. Demirkol M, Baykal T, Hüner G, Yalvaç S, Kurdoğlu G. The problems of newborn screening in a developing country. In: New horizons in neonatal screening. Farriaux JP and Dhondt JL (eds). Amsterdam: Elsevier Science BV, Excerpta Medica, 1994, 309.
4. Boat TF. Cystic fibrosis. In: Nelson's textbook of pediatrics. 14th edition. Behrman RE, Nelson WE (eds). Philadelphia: W.B. Saunders Company, 1992, 1106.
5. Gibson LE, Cooke RE. A test for concentration of electrolytes in sweat in cystic fibrosis of the pancreas utilizing pilocarpine by iontophoresis. Pediatrics 1959; 23: 545–549.
6. Jackson ADM. The natural history of cystic fibrosis. In: Cystic Fibrosis. Peter Goodfellow (editor). Oxford: Oxford University Press, 1989, 1.
7. Fitzsimmonds SC. The changing epidemiology of cystic fibrosis. J Pediatr 1993; 122: 1–9.
8. Ramsey BW, Boat TF. Outcome measures for clinical trials in CF. Summary of a Cystic Fibrosis Foundation Consensus Conference. J Pediatr 1994; 124: 177–192.
9. Hammerschlag MR, Harding L, Macone A, Smith AL, Goldman DA. Bacteriology of sputum in cystic fibrosis: Evaluation of dithiotheritol as mucolytic agent. J Clin Microbiol 1980; 11: 552–557.
10. NCCLS. Performance standards for antimicrobial disc susceptibility tests. 5. edition approved standard M2-A5 NCCLS, Villanova PA, 1993.

11. Bauernfeind A, Bertele RM, Harms K, Hörl G, Jungwirth R, Petermüller C, Przyklenk B, Weisslein-Pfister C. Qualitative and quantitative microbiological analysis of sputa of 102 patients with cystic fibrosis. Infection 1987; 15: 270–277.

12. Dodge JA. Management of cystic fibrosis. In: Cystic fibrosis. Peter Goodfellow (editor). Oxford: Oxford Univeristy Press 1989, 12.

13. Tizzano EF, Buchwald M. Cystic fibrosis: Beyond the gene to therapy. The J Pediatr 1992; 120: 337–349.

14. Dodge JA, O'Rawe A, Metabolism and hyperalimentation in cystic fibrosis: An overview. In: Cystic fibrosis basic and clinical research. Høiby N and Pedersen SS (editors). Amsterdam: Elsevier Science Publishers B.V., Excerpta Medica, 1992, 59.

15. Moore MC. Enternal-tube feeding as adjunct therapy in malnourished patients with cystic fibrosis: clinical study and literature review. Am J Clin Nutr 1986; 44: 33–41.

16. Steinkamp G, von der Hardt H. Improvement of nutritional status and lung function after long-term nocturnal gastrostomie feeding in cystic fibrosis. J Pediatr 1994; 124: 244–249.

17. Galabert C, Montet JC, Lengrand D ets. Effects of ursodeoxycholic acid on liver function in patients with cystic fibrosis and chronic cholestasis. J Pediatr 1992; 121: 138–141.

18. Demirkol M, Baykal T, Hüner G, Tosun N, Kurdoğlu G. Cystic fibrosis: Does an undiagnosed patient group still exist in Turkey? Proceedings of XIth International Cystic Fibrosis Congress, Cystic Fibrosis Association (ed). Dublin: Trinity College Press, 1992, 108.

Cystic Fibrosis Pulmonary Infections:
Lessons from Around the World
ed. by A. Bauernfeind, M. I. Marks and B. Strandvik
© 1996 Birkhäuser Verlag Basel/Switzerland

CHAPTER 16
The General Approach to Cystic Fibrosis Pulmonary Infection in Greece

George S. Adam

Director of Cystic Fibrosis Centre "Aghia Sophia" Children's Hospital, 11527 Athens, Greece

Summary. Cystic Fibrosis is the second most common autosomal recessive genetic disorder in Greece next to Mediterranean Anaemia (thalassaemia). There are about 50–60 affected neonates expected each year. The carrier frequency is estimated at 5% of the general population. There are 287 CF patients attending the CF Centre which was started in 1966 at the Aghia Sophia Children's Hospital in Athens. 25% of the patients are older than 16 years and the oldest known patient in Greece is 46 years old. From a group of 211 patients regularly followed at the Centre 101 are free from microbial colonization and 110 have positive sputum culture, in 88 of which *P. aeruginosa* has been cultured. *B. cepacia* has never been cultured in this series. Therapeutic approach to chest infection consists of oral or IV antibiotics according to the sensitivity of microorganisms cultured in the sputum; home IV therapy is not applied. Some patients are given antibiotics by inhalation and all have intensive physiotherapy. In the majority of patients clinical progress is good: as evaluated by the Shwachman-Kulczycki score 73% are in very good or excellent condition and only 11.8% are in moderate or poor condition. School-age children are attending regular school with low absence rate and good performance. Some of the adult patients are pursuing higher education and the rest are engaged in various professions. Our experience is that the introduction of a programme of aggressive and intensive therapy has had a positive effect on survival and clinical condition and has reduced hospitalization.

Cystic Fibrosis (CF) is the second most common autosomal recessive genetic disorder in Greece, next to Mediterranean Anaemia. The carrier frequency is estimated at 5%, resulting in the birth of 50–60 affected newborns per year. Recent genotype studies of CF families showed an incidence of mutations ΔF508: 51.3%, G542X: 4.3%, N1303K 4.3%, 621 + 1G > T: 3.5% and 35.7% of CF alleles remain uncharacterized [1, 2]. Use of the known mutations can identify 65.6% of carriers in the general population. A programme for prenatal diagnosis in CF families implemented soon after identification of the CF gene has resulted in the birth of 51 unaffected children in these families.

Systematic study of CF cases started in Greece in 1966 with the opening of the CF Centre at the Aghia Sophia Children's Hospital in Athens. In 1980 a clinic was opened in Thessaloniki, the second most populous city of Greece. As the diagnostic skills of pediatricians and general practitioners developed gradually, the number of diagnosed cases increased and has for the last five years stabilized at about 30 new cases out of 1800–1900 sweat tests performed per year in our Centre. Sweat electrolyte estimations are performed by pilocarpine iontophoresis.

There are about 380 known cases of CF in Greece. Of these 287 are followed in our centre at Aghia Sophia Children's Hospital and 93 at the Thessaloniki clinic.

In our group of patients 211 attend the out-patient clinic regularly and 60 at variable and irregular intervals. There are 143 males and 128 females aged 0–32 years, with an age distribution of 0–5 years: 28.6%, 6–10 years: 24%, 11–15 years: 22.4%, 16–20 years: 14.4%, >20 years: 10.6%. (A 46 year old patient is seen by a pneumonologist). The clinical symptoms which led to the patients' referral for sweat test vary (Table 1). The mean age at diagnosis is 11 months. During the last five years there has been an increase of cases diagnosed in adulthood.

Patients are seen at the out-patient CF clinic every 4–8 weeks depending on their age and clinical condition. Treatment is adapted to the needs of each case and includes physiotherapy, mucolytic and bronchodilating medication, pancreatic enzymes, vitamin supplements (A, D, E, K.) and NaCl supplements during summer months. Antibiotics are prescribed only in cases of active infection and of positive sputum culture and are not given prophylactically.

Sputum culture is performed at every visit. All patients have chest X-rays, blood counts, liver function tests, blood glucose, urea and serum creatinine estimations routinely performed once a year. In patients older than seven years lung function tests are carried out on a yearly basis.

Patients with lung infection identified by a) clinical symptoms (fever, increased cough and sputum production, dyspnoea or cyanosis, poor appetite, loss of weight), b) laboratory tests (chest X-rays, sputum culture, full blood count, ESR, CRP) are admitted to hospital and receive IV antibiotics for 12–15 days according to the *in vitro* sensitivity of the micro-organisms cultured in their sputum [3, 4].

Patients with sputum cultures positive for *Pseudomonas aerguinosa* receive a course of IV antipseudomonas antibiotics one to four times a year [5]. The therapeutic scheme administered is a combination of

Table 1. Clinical features which led to referral for sweat test in 213 CF patients

Respiratory and digestive system	126	(60%)
Digestive system	43	(20%)
Meconeum ileus	15	(7%)
Severe dehydration	10	(4%)
Nasal polyps	2	(1%)
Affected siblings	17	(8%)

aminoglycosides and a third generation cephalosporin or aminoglycoside and antipseudomonas penicillin.

Adolescents and young adults receive quinolones with a view to a
reduction of hospitalizations [6]. In some patients older than seven
years with persistent *Pseudomonas aeruginosa* colonization gentamicin
inhalation is administered [7–9].

The dieticians of the CF Centre see that patients comply with a
balanced maximum calorie intake diet and try to adapt this diet to the
personality of the child and the capabilities of the family.

The physiotherapists try to establish satisfactory compliance of the
children to regular intensive physiotherapy and to train the parents for
home physiotherapy programmes [10].

Influenza vaccine is administered every year. All other immunizations
are given in compliance with the Greek scheme for the general population (DiTePer, OPV, MMR, BCG).

The nutrition of patients regularly attending the out-patient CF clinic
before and after intervention is shown in Table 2. Implementation of an
aggressive dietary intervention programme showed a marked increase in
weight gain. Dietary intervention consists of a caloric intake above
120% of basic requirements for age and sex and intensive support for
compliance.

Evaluation of the patients' condition by Shwachman-Kulczycki clinical score (clinical examinations, chest X-rays, activity, nutrition) shows
good progress in the majority of cases: 150 patients (73%) are in very
good or excellent condition and only 25 (11.8%) are in moderate or
poor condition (Table 3).

Table 2. Distribution of weight centiles before and after dietary intervention

Centile	Males %		Females %	
	Pre	Post	Pre	Post
< 3	13	8	15	7
3–25	35	18	34	18
25–50	32	44	23	45
> 50	20	30	28	30

Table 3. Shwachman-Kulzcycki (S-K) score and *Pseudomonas aeruginosa* colonization

S-K score	*P. aeruginosa* (+)	*P. aeruginosa* (−)	Totals
Excellent 86–100	12 (14%)	75 (63%)	87 (44%)
Very good 71–85	28 (33%)	33 (28%)	61 (29%)
Good 56–70	21 (25%)	10 (8.5%)	31 (15%)
Moderate 41–55	12 (14%)	1 (0.3%)	13 (6%)
Poor < 40	12 (14%)	—	12 (5.8%)

All patients of school age attend regular school successfully. Only in very rare cases has the absence rate exceeded the average allowed to Greek students. School performance and participation in usual school activities is above average. Adult patients are pursuing higher education or are employed in a variety of jobs (teaching, law, shop attendants, office clerks, farmers).

Of the group 211 patients regularly followed in the CF Centre, 101 are free from microbial colonization and 110 have had positive sputum cultures: 88 *Pseudomonas aeruginosa*, 17 *Staphylococcus aureus* and 5 *S. aureus* + *Haemophilius influenzae*. *Burkholderia cepacia* has not been isolated in this group although meticulously sought [11, 12]. The age at colonization for both sexes ranges between 3–18 years for *P. aeruginosa* and 2–10 years for *Staph. aureus*. Of the 110 sputum positive patients 53 needed hospitalization because of increased respiratory symptoms, fever, increased cough and secretions, poor appetite, loss of weight dyspnoea (Table 4). Admission more than once yearly for IV therapy was needed only in patients colonized with *Pseudomonas aeruginosa*. The one patient with multiple admissions had severe pulmonary haemorrhage on several occasions. She was treated with aggressive chemotherapy. Therapeutic bronchial artery embolization was tried without success.

The results of lung function tests in 116 patients are shown in Table 5. The patients with *P. aeruginosa* colonization and FVC, FEV1 <40% of predicted values for height and weight (ages 11–32 years, mean age 19.5) had all been colonized for more than 7 years. They all have pancreatic insufficiency and Shwachman-Kulczycki clinical score <55.

Table 4. Number of admissions per year for IV therapy for colonization with *P. aeruginosa*

Admissions per year	Patients	*P. aeruginosa* (+)
1	37	30
2	9	9
3	6	6
>4	1	1

Table 5. Lung function tests (% of FVC, FEV1 predicted for height and weight) and microbial colonization

FVC, FEV1	*P. aeruginosa* (+)	*P. aeruginosa* (−)
>80	22 (28.9%)	28 (70.0%)
56–80	24 (31.5%)	8 (20.0%)
41–55	16 (21.0%)	3 (7.5%)
>40	14 (18.4%)	1 (2.5%)
Total	76 (100)	40 (100)

All but one are on antibiotic inhalation once or twice per day and have an IV course of antibiotics 1–3 times a year [7–9]. In the group of 22 patients with lung function tests better than 80% of predicted values (ages 8–24 years, mean age 13.4 years), 11 had been colonized with *P. aeruginosa* for less than 3 years, 9 for 4–5 years and 2 for 6 and 10 years. All had Shwachman-Kulczycki scores >55. Specifically: 12 have scores 86–100, 8 had 71–85 and 2 have 56–70 (Table 3). The two patients with the lowest Shwachman-Kulczycki score have also the longest standing colonization. They are treated with daily antibiotic inhalations and are given a course of IV antipseudomonas therapy twice a year. All other patients in this group have an IV course once a year and on the appearance of clinical symptoms they are given antipseudomonas drugs *per os*.

Our approach to pulmonary infection in CF patients has developed during the last 15 years into a more aggressive treatment consisting of IV antibiotics upon colonization with a microorganism, intensive physiotherapy and intensive nutrition monitoring [13–15]. Our impression is that the observed improvement in survival and clinical condition is accompanied by a marked improvement in the quality of life, all patients being able to participate in the usual life activities. It was with reluctance that we introduced the policy of regular visits the CF Centre at such short intervals as 4–8 weeks, because this could create feelings of dependence on the health services and have untoward psychological effects. However, we realized over the years that this policy leads to a very good contact of the patients and their families with the physician and all other members of the CF team which results in good compliance with every aspect of the agressive therapy which we apply.

References

1. The Cystic Fibrosis Genetic Analysis Consortium. Worldwide survey of the ΔF508 mutation. Amer J Hurn Genet 1990; 47: 354–359.
2. Tsul LC. The spectrum of cystic fibrosis mutations. Trends Genet 1992; 8: 392–398.
3. Thomasson MJ, Demko CA, Doershuk C. The Cystic Fibrosis. A review of pulmonary infections and interventions. Pediatr Pulmon 1987; 3: 334–351.
4. Zach MS. Lung disease in cystic fibrosis – an updated concept. Pediatr Pulmon 1990; 8: 188–202.
5. Szaff M, Holby N, Flensborg EW. Frequent antibiotic therapy improves survival of cystic fibrosis patients with chronic *Pseudomonas aeruginosa* infection. Acta Pediatr Scand 1983; 72: 651–657.
6. Rubio TT. Ciprofloxacin in the treatment of Pseudomonas infection in children with cystic fibrosis. Diagn Microb Infect Dis 1990; 13: 153–155.
7. Hodson M, Penratti A, Batten J. Aerosol carbenican and gentamycin treatment of *Pseudomonas aeruginosa* infection in patients with cystic fibrosis. Lancet 1981; 1: 1137–1139.
8. MacLusky I, Levison H, Goldman R, McLaughlin FJ. Inhaled antibiotics in cystic fibrosis: Is there a therapeutic effect? J M Pediatr 1986; 108: 861–865.
9. Hodson ME. Aerosol antibiotic therapy. Pediatr Pulmonol 1991: 6(Suppl): 76–78.

10. Desmond KJ, Schwenk WF, Thomas E, Bewdry PH, Coates AL. Immediate and long term effects of chest physiotherapy in patients with cystic fibrosis. J of Pediatr (1983) 103: 538–542.
11. Moams MB, Hunt GH, Rushworth R. Bacterial flora of the respiratory tract in patients with cystic fibrosis 1950–1971. Arch Dis Child 1972; 47:902–907.
12. Hoiby N. Microbiology of lung infections in cystic fibrosis patients. Acta Ped Scand 1982; suppl 301: 33–54.
13. Marks MI. The pathogenesis and treatment of pulmonary infection in patients with cystic fibrosis. J M Pediatr 1981; 98: 172–179.
14. Wood RE. Treatment of CF lung disease in the first two years. Pediatr Pulmon 1989; 4 suppl: 68–70.
15. Regelmann WE, Elliott GR, Warwick WJ, Clawson CC. Reduction of sputum *Pseudomonas aeruginosa* density by antibiotics improves lung function in cystic fibrosis more than bronchodilators and chest physiotherapy alone. Amer Rev Respir Dis 1990; 141: 914–921.

Cystic Fibrosis Pulmonary Infections.
Lessons from Around the World
ed. by A. Bauernfeind, M. I. Marks and B. Strandvik
© 1996 Birkhäuser Verlag Basel/Switzerland

CHAPTER 17
The General Approach to Cystic Fibrosis Pulmonary Infection in Italy

Rita Padoan, Alessandra Pianaroli and Annamaria Giunta

*Centre for the Diagnosis, Prevention and Therapy of Cystic Fibrosis, "De Marchi"
Pediatric Clinic, University of Milan, 20122 Milan, Italy*

Summary. Epidemiological data of the Italian CF population followed at Regional Health Care Centres are available from the Italian National Cystic Fibrosis Register. Data updated at 31.12.1994 are presented. It is important to note that over 29% of patients are older than 18 years, the cumulative survival probability being equal to 0.58 at 25 years. Both structures for the care of Italian CF patients (16 Regional CF Centres and CF support services) and the new laws passed in 1993 to facilitate care for CF patients are presented. Prevalence of *P. aeruginosa* and *B. cepacia* are shown together with various aspects of prevention of viral infections, and of *Pseudomonal* cross-infection. Therapy strategies against lung infection (early colonization, chronic infection; criteria for inhospital or home therapy) adopted in the different Italian centres are also presented. Prognosis and quality of life of Italian CF patients are improving thanks to this global approach to the disease.

Introduction

Over the last twenty years, the fact that the prognosis in patients with cystic fibrosis (CF) has certainly improved is due to the greater specialisation of Referral Centres and an improved approach towards nutrition and the treatment of respiratory infections. The greater physiopathological understanding brought about by the discovery of the gene, as well as the consequent adoption of more appropriate therapies for combatting the evolution of the underlying disease, are both factors which will surely lead to a further improvement in the prognosis of CF patients in the near future.

Over the last ten years, the epidemiology of CF has also changed. This study presents:

1) the epidemiological and survival data of the Italian CF patient population and information concerning the structure of CF health care services in Italy;
2) data concerning the incidence and prevalence of respiratory infections in the principal 'Italian CF Centres;

Correspondence address: Prof.ssa Annamaria Giunta and Dr.ssa Rita Padoan, Centro Fibrosi Cistica, Clinica Pediatrica "DE MARCHI", via Commenda 9, 20122 Milano, Italy.

3) information concerning the various approaches to the treatment of bronchopulmonary infections in the different Centres.

A further aim of the study is to describe the most recent laws approved in Italy in order to confront the problem of the prevention and treatment of CF.

Italian Epidemiological Data

The Italian National CF Register was founded on 1 January 1988 with the aim of making a census of all of the CF patients attending regional health care centres or support services. The register provides epidemiological data relating to the Italian CF population known to the Centres, but does not include those diagnosed patients who are being treated in pneumology departments and have never been referred to regional centres themselves [1].

By 31 December 1994, a total of 3046 monitored patients (males: 1582 (51.9%) and females: 1464 (48%)) had been reported to the national register. At that time, 2733 (90.9%) were living and 265 (8.8%) had died. The median age of the patients was 13.5 years.

Since 1988, the annual number of new CF diagnoses has been fairly constant at about 160, for a total of 1111 patients. Their age at diagnosis ranged from birth to 43 years, the mean being about 4 years. Fiftytwo percent of all of the patients were diagnosed during their first year of life; 5% at an age of more than 18 years. Neonatal screening had identified 21.2% patients and in a further 10.4% the diagnosis was based on the presence of meconium ileus.

Over the last few years, a great number of patients (most of whom were pancreatic sufficient) have been diagnosed during adolescence or adulthood. In many of these cases, the absence of pancreatic insufficiency undoubtedly delayed correct diagnosis, underlying the need for greater diagnostic sensitivity on the part of pneumologists treating adults: 40% of the adult CF patients diagnosed in Lombardy and referred to our centre were due to the diagnostic suspicion of only one single pneumologist.

At the present time, the national register does not collect data concerning the whole Italian CF population.

There are a number of reasons for the large number of "missing patients" (i.e. expected minus diagnosed patients):

1) only the patients referred to CF Centres were registered
2) the mean age at the time of diagnosis is 4 years, so many patients born after 1988 have yet to be diagnosed
3) a certain number of potential patients presumably died during their first months of life before CF was diagnosed (i.e. those who presented meconium ileus).

However, it is worth noting that the percentage of missing patients is lower in the few regions where a neonatal CF screening program for CF has been operating for several years (Veneto, Trentino Alto Adige, Lombardy); consequently, in 1992, a law was passed in Italy making neonatal CF screening obligatory also in those regions which had not already instituted such a programme (Law No. 104 – February 5, 1992).

The age and sex distribution of the patients who were alive on 31 December 1994 are shown in Table 1. It is worth noting that 29% of the patients were older than 18 years; there was no significant reduction with increasing age in the number of females. The median age at death increased from 13.7 years in 1988, to 20.7 in 1994. The rate of mortality reported by the Italian CF Register is 37 patients per year.

The Italian CF Register was started only a few years ago and current experience is limited; as a result, survival statistics will not be available until the next few years. However, in order to assess cumulative survival rates (using the actuarial life table method) in a large Italian CF population, a multicentre study was carried out in 1992 using data relating to 1650 patients (857 males) born between 1945 and 1991 collected in 10 regional CF Centres [2] by means of Cystic Fibrosis Data Base (CFDB) [3]. The diagnoses were made between 1952 and December 1991.

For the population as a whole, the cumulative survival probability was 0.91 at 5 years, 0.84 at 10 years, 0.75 at 15 years, 0.65 at 20 years and 0.58 at 25 years. However, a better survival curve was obtained when the patients born after 1980 are extrapolated from the whole population. The different distribution by age of the studied population at the end of 1979 and the end of 1991 is shown in Figure 1. During this 12 year period, the median age increased from 6.9 to 12 years, the change in age distribution being more apparent in teenage and adult patients.

The genetic analyses performed in 758 patients (46%) made it possible to calculate a 56% frequency of the ΔF508 mutation, with only 27.6% being ΔF508 homozygote and up to 24.4% carrying other or unknown mutations.

Table 1. Age and sex distribution of CF patients alive at 31 December 1994

Age	Males (%)		Females (%)	
0– ≤1 y	35	(2.45)	36	(2.76)
>1 y–5 y	274	(19.17)	271	(20.78)
6 y–10 y	266	(18.61)	252	(19.33)
11 y–15 y	274	(19.17)	234	(17.94)
16 y–18 y	178	(12.46)	129	(9.89)
>18 y	402	(28.13)	382	(29.29)
Total	1429	(52.28)	1304	(47.41)

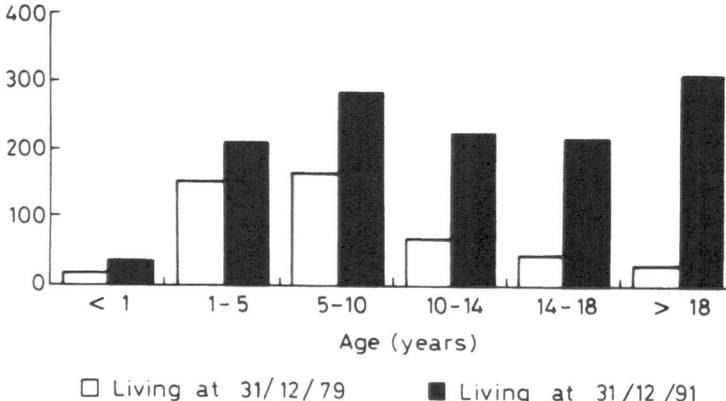

Figure 1. Age distribution of Italian CF patients living on 31/12/79 and on 31/12/91.

Structures for the Care of Italian Cystic Fibrosis Patients

At present, 12 of Italy's 19 Regions have Centres for the diagnosis, prevention and care of CF patients of pediatric age (Table 2); in the other regions, there are CF support services.

Only three regions have Referral Centres for adult patients; the adult CF patients resident in the other regions are referred to the specialist centres or support services organised in the pediatric hospitals.

Table 2. Structures for the care of cystic fibrosis in Italy in December 1994

Italian region	Operative units
(No. of resident CF patients*)	
Veneto (305)	2 Pediatric CF Centres
	1 Adult CF Centre
Lombardy (392)	1 Pediatric CF Centre
Piemonte/Val d'Aosta (163)	1 Adult CF Centre
Emilia Romagna (177) Lazio (273)	2 Pediatric CF Centres**
Sicilia (256)	
Tuscany$ (158) Marche (52)	
Campania (209) Puglie$ (142)	1 Pediatric CF Centre**
Sardinia (58) Liguria (71)	
Trentino Alto Adige (43)	
Umbria (17) Basilicata (34)	
Calabria (79) Friuli (58)	1 CF Support Service**
Abruzzi (50) Molise (12)	

*National Register data as of 31/12/92.
**Adult patients also accepted.
$Support Services also present.

Furthermore, the Italian Society of Pediatrics has, for many years, organised the Italian CF Working Group (ICFWG) of doctors involved in the care of CF patients in the various Regional Centres.

The ICFWG organises scientific meetings and national congresses on particular aspects of CF diagnosis, prevention and care, and has been responsible for numerous publications [4, 5] aimed at improving the standards of CF care in Italy. Other meetings with the same aims are organised on a regional or national basis by the various regional centres.

All of this allows a comparison to be made of the different policies and strategies adopted in the different regions and also makes feasible the possibility of setting up multicentre collaborative studies.

Respiratory Infections

The reported data were collected by means of a questionnaire sent to nine Italian Centres and subsequent telephone interviews on the part of two of the authors (RP and AP) designed to obtain as much information as possible concerning their different preventive strategies and treatment policies.

In the field of CF care, the treatment of respiratory infections plays a particular role. It has been widely demonstrated that the morbidity and mortality of the disease (i.e. the quality of life and prognosis) are largely determined by the evolution of chronic bronchopneumonia. Chronic lung infection by *P. aeruginosa* is the major therapeutic challenge in these patients.

However, such infections represent only the advanced stage of an evolutionary process which may begin immediately after birth with the onset of viral infections [6, 7]. Although CF lungs are histologically normal at birth, it has been shown that, in groups of patients genetically characterised as homozygotes for the presence of the DeltaF508 mutation, alterations are present as early as the time of diagnosis by positive neonatal screening. [8].

Furthermore, in our own experience at the Milan Centre, 7 out of 20 DeltaF508 homozygote patients (35%) diagnosed by means of neonatal screening between January 1990 and December 1993 needed prolonged hospitalisation in our CF centre for early and severe respiratory symptoms (lobar actelectasia, bronchiolitis) into the third month of life. Therefore, the early diagnosis of CF by means of screening not only allows prompt initiation of physiotherapy and the appropriate treatment of respiratory infections, but also the initiation of preventive strategies against viral infections.

Vaccination

Anti-pertussoid vaccination (which is not obligatory in Italy) is recommended in all patients during the first years of life; they are also immunised against measles. It is further recommended that they be given anti-influenza vaccinations with split virus antigens. For some years now, CF infants with RSV bronchiolitis have been prescribed aerosol-administered ribavirine according to the recent recommendations of the Committee on Infectious Diseases [9], but our still limited experience does not allow any evaluation of long-term prognosis in these patients. As far as varicella/herpes zoster infection is concerned, it seems to be opportune to administer a specific immunepassive prophylaxis or an antiviral treatment (acyclovir).

In any case, the usual praxis is to initiate antibiotic therapy (guided by the examination of sputum cultures and *in vitro* drug sensitivity) during the course of every viral infection.

Pseudomonas Infections: Prevention and Treatment

After the reports from Hoiby's group (Copenhagen CF Centre) [10–11], the problem of patient-to-patient transmission of *Pseudomonas* infection has been confronted by all of the Italian Centres. Particular attention is given to separating the patients with and without *B. cepacia*: the former are examined on different days in the Outpatients' Department or Day Hospital, or even in different Departments; they are usually admitted to single hospital rooms; spirometers and the aerosol devices for treatment administration are not the same as those used for the other patients; and the doctors and nursing staff wear disposable gloves and coats. In the majority of centres the patients with and without *P. aeruginosa* infection are also carefully separated, with visits to the Day Hospital or Outpatients' Department on different days. In addition to the recommended hygienic measures (frequent hand washing, coat changes, no coughing of patients in the Outpatients' Department if possible, and the use of masks during hospitalisation), some centres also carry out daily disinfections using a chloride solution for furniture and bleach for sinks.

Table 3 shows the prevalence of chronic *S. aureus* and *P. aeruginosa* infection in the CF patients attending the Milan Centre. As has already been reported in the literature [12], chronic *Staphyloccocus* infection is the most precocious, about 90% of the patients being colonised by the age of 5–9 years; but an approximately 85% prevalence of chronic *S. aureus* infection is also reported (Verona, Milan).

In the case of exacerbation, *S. aureus* and *H. influenzae* infections are treated with therapeutic cycles of 14–21 days. No prophylaxis against

Table 3. Prevalence of *P. aeruginosa* and *S. aureus* infection by age in the Milan CF Centre in 1993

Age group (years)	No. of pts	P. aer. (%)	S. aur. (%)
<1	16	6.25	50
1–4	58	24	74
5–9	67	45	93
10–14	62	52	92
15–18	61	59	90
19–30	58	67	84
>30	4	75	100

S. aureus is prescribed, and only in the case of chronic infection in severely compromised patients are short cycles or continuous treatment adopted. The drugs used to combat these infections are macrolides, cephalosporins and beta-lactamase resistant broad-spectrum penicillins (at the doses recommended for CF patients) [13].

The prevalence of chronic *P. aeruginosa* infection in the different age groups increases with age. In patients of >10 years, 50% of our patients show chronic infection; nevertheless it is interesting to note that a good 25% of the patients above the age of 30 years are free of *P. aeruginosa*. A possible explanation for this could be the fair number of CF patients with mild pulmonary disease and pancreas sufficiency diagnosed as adults and referred to the Milan Centre between 1990 and 1993 [14].

Table 4 shows the prevalence of chronic *P. aeruginosa* and *B. cepacia* infections in the different Italian Centres. The prevalence of *P. aeruginosa* infection varies from 45% to 68%, with an average age at onset of 7–12 years. The prevalence of *B. cepacia* in Italy varies from 0% to 14.5%, with an average age at onset of 12–17 years. At the Milan Centre, the prevalence of chronic *P. aeruginosa* infection over the last ten years has remained constant at 45–58%, the annual incidence being about 30% (reduced to 13.8% in 1993, 12 months after the policy of segregating patients with and without *P. aeruginosa* was adopted).

Early treatment at the first onset of *P. aeruginosa* infection has the greatest chance of eradicating the organism and therefore of delaying the onset of chronic infection. The adopted treatment regimens are substantially the same as those proposed by the Danish group [15], with quinolonic agents combined with aerosol-administered colimycin. The treatment is prescribed for home use, intravenous therapy and hospitalisation being reserved for the more clinically compromised patients.

For patients with chronic *P. aeruginosa* infection and moderate–severe respiratory impairment, the therapeutic protocols include intravenous treatment every 3–4 months and during pulmonary exacerbations. In the case of patients with moderate respiratory impairment ($FEV_1 > 70\%$) intravenous anti-*P. aeruginosa* treatment is used

Table 4. Prevalence of chronic *P. cepacia* and *P. aeruginosa* infections in some Italian CF Centres

CF Centre (Region)	No. of pts in follow-up (range of age)	Prevalence of *P. aeruginosa*	Mean age at chronic infection	Prevalence of *P. cepacia*	Mean age at onset
VERONA (Veneto)	654 (2 m – 44 y)	68%	6 y*	7%	17 y
MILAN (Lombardy)	327 (2 m – 43 y)	47%	10 y 7 m	1%	12 y
ROME (Lazio) Universita' La Sapienza	243 (1 m – 44 y)	60%	12 y	4.5%	15 y
ROME (Lazio) Osp. Bambino Gesu'	94 (2 m – 23 y)	4% < 6 y 77% > 6 y	7 y	2%	15 y
PARMA (Emilia Romagna)	104 (2 m – 34 y)	64%	8 y 11 m	1%	14 y
CESENA (Emilia Romagna)	73 (2 m – 33 y)	—	—	9%	
PALERMO (Sicily)	153 (2 m 41 y)	60%	—	0.65%	14 y
FLORENCE (Tuscany)	118 (4 m – 41 y)	47%	10 y	0	
GENOA (Liguria)	210 (4 m – 43 y)	56.5%	14 y 6 m	14.5%	15 y

*Sample of 44 patients diagnosed by positive newborn screening.
—Unknown.

only during clinical exacerbations. The antibiotics used are an amino-glycoside plus a beta-lactam, the dosage are those recommended for CF patients [16].

Although vigorous and frequent intravenous antibiotic courses have thus become the norm in the management of chronic pulmonary *P. aeruginosa* infections, frequent hospitalisations can lead to a poor quality of life for CF patients and may increase the risk of cross-infection from resistant strains. Consequently, the majority of Italian CF Centres have instituted home intravenous antibiotic therapy programmes in an attempt to reduce some of the problems associated with in-hospital treatment (stress, and the time spent away from school or work).

The Milan Centre began using home therapy for carefully selected patients in 1990 [17]. The selection criteria used are as follows: the presence of moderate–severe pulmonary disease requiring regular anti-*P. aeruginosa* therapy every three months; previous treatment in our hospital department with intravenous anti-*P. aeruginosa* therapy; familiarity on the part of patients and their families with intravenous drug administration and the problem of venous access, as well as their preference for home therapy; help and support, and no objection to home treatment on the part of the family doctor or the need for long-term antibiotic therapy (4–6 weeks).

We exclude home therapy in the case of patients with acute severe lung infections or complications (new atelectasias, emphysema or suspected ABPA) and/or the worsening of clinical condition with respiratory insufficiency; a history of allergy to beta-lactams; the need for invasive nutritional supplementation; families poorly compliant to the global CF therapy; and, of course, a preference for in-hospital treatment (those living a long way from the CF Centre, or who receive no help or support from their general practitioner).

For the intravenous access, we use either an intravenous cannula inserted into the forearm (flushed with 20 units of heparin/ml of saline in order to maintain patency between drug administrations) or, in patients who need continuous antibiotic therapy and nutritional supplementation, totally implantable intravenous access devices.

The patients and their families are trained in our CF Day Hospital, where the first antibiotic is administered; the therapy is continued at home by the patients themselves or their parents.

Antibiotics are prescribed for at least 14 days on the basis of sputum cultures and their antibiotic sensitivity. The availability of new elastomeric infusion devices saves time in drug preparation and eliminates possible errors and contamination.

Between January 1990 and April 1993, 52 CF patients aged 2–34 years (median 17 years), with a mean chest X-ray score (Chrispin–Norman score) of 22 (range 11–31) [18], underwent a total of 104 i.v.

Table 5. Efficacy and safety in home therapy (34 antibiotic courses, January–April 1993)

	Pre-treatment	Post-treatment	P(*)
ESR (mean)	41.8	27.4	<0.001
(range)	(2–90)	(3–102)	
PCR (mean)	21.7	11.1	<0.001
(range)	(<3–74)	(<2–49)	
WBC × 10^3/mm^3	9.976	9.592	n.s.
(range)	(4.3–16.15)	(4.7–21.2)	
Serum creatinine	0.74	0.74	n.s.
(range)	(0.42–1)	(0.51–1.01)	
AST U/l	17.3	20	n.s.
(range)	(7–34)	(7–35)	
ALT U/l	17.6	23.3	n.s.
(range)	(6–45)	(4–64)	

(*) Paired t test.

antibiotic courses. Home treatment has so far proved safe and clinically efficacious in the majority of cases (Table 5).

As regard to quality of life, as part of a study concerning the clinical characteristics of adult patients, which was carried out by the Milan Centre [14], the review of 55 adult patients diagnosed during the first years of life and regularly followed by the centre shows the satisfactory clinical condition of a population which has received such aggressive treatment over a period of years. Despite the fact that 42 of the 55 patients were chronically infected with *P. aeruginosa* (76.4%) mean FEV$_1$ (SD) and mean FVC (SD) were respectively 65.2% (23) and 80.6% (21) of predicted values. Most of them have a normal life, 80% working or attending a school.

Among the female patients, three pregnancies have led to the birth of healthy children with no post-birth deterioration in clinical condition.

We are currently carrying out a study aimed at comparing the quality of life of school-aged CF patients and that of their disease-free contemporaries with similar socio-economic backgrounds.

New Laws in Italy

On 23 December 1993, the Italian Parliament passed Law No. 548 "Provisions for the prevention and care of cystic fibrosis". This law, which was published in the Official Gazzette on 30 December and came into force on 1 January 1994, requires the Regions to institute a number of provisions, a summary of which is given below.

Law No. 548
Article 1
. . .
2. Regional interventions . . . are aimed at:

   a) the primary prevention and prenatal/early diagnosis of cystic
      fibrosis;
   b) the care and rehabilitation of patients with cystic fibrosis;
   c) encouraging the provision of health information and education
      to patients, patients' families and the population as a whole
      concerning the care and prevention of cystic fibrosis;
   d) providing for the education and continuing professional train-
      ing of health-care and social welfare personnel;
   e) promoting research programmes designed to improve basic and
      clinical knowledge of the disease in order to update the possi-
      bilities of prevention, early diagnosis, care and rehabilitation.

Article 3
   1. The Regions shall provide free of charge the medical, technical and
      pharmaceutical materials necessary for aerosol therapy, physio-
      therapy and rehabilitation, enteral and parenteral nutritional ther-
      apy, and whatever else is considered essential for the home care
      and rehabilitation of cystic fibrosis patients.
   2. The Regions shall institute a specialised Regional Referral Centre
      which shall have the functions of prevention, diagnosis, the care
      and rehabilitation of patients, the direction and coordination of
      informational, educational, social and health activities, as well as
      of research into cystic fibrosis . . . with sufficient personnel and
      equipment in relation to the number of treated patients and the
      residential population as determined on the basis of epidemiologi-
      cal evaluations.

Article 5
   1. The Centres referred to in comma 2 of Article 3 shall provide for
      the care and rehabilitation of hospitalised, ambulatory, Day Hos-
      pital and home-treated cystic fibrosis patients.

Furthermore, the law sanctions the right of CF patients to be exoner-
ated from military service and the right to be authorised to practise
sporting activities (Art.8.7).

This law has the virtue that it considers the problems of providing CF
patients with health care as a whole, not only by unifying the albeit
partial and fragmentary existing provisions concerning patient care, but
particularly by guaranteeing the necessary flexibility for the acquisition
of the new methods made available to us by the continuous updating of

health techniques (especially the regulations governing home oxygen therapy and artificial nutrition which only a few Regions had previously controlled).

Conclusions

As the Italian population as a whole is increasing in number and becoming older, so the number of Italian CF patients is also increasing and their mean life expectancy is good. The prognosis and quality of life of the patients is improving and there is a good chance that new treatments will lead to further improvements.

As we see it, important aspects are the prevention of *Pseudomonas* cross-infections and early and regular treatment of chronic *Pseudomonas* infection. It is clear that the containment of the prevalence of *B. cepacia* infection to only 3 cases (about 1%) in the Milan Centre is a result of the careful separation of these patients.

One of the great advantages of the availability of a home therapy programme is the fact that antibiotic treatment can be initiated very early. It is our opinion that the careful selection of the patients, the training that they are given and their free access to the Home Care Service when necessary has improved their treatment (as can be seen by the fact that home therapy is preferred by the majority of them).

For the majority of CF Centres, the provision of adequate structures that guarantee the continuing care of adult patients remains an unresolved problem.

Nevertheless, the fact that almost all CF patients now have the possibility of attending a specialised Regional Centre, that neonatal screening makes early diagnosis possible and that, thanks to the recent Italian law, patients and their families no longer have to bear all of the frequently high costs of care will undoubtedly lead to a further improvement in the prognosis of Italian CF patients.

Acknowledgements

The authors would like to thank Dr. Miano (Cesena) Prof.ssa Marianelli (Florence), Dott.ssa Minicucci (Genoa), Dott.ssa Pardo (Palermo), Prof. Grzincich (Parma), Prof. Antonelli (Rome), Prof. Castro (Rome), Dr. Cazzola (Verona) for their cooperation.

References

1. Bossi A, Gagliardini R, Manca A, Zanda A, Miano A, Marianelli L et al. Experience of the Italian Register for Cystic Fibrosis. In: H Escobar, F Baquero, L Suarez, editors: Clinical ecology of cystic fibrosis. Proceedings of the 18th European Cystic Fibrosis Conference; 1993 May 21–26; Madrid (Spain). Amsterdam: Elsevier Science, 1993; 305–307.

2. Padoan R, Arban D, Cesana B, Gagliardini R, Manca A, Zanda M et al. Prognostic factors influencing cystic fibrosis survival in a large Italian population (1650 patients). Proceedings of the XIth International CF Congress; 1992 Aug 23–27; Dublin (Ireland) Book of abstracts MS6.
3. Bettinelli ME, Ceri S, Cancarini F, "Basi di dati." In: Informatica di base per la medicina. Ed Uses, 1990.
4. Gruppo di Lavoro per la fibrosi cistica della Societa' Italiana di Pediatria. Guida alla Terapia della Fibrosi Cistica. Milano, Giugno, 1990.
5. Gruppo di Lavoro per la fibrosi cistica della Societa' Italiana di Pediatria. La terapia delle complicanze meno comuni, gravi della Fibrosi Cistica. Firenze, Febbraio, 1986.
6. Wang EEL et al. Association of respiratory viral infections with pulmonary deterioration in patients with cystic fibrosis. N Engl J Med 1984; 311: 1653–1656.
7. Abman SH, Ogle JW, Butler-Simon N et al. Role of respiratory syncytial virus in early hospitalizations for respiratory distress in young infants with cystic fibrosis. J Pediatr 1988; 113: 826–830.
8. Mohon RT, Wagener JS, Abman SH, Seltzer WK, Accurso FJ. Relationship of genotype to early pulmonary function in infants with cystic fibrosis identified through neonatal screening. J Pediatr 1993; 122: 550–555.
9. Committee on Infection Disease. Use of Ribavirin in the Treatment of Respiratory Syncytial Virus Infection. Pediatrics 1993; 92: 501–504.
10. Pedersen SS, Koch C, Hoiby N, Rosendal K. An epidemic spread of multiresistant *Pseudomonas Aeruginosa* in a Cystic Fibrosis Center. J Antimicrob Chemoter 1986; 17: 505–509.
11. Hoiby N, Pedersen SS. Estimated risk of cross infection with *Pseudomonas aeruginosa* in Danish Cystic Fibrosis patients. Acta Paediatr Scand 1989; 78: 395–404.
12. Hoiby N. Haemophilus influenzae, *Staphylococcus aureus*, *Pseudomonas cepacia*, and *Pseudomonas aeruginosa* in patients with cystic fibrosis. Chest 1988; 94: 97–102 (Suppl.).
13. Strandvik B. Antibiotic therapy of pulmonary infections in Cystic Fibrosis. Chest 1988; 94: 146–149 (Suppl.).
14. Padoan R, Arban D, Costantini D, Marzano MT, Madonini E, Giunta A. Diagnosis of Cystic Fibrosis in the adult life. Proceedings of the 18th European Cystic Fibrosis Conference; 1993, May 21–26; Madrid (Spain); Book of abstracts PD75.
15. Pedersen SS, Koch C, Hoiby N. Prevention and early treatment of Pseudomonas Aeruginosa infection. In: SS Pedersen, N Hoiby, editors: Cystic Fibrosis, basic and clinical research. Proceedings of the 17th Annual Meeting of the European Working Group for Cystic Fibrosis; 1991 June 17–21; Copenhagen (Denmark), 135–144. Amsterdam: Elsevier Science.
16. Koch C, Pedersen SS, Hoiby N. Treatment of chronic Pseudomonas aeruginosa infection in cystic fibrosis: Effects and side-effects of antibiotic. A brief survey of the experience at the Danish CF Center. In: SS Pedersen, N Hoiby, editors: Cystic Fibrosis, basic and clinical research. Proceedings of the 17th Annual Meeting of the European Working Group for Cystic Fibrosis; 1991 June 17–21; Copenhagen (Denmark), 147–156. Amsterdam: Elsevier Science.
17. Padoan R, Marzano MT, Pianaroli A et al. Home care in patients with cystic fibrosis: intravenous antipseudomonas antibiotic therapy. Proceedings of the 2nd International Conference on Advances in Pulmonary Rehabilitation; 1992 November 2–4; Venice, 147.
18. Chrispin AR, Norman AP. The systematic evaluation of the chest radiograph in Cystic Fibrosis. Pediatr Radiol 1974; 2: 101–104.

Cystic Fibrosis Pulmonary Infections:
Lessons from Around the World
ed. by A. Bauernfeind, M. I. Marks and B. Strandvik
© 1996 Birkhäuser Verlag Basel/Switzerland

CHAPTER 18
The General Approach to Cystic Fibrosis Pulmonary Infection in Spain

Sira Carrasco[1] and Fernando Baquero[2]

[1]*Cystic Fibrosis Unit of the La Paz Children Hospital, 28046 Madrid.*
[2]*Cystic Fibrosis Unit of the Ramón y Cajal Hospital, 28034 Madrid, Spain*

Demography

The ACLFQ (Asociación Científica de Lucha contra la Fibrosis Quística) organization was generally working on the assumption of a total number of about 2000 patients for the whole country. The real number of well-identified patients currently registered in the different CF Units is 996. This figure is based on the data obtained by us from fifteen reference hospitals where the cases of smaller institutions are collected. The Social Security organization in Spain assures a practical 100% coverage of the population, so that only few clinically relevant cases are expected to remain undetected in children. The real number of cases needs to be documented by an extensive neonatal screening at national level.

Diagnosis

Neonatal screening with the serum immunoreactive trypsin test was only applied in short series. The discussion is still active on the interest of applying such technique at the country-scale. Suspected patients are submitted to hospitals by general pediatricians. Confirmatory CF diagnosis is always accomplished in large university hospitals by highly specialized personnel. Diagnosis is based on the presence of respiratory involvement, pancreatic insufficiency and/or familiar history, and a repeatedly (at least two times) positive sweat test (> 70 mEq/1), carried out by the Gibson and Cooke or more recently by the Wescor method. Prenatal diagnosis was only available from 1987 in Madrid and Barcelona [1]. In the La Paz Hospital series, the number of families with prenatal diagnosis was only 6/145.

Correspondence address: Sira Carrasco, Gastroenterology and Nutritional Service, Hospital Infantil La Paz, Paseo de la Castellana 261, 28046 Madrid, Spain.

Organization of Assistance to Cystic Fibrosis Patients

It has become clear that one of the most important factors in improving survival of CF patients has been the development of specialized units [2]. The location of these units in large hospitals is generally recommended, because a highly interdisciplinary team and accessibility to a wide variety of technology should be assured. One of the main advantages of the units is to provide a continuum in management from childhood to adolescence and into adult life. In Spain, nine official CF-Units have been appointed, four of them in Madrid. The largest are located in the La Paz Hospital in Madrid (157 patients), followed by the Valle de Hebrón Hospital in Barcelona (130) and Ramón y Cajal Hospital in Madrid (100). As an example, the CF-Unit in La Paz Children's Hospital is currently composed of paediatric pneumologists, and gastroenterologists; microbiologists, physiotherapists, dietists, psychologists and geneticists, and availability of consultation with cardiologists, endocrinologists and surgeons is assured. Only recently (two years ago) adult pneumologists were included in the unit. The leadership of most units is based on a paediatric gastroenterologist or pneumologist.

The patient's follow-up is generally provided every two-three months, but patients with acute problems are assisted immediately. Clinical evaluation, analytical and radiological studies are available the same day. Drugs used in therapy are provided free of cost at the hospital pharmacy: the current average yearly cost per patient has been calculated in the La Paz Hospital series to be about 1700 ECUs.

Microbiology

Sixty-five percent of the patients reviewed in this work were chronically colonized (more than three significantly positive cultures separated by at least 1-month interval) by *Pseudomonas aeruginosa*. This rate was not modified during the last five years. A worse clinical condition in patients colonized with mucoid *P. aeruginosa* if compared with those with non-mucoid isolates (FEV 51.8 versus 74.8; $p < 0.05$) was found in one of our hospitals (3). The more frequently found serotypes were 0:6 (27%), 0:3 (14%), 0:1 (10%) and 0:11 (8%). In this hospital, a relation of high-bacterial counts of *P. aeruginosa* colonization and clincal evolution was found. Four groups were established: 1) with bacterial counts never exceeding 10^6; 2) 1–3 sputum samples/year with more than 10^6; 3) 4–6 sputum samples/year with more than 10^6 and 4) persistently colonized with more than 10^6 *Pseudomonas aeruginosa*. The corresponding Tiffenau indexes were 75.7, 87.2, 66 and 45 respectively; which again suggests the importance of the bacterial charge in the pulmonary lung damage.

Sixty percent of the patients were chronically colonized by *Staphylococcus aureus*, being more frequently found among younger children. The percentage of chronic colonization by *Haemophilus influenzae* was 10%. The incidence of patients chronically colonized by *Burkholderia cepacia* was only 2%, but this organism was sporadically recovered in 15% of them, particularly among late adolescent or adult patients. *Stenotrophomonas maltophilia* was isolated in 31% of our patients, and chronic colonization was found in 9.6% of them. *Aspergillus* colonization is extremely frequent, particularly in the northern part of the country, where more than 50% of the patients are colonized (C. Vazquez, personal communication); in Madrid and Barcelona the rates are nearly 30% and lesser rates (below 10%) are found in the south and eastern regions. Most contributors to the national survey done to document these data attribute such high incidence to the use of aerosol therapy. In fact bronchopulmonar aspergillosis has increased in Spanish cystic fibrosis patients [4, 5].

Antibiotics

To document the current policy of use of antibiotics in cystic fibrosis in Spain, a survey was carried out in the Spanish cystic fibrosis units. In young children colonized by *Haemophilus*, the more frequently antibiotics used were amoxycillin-clavulanate, cefuroxime and cotrimoxazole; if *S. aureus* is present, amoxycillin–clavulanate, isoxazolyl–penicillins and cefuroxime. In some severe cases, fusidic acid was used with success. Most units prefer (in *P. aeruginosa* infection) antibiotic aerosol therapy with a CR60 high-pressure inhalation device. Antibiotics included in aerosol therapy are: colistin or ceftazidime or aztreonam in combination with tobramicin or gentamicin. Aerosol therapy is generally used continuously. In some Cystic Fibrosis Units, as in the Ramón y Cajal Hospital, the prescription of antibiotics is based on the results of quantitative bacterial cultures of bronchial secretions carried out in each patient once every three weeks. When the amounts of *P. aeruginosa* exceed 10^6 or 10^5 for *S. aureus* or *H. influenzae*, antibiotic therapy is instituted. Only a single Unit periodically uses intravenous ceftazidime treatment, every three months. Intravenous antibiotic therapy is only applied in the other Units in acute exacerbations. Fluoroquinolones were used from 1985, generally in children of more than five years, with excellent results and without major secondary effects.

The quantitative evolution of bacterial resistance to antimicrobial agents is regularly monitored in the patients. The main trend observed in recent years was the increase in *P. aeruginosa* isolates showing a derepressed chromosomal β-lactamase, and therefore with ceftazidime-aztreonam minimal inhibitory concentrations $> 16 \mu g/ml$: (14.9% in

1988 and 21.1% in 1992). One-tenth of the strains show imipenem resistance, mainly by the association of loss of outer membrane proteins and chromosomal β-lactamase derepression. Fluoroquinolone suscepti-bility was severely reduced (nearly 25% of resistant strains in 1992). On the contrary, tobramycin susceptibility rates remained stable (8% of resistance) during the last years. The susceptibility of *B. cepacia* isolates remained at rates of nearly 40% for ceftazidime, imipenem and to-bramycin, and higher (75%) for cotrimoxazole [6].

Clinical Aspects

The current clinical situation of CF-patients in Spain was analysed in a sample of 197 patients from two large Units in Madrid. The mean age was 12.12 years, with a range from 6 months to 48 years, and the male/female proportion of 1.18. The current Shwachman scores and the corresponding distribution by age groups are presented in Figure 1. Almost two-thirds of patients below 10 years old show an excellent Shwachman score, and this situation is maintained for at least 40% of patients even in the 15–20 years group. In adult patients, the increase in lower Shwachman scores becomes patent, but still most patients are located in the moderate degree of impairment.

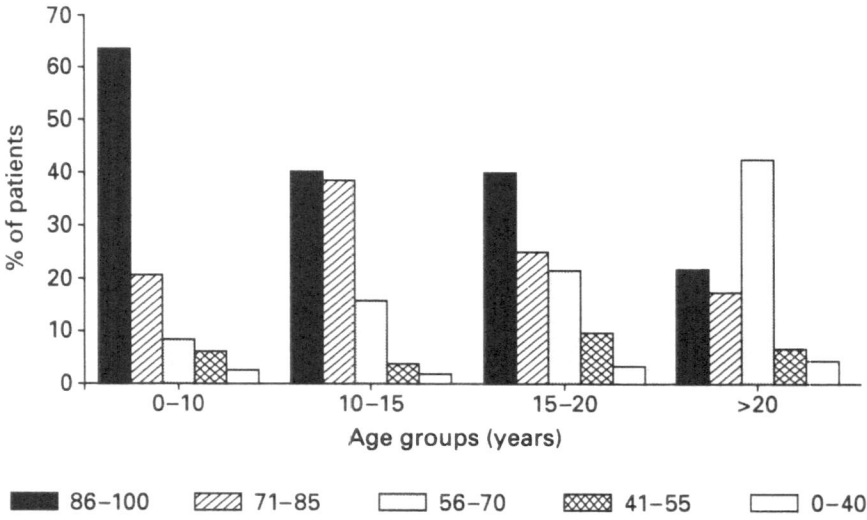

Figure 1. Shwachman scores in four age groups in 197 patients from two Cystic Fibrosis Units in Madrid.

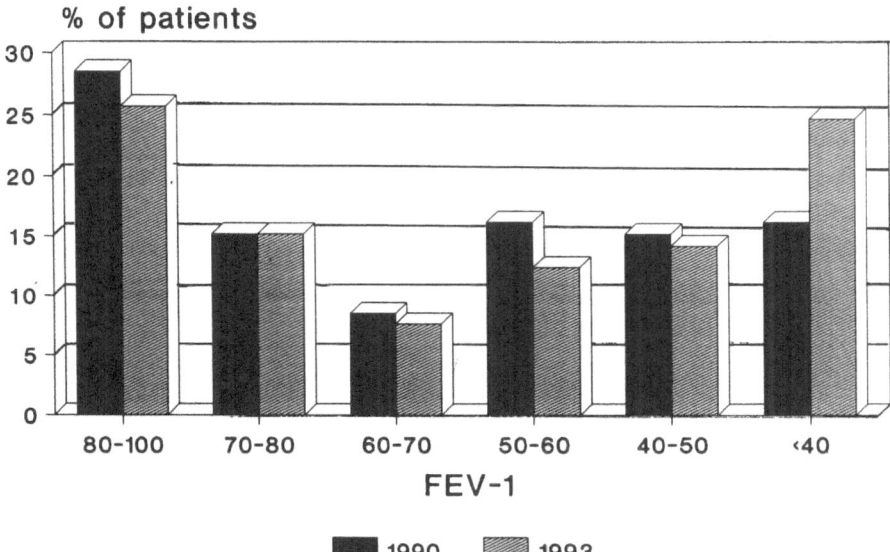

Figure 2. Three-years evolution of pulmonary function in 197 patients (see Figure 1), evaluated by the FEV_1.

Effort has been directed at maintaining the patients in the best possible nutritional status. Nutrition should be condsidered as one of the main factors contributing to a positive evolution and survival in these patients. The protocol of nutritional status evaluation includes weight and height measurements, skin fold and arm perimeter. In the La Paz Unit, 80% of the patients are located above the 10-percentile of height and weight.

The results of pulmonary function (FEV_1) evolution during three years in the same group of patients is presented in Figure 2. As is expected, a slow trend towards pulmonary deterioration occurs.

Most patients (144/157; 91.7%) never required hospitalization. From hospitalized patients, the average number of hospitalizations/year was 1.37, with a mean stay of 16.8 days. The more frequent indication for hospitalization was pulmonary infection exacerbation, but abdominal pain (DIORS) or gastrointestinal bleeding by oesophageal varices were others.

Quality of Life

The average quality of life of most Spanish CF-patients is considered as good or very good. Less than 5% of the patients maintain Shwachman scores under 30. These patients may require continuous monitoring at the hospital and have a substantial school or work loss. The rest usually attend regularly their academic or professional activities, with an average loss of seven days/year.

Acknowledgements

We would like to acknowledge the contributions of the Spanish cystic fibrosis units to this work, and are grateful in particular to the following investigators: Cobos N, Escobar H, Antelo MC, Vasquez C, Ferrer J, Sequeiros A, Perez Frias J, Perez Ruiz E, Sirvet, J. We would like to thank all those who provided us with data and opinions to be included in this work.

References

1. Casals T, Nunes V, Giménez J, Parra G, Estivill X. Diagnóstico prenatal de fibrosis quística en familias españolas utilizando marcadores del DNA: nuestra experiencia 1987–1989. An Esp Ped 1990; 32: 287–92.
2. Nielsen OH, Thomsen BL, Green A, Andersen PK, Hauge M, Schiotz PO. Cystic fibrosis in Denmark 1945 to 1985. Acta Paediatr Scand 1988; 77: 836–841.
3. Ballestero S, Escobar H, Villaverde R, Negredo P, Elia M, Ojeda-Vargas M, Baquero F. Microbiological parameters and clinical evolution in cystic fibrosis. 1993. In: H. Escobar, F. Baquero and L. Suarez, editors. Clinical Ecology of Cystic Fibrosis, Excerpta Medica, Amsterdam, p. 55–62.
4. Vazquez C, Elorz J, Gaztelurrutia I, Baranda F, Sojo A, Vitoria JC et al. Allergic bronchopulmonary aspergillosis in CF: increased prevalence associated with long-term antibiotic aerosol therapy. Proceedings of the Eighteenth European Cystic Fibrosis Conference; 1993 May 21–26: Madrid; p. 122.
5. Antelo MC, Barrio MI, Marin M, Carrasco S. Allergic bronchopulmonary aspergillosis in 12 patients with cystic fibrosis. Proceedings of the Eighteenth European Cystic Fibrosis Conference; 1993 May 21–26: Madrid; p. 118.
6. Ballestero S, Escobar H, Villaverde R, Elia M, Ojeda-Vargas M, Baquero F. Continuous monitoring of antimicrobial resistance in cystic fibrosis patients. 1993. In: H. Escobar, F. Baquero and L. Suarez, editors. Clinical Ecology of Cystic Fibrosis, Excerpta Medica, Amsterdam, p. 63–72.

Cystic Fibrosis Pulmonary Infections:
Lessons from Around the World
ed. by A. Bauernfeind, M. I. Marks and B. Strandvik
© 1996 Birkhäuser Verlag Basel/Switzerland

CHAPTER 19
Cystic Fibrosis in the Western Part of Germany: A General Review about Cystic Fibrosis Management

H.-G. Posselt

Zentrum der Kinderheilkunde, Abteilung für Allgemeine Pädiatrie I, Pädiatrische Gastroenterologie und Mukoviszidose, Klinikum der Johann Wolfgang Goethe-Universität, D-60590 Frankfurt/M, Germany

Introduction

In 1964 the German CF Association (Deutsche Gesellschaft zur Bekämpfung der Mukoviszidose e.V.) was founded in Erlangen. In the same year the first CF centers were set up in some university hospitals. Regular conventions of the CF Association led to a better education of German pediatricians and stimulated the founding of further CF centers throughout the former FRG, preferably in the university pediatric medical centers. In addition to these conventions directed both to doctors and lay people, regular scientific meetings for physicians interested in CF have taken place every year in Titisee/Black Forest since 1979. The aim of these meetings is to train young doctors in CF management, to standardize the medical care of CF patients in Germany and to discuss new therapeutic concepts. These Titisee meetings also initiated the start of a CF register of all patients treated in the participating CF centers.

Intensive contact was made with the International CF Association and in 1972 the annual meeting of the EC CF was organized in Schloss Reinhardshausen near Wiesbaden by Prof. U. Stephan, president of the German CF Association. Since 1980, every second year an international scientific CF meeting has been organized in Germany. This international meeting was initiated by Pforzheim D. Kaiser, the president of the German CF Association.

At present 53 specialized CF centers are engaged in the medical care of CF patients in the former FRG. Together with 23 in the former GDR, a total of 76 centers covers Germany with a dense network. (Figure 1).

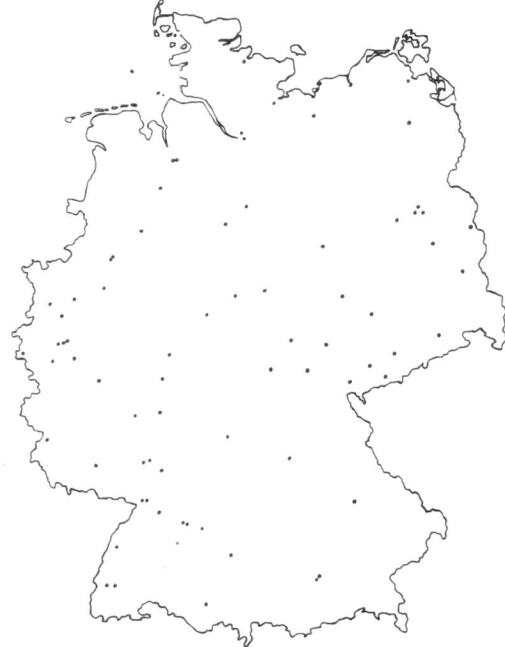

Figure 1. Cystic fibrosis outpatient wards in Germany as per 1 July 1991.

The Professional Care System for Cystic Fibrosis Patients in Germany

An intensive interaction exists between the German CF Association (Deutsche Gesellschaft zur Bekämpfung der Mukoviszidose) as a lay organization in which CF physicians have been engaged since the organization's foundation and the CF centers. As a part of the German CF Association there are specialized working groups in the field of physiotherapy, psychosocial care, nutrition and an advisory board on medical research.

The adult German CF patients are organized in the working group "living with CF" as a subgroup of the German CF organization.

In addition to the German CF Association there is a second CF association (CF-Selbsthilfe). This association is more engaged in psychosocial topics and local "self-help".

The German CF centers are mainly organized in association with university pediatric hospitals. There are also few centers in regional district hospitals and some specialized outpatient clinics in private practices. Experience with centers for adult patients has been gained in Hannover and Saarbrücken and such centers are being organized in München, Würzburg and Frankfurt. More than 90% of the adult German CF patients are still treated in pediatric hospitals. The number of patients,

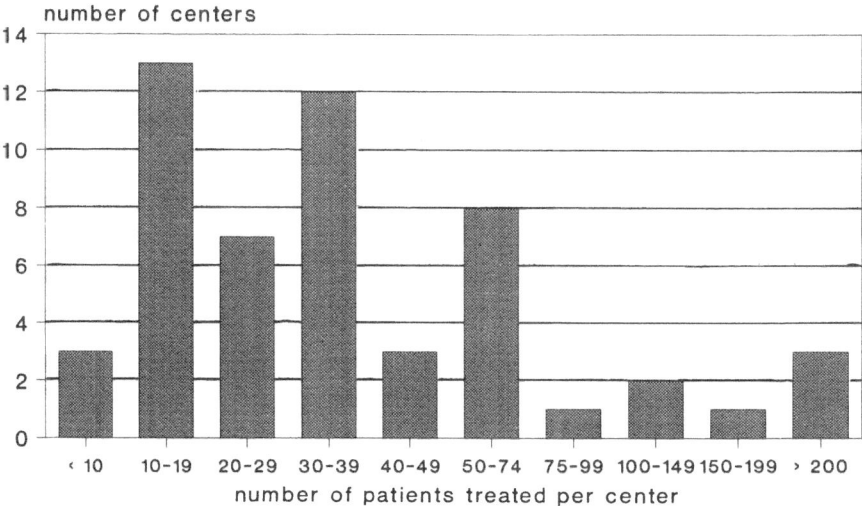

Figure 2. Number of patients treated in CF-centers. 53 centers from the former FRG as per 1 July 1993.

treated in each center, differs very widely from CF center to CF center. Figure 2 shows the size of 53 CF centers of the former FRG with the exception of West Berlin. There are six centers with more than 100 patients under regular care and three of them have more than 200 patients. The major five CF centers have been organized in a special working group for the last four years and some of the results will be presented and discussed in this paper. This working group was supported by the German ministry of research and technology.

The Monitoring System

For the German CF centers, the following has been accepted as a routine control system: Every patient should be monitored regularly by his CF center every three months, disregarding the natural course of the disease. In addition, acute checks are possible if necessary, depending upon the individual situation.

This concept has been accepted by all CF centers. The routine checks and their time intervals are given in Table 1.

Therapeutic Concepts

Medical treatment is paid for by patient's health insurance, irrespective of cost. The costs of mechanical aids like inhalation apparatus, oxygen concentrators etc. are also covered by the insurance.

Table 1.

Type of investigation	No. of controls per year
Hemoglobulin, WBC-count, ESR, CRP	by any control
AST, ALT, AP, GLDH, CHE	b.i.d.
Na^+, K^+, Ca^{2+}, Cl^-, P^{3-}	b.i.d.
Creatinine, urea, uric, acid	b.i.d.
Vitamin A, E, B; TPZ, PTT, Fibrinogen	1x
Blood sugar, HbA1c	b.i.d.
Serum IgA, $-$ G, $-$ M, $-$ E	1x
Blood gase analysis	b.i.d.
Urine analysis	1x
Spirometry	b.i.d.
Body plethysmography	1x
Sonography of abdominal organs	1x
Chest x-ray (frontal and lateral)	1x
x-ray of the left hand	1x (during growth)
Sputum analysis (microbiological)	by any control

Routine medication consists of pancreatic enzyme supplementation with enteric coated capsules or pellets for all pediatric insufficient patients, multivitamin supplementation, secretolytic therapy with oral administration of (Ambroxol or N-acetylcysteine) secretolytic chest physiotherapy, inhalation therapy with betamimetics and antibiotic treatment. In most centers, pancreatic enzyme supplementation is adapted to the need based upon stool-fat exretion. The daily dosage of enzymes is less than 10 000 U lipase/kg body weight in about 70% of all German patients. According to the results of a questionnaire analyzed in 1994, only 7.1% of all German patients are treated with more than 20 000 U lipase kg/body weight and day. Under this treatment regimen no colonic structure has so far been observed in Germany [1].

Oral secretolytic therapy is performed in most centers. Inhalation therapy with these medications is considered obsolete. In addition to the regular chest physiotherapy, inhalation with betamimetics is well accepted in most centers. The physiotherapy program is adapted to the individual situation of each patient and his age. Chest clapping and postural drainage is done only in selected cases. Most common is chest vibration with smaller infants, positioning of the chest and body with gymnastic (Keil'sche Körperstellungen), autogenic drainage and sport. In addition, inhalation with the pep-mask is accepted. Inhalation of amiloride and rh-DNase (human recombinant) is as yet done on an experimental basis or under study control.

The antibiotic therapy regimen differs from center to center. Only a few centers treat their patients continuously with a S. aureus oriented medication since diagnosis. This regimen has been favoured by one Munich center (Dr. V. Haunersches Kinderspital).

More accepted is an interval medication of acute infection guided by sputum analysis. In more advanced diseases and in patients colonized with *Pseudomonas aeruginosa* the regular intravenous treatment with antibiotics is becoming more accepted in Germany.

This therapy is becoming more common on an outpatient basis. The Intermate[R]-system provides a safe and time-saving possibility of home-parenteral antibiotic therapy for patients and their physicians. This system has been used in the Frankfurt CF center since July 1993 in more than 150 treatment courses without problems and is well accepted by patients and their parents.

Antibiotic inhalation therapy mostly with tobramycin and in some patients with colomycin or ceftazidim is a routine therapy in patients with more advanced lung damage. About 40% of the elder patients are on regular inhalation therapy according to the results of the German multicenter-study [2]. In a double-blind placebo-controlled study, the German CF multicenter study group could demonstrate a benefit of tobramycin inhalation in patients newly colonized with *Pseudomonas aeruginosa* in eradication of this bacterium from the lung [3]. These results have to be confirmed by other studies with a larger patient group.

The therapy concepts for CF-related complications like pneumothorax, distal intestinal obstruction syndrome, diabetes and others are similar to the regimens accepted worldwide.

Complications of the hepatobiliary system were for a long time considered untreatable [4]. The incidence of these complications is controversial and depends on intensity of diagnostic procedures and terms of definition. Since 1989 treatment of these patients with ursodeoxycholic acids has been proposed [5].

Table 2. Changes in standard liver function tests under 6-month treatment with UDCA (10 mg/kg/Day) mean ± sem

Parameter	Number of patients	Before UDCA	After UDCA	Improvement (%)	Significance (p <)
GLDH (U/l)	18	29.9 ± 5.5	12.5 ± 3.6	58	0.006
GGT (U/l)	20	90.7 ± 16.1	40.3 ± 5.1	56	0.059
ASAT (U/l)	20	35.8 ± 3.5	22.8 ± 3.0	36	0.006
ALAT (U/l)	20	45.2 ± 7.7	28.2 ± 4.1	38	0.032
AP (U/l)	20	738 ± 114.2	534 ± 47.5	28	0.021
CHE (U/l)	18	4907 ± 341	4417 ± 384	10	0.09

In a randomized double-blind, placebo-controlled multicenter study we could demonstrate the benefit of 20 patients treated with the verum in comparison to the placebo-group [6]. As far as we know, this is the first placebo-controlled study in this field.

Since that time all patients in the Frankfurt center and most of the patients in Germany have been treated with ursodeoxycholic acid in a dosage of 15 mg/kg if signs of alterations of the hepatobiliary system are present. Since that time no further patients with advanced liver damage or portal hypertension could be detected in the Frankfurt cohort and even the liver injury of those patients with advanced liver disease remained unchanged in a stable phase. Table 2 shows the significant change in liver function tests under URSO-Therapy during the placebo-controlled double blind study.

Diagnostic Situation and Age Distribution

The prognosis of CF patients depends upon genetics and age at diagnosis but mostly upon the regular care in an experienced CF center. The intensity of daily therapy including encouraged self-treatment in physiotherapy, intensive nutritional therapy and antibiotic therapy, plays the most important role in the battle for a better prognosis of these patients. During the last ten years of regular analysis no change was possible with regard to the age of newly diagnosed patients. Only for a short period was the BM-Test (meconium test for albumin analysis) performed in Germany. Table 3 illustrates the diagnostic situation of the CF patients during the last ten years. Only about 55% of the patients were diagnosed before the age of six months, approx. 75% to 78% diagnosed at

Table 3. Diagnosis of CF in the former FRG

Year of diagnosis	Number of patients	Age at diagnosis		
		< 6 months	< 3 years	< 10 years
1982/83	144	56%	82%	97%
1983/84	159	50%	75%	87%
1984/85	138	58%	80%	95%
1985/86	162	53%	81%	96%
1986/87	181	50%	78%	89%
1987/88	152	51%	76%	92%
1988/89	157	57%	81%	93%
1989/90	168	45%	70%	88%
1990/91	167	50%	77%	94%
1991/92	76	63%	89%	95%
1992/93	73	48%	82%	93%

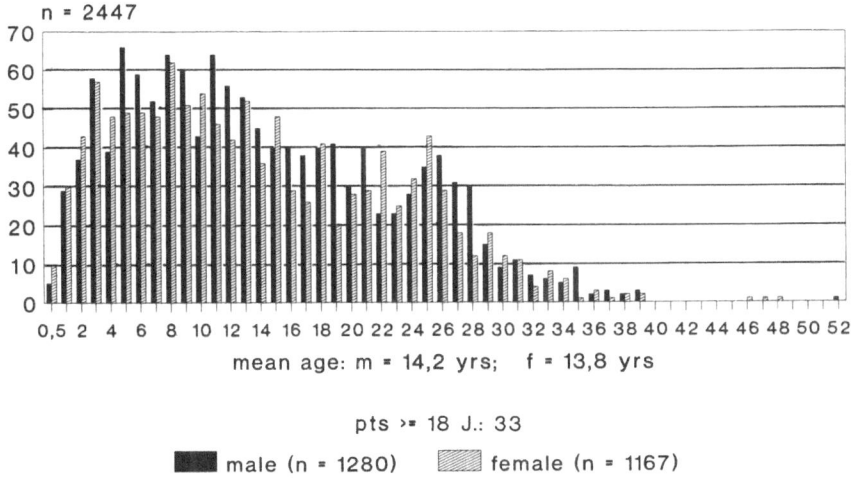

Figure 3. Age distribution of CF patients under regular care in 53 centers as per 1 July 1993.

the end of the third year of life and every year about 8% of all newly diagnosed patients are older than ten years. This situation is certainly unsatisfactory.

Also for the German CF patients, the goal to treat all or most patients in specialized CF centers has not been obtained. Calculated on the basis of the well accepted incidence of CF (1:2500 newborns) and calculated on the CF patients' expectation of life in the CF centers of München and Frankfurt we could demonstrate that only one 50% of the postulated patients were under regular care in the specialized CF centers in 1984 [7]. This situation has not changed over the last few years. On the other hand a great fluctuation of patients was noted. Thus 1229 living patients were lost from regular care of the CF centers during the last ten years. The need for regular care in specialized centers has not been accepted by all German pediatricians.

Over the last decade the number of continuously controlled patients increased from 1548 to 2447, while that of the number of specialized CF centers increased from 44 to 53. During this time there remained a slight difference between the percentage of female and male patients (approx. 45% female and 55% male).

The mean age of both sex groups was similar: in 1993 13.8 years for females and 14.2 years for males. The percentage of adult patients treated in the CF centers increased steadily from 16.3% in 1983 to 33.5% in 1993. Figure 3 demonstrates the age distribution of 2447 regularly controlled patients from the CF centers of the former FRG.

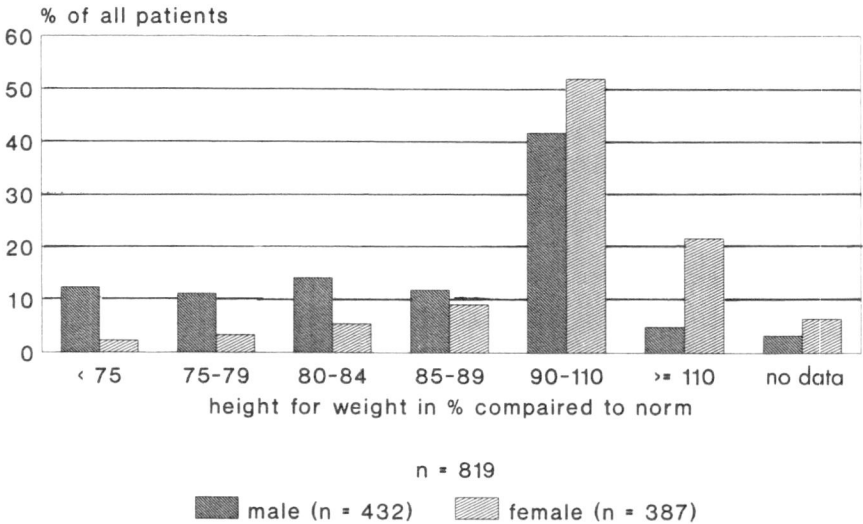

Figure 4. Weight for height distribution in adult CF patients.

Health and Psychological Status of German Cystic Fibrosis Patients

A more or less expressed malnutrition reflects the pulmonary situation in most patients — even when nutritional interventions have been maximised during the last years to prevent malnutrition. Analysis of the nutritional status shows that *ca* 60% of all CF patients are well nourished whilst the remaining 40% show different stages of malnutrition. The analysis of 819 adult patients presented a surprising result: Approximately 80% of the adult females were within the normal range compared to 50% of adult males. Consequently three times more male patients showed a more or less expressed marasmic malnutrition (Figure 4).

Lung function tests (FEV₁) showed normal results in 40% of all patients and 13.8% showed severe pulmonary damage with extremely reduced lung function, i.e. less than 35% of the predicted normal range. Exact analysis of lung function in the German multicenter study confirmed these results. The varying percentage of malnourished patients of the participating centers did not correlate with the lung function tests of those patients.

These results confirm the observation that nutritional concepts may reduce malnutrition in patients even with severe lung damage but the pulmonary function remains poor.

The percentage of CF patients in the former FRG colonized with *Pseudomonas aeruginosa* differs from those in the former GDR. 60.4%

of all patients from the former FRG are colonized with *P. aeruginosa* and the perentage increased to 77.4% in the cohort of adult patients. These results are comparable to other countries of the Western hemisphere.

In addition to *P. aeruginosa* other species of *Pseudomonas* were detected in about 15% of all patients. *Pseudomonas cepacia* plays a minor role in German patients and epidemics with this have so far not been reported from German centers.

In contrast to the increasing percentage of *P. aeruginosa*-positive patients with age, the German multicenter study could show that the colonization with *S. aureus* remained stable with about 40% for all age-groups. Our own experience is that many CF patients treated with *S. aureus* orientated antibiotics showed persistent colonization with this type of bacterium even after several treatment courses. So the question arises whether some patients should be declared as having a chronic colonization with *S. aureus* like the older patients colonized with *Pseudomonas aeruginosa*. It is also questionable whether these patients benefit from continuous medication with antibiotics directed against *S. aureus*.

The German multicenter study could demonstrate a markedly reduced number of patients with elevated serum IgG levels in this center which performed a consequent *S. aureus*-directed prophylaxis with antibiotics. On the other hand the percentage of *Pseudomonas aeruginosa*-colonized patients in the younger age groups was slightly increased compared to the other centers. These data remain to be interpreted.

The prognosis of CF patients has continuously increased in the last decades. Corresponding to this observation the mean age of death increased in German CF patients from 13.4 years in 1985 to about 20 years in 1993. Even if most patients died as adults, there remains a number of patients with a very fulminant disease course.

On the other hand several patients come too late with early severe lung damage under regular care caused by delayed diagnosis and/or several years of inadequate therapy.

Living Conditions, Family Status and Educational and Occupational Status of Adult Cystic Fibrosis Patients in Germany

From 819 adult patients out of the 2447 patients from 53 CF centers data exist about the family status. 80.3% of females and 91.4% of males are single and 18.1% of females and 7.2% of males are married. 1.3% of females and 0.7% or males were divorced. In 22 families one or more healthy children were born to women with CF. From the group of adult patients, 60% of females and 66% of males live with their parents; on the other hand 39% of females and 31% of males are living on their own. This might reflect a difference in self-confidence between both sexes and might reflect greater problems in males in forming a solid partnership.

The educational and occupational situation of the adult patients reflects the policy of the German CF centers. First implication is to give the best education to the patients so that they can learn the so-called "white-collar professions". So it is not surprising that about 45% of all adults are at school, university or in other education. About 35% are professionally qualified. Only 2.5% of all patients are pensioners and 11.4% are unemployed. The percentage of unemployment is higher than in the normal German population but is similar to other patient-groups with chronic diseases.

Conclusions

In total the statistical analysis shows a situation of the German CF centers similar to other countries of the Western hemisphere. Medical care and life expectation is comparable with other countries. More effort should be made to reach all CF patients and to maintain them under regular care in specialized CF centers. In addition, it is time to create CF centers for adult patients throughout the FRG to offer adequate care for this patient group.

References

1. Posselt H.-G. Colonic structures in CF-patients in Germany. Results of a questionnaire. Consensus Conference on the Management of Cystic Fibrosis. Berlin, Heidelberg: Springer-Verlag, 1995, pp. 3–5.
2. Von der Hardt H, Kühn L. The multicenter cystic fibrosis database – clinical status and laboratory data. Poster: presented at the Cystic Fibrosis Symposium, March 1994.
3. Ratjen F, Steinkamp G, Döring G, Bauernfeind A, Wiesemann HG, Von der Hardt, H. Prevention of chronic *Pseudomonas aeruginosa* colonization in cystic fibrosis by early Tobramycin-inhalation therapy. Results of a placebo controlled double-blind multicenter study. Pediatric Pulmonology, Suppl. 10, Sept. 1994, p. 255.
4. di Sant' Agnese PA, Hubbard VS: The hepatobiliary system. In: Cystic Fibrosis. Lynn M. Taussig, Editor. New York: Thieme-Stratton Inc, 1984.
5. Colombo C, Setchell K, Podda M *et al*. Effects of ursodeoxycholic acid therapy for liver disease associated with cystic fibrosis. J. Pediatr.: 1990; 117: 482–489.
6. Bittner P, Bender SW, Bertele-Harms RM, Ott H, *et al*.: Efficacy of ursodeoxycholic acid in cystic fibrosis: A placebo-controlled double-blind trial. Lancet (In press).
7. Posselt H.-G, Bender SW. Zur Situation der Mukoviszidose in der Bundesrepublik Deutschland. Atemw.-Lungenkrkh. 1984; 10: 345–350.

Cystic Fibrosis Pulmonary Infections:
Lessons from Around the World
ed. by A. Bauernfeind, M. I. Marks and B. Strandvik

CHAPTER 20

The General Approach to Cystic Fibrosis Pulmonary Infection in the Eastern Part of Germany: Patients' Register and Clinical Research

Peter Wunderlich[1], Klaus-Dieter Paul[1] and Bärbel Wiedemann[2]

[1]*Children's Hospital and* [2]*Institute of Medical Informatics and Biometry of the Faculty of Medicine "Carl Gustav Carus" of the Technical University of Dresden, D-01307 Dresden, Germany*

Summary. This chapter presents a summary about the patients' register of cystic fibrosis in the former German Democratic Republic in Dresden. It includes data of 1482 persons, among them 1060 living CF patients. The proportion of *Pseudomonas aeruginosa* positive findings increased steadily from year to year and amounts now to 32.9%. Of the *P. aeruginosa* positive patients, 50% were infected up to the age of 12.55 years. Besides these register data the authors summarize clinical studies which were performed at the Children's Hospitals of Dresden and Leipzig. These concerned neonatal screening, a follow-up study of CF-patients detected by this screening, genetic diagnostics, inhalation therapy with azlocillin and the retrospective study of a group of patients from Leipzig.

Introduction

Living and working in Eastern Germany, the former German Democratic Republic (GDR) – a separated, so called socialist country – was impaired by the lack of personal and scientific communication. This was true also for CF research.

Only a few doctors and scientists were allowed to travel abroad and to take part in scientific meetings in foreign countries, including Western Germany. They reported the latest news.

We have seen the advantages and disadvantages of a centralized state health care system. We have to make the best of our specific situation [1]. On the one side it was very difficult to overcome the overwhelming deficiencies and to get new drugs or new apparatus. This led to the development of a specific medical subculture, a situation which often required improvisation or new methods for the same goal.

On the other hand we could get official support for special research projects which corresponded to the official domination of organisation and statistics. There were for example no problems with individual

Correspondence address: Prof. Dr. med. habil. Peter Wunderlich, Children's University Hospital, Dept. of Bronchopneumology, Fetscherstr. 74, D-01307 Dresden, Germany.

rights concerning the privacy of statistic data. So we could get without difficulty the authorities' approval for a planned national patients register which was started in 1978.

The organization of a country-wide neonatal screening test was another project which would have been impossible without the strong aid of the state authorities in a centralized state.

There was a strong hierarchy, from the GDR Ministry of Health to every scientific association (e.g. the Paediatric Association) and its subgroups. The "Arbeitsgemeinschaft zur Bekämpfung der Mukoviszidose" (Working Group to Combat Cystic Fibrosis) was founded in 1968. It organized many scientific activities and annual conventions. In 1972 it became a member of the European Working Group (EWGCF) and invited it to the 7th Annual Meeting in Dresden in 1977. H.-J. Dietzsch was the president of this major event. The very stimulating meeting became a starting point for personal contacts over the "wall" and for further research projects, among them tests with new drugs, especially antibiotics.

The Cystic Fibrosis Patients' Register

The central patients' register of the former GDR was started in 1978. The results have been reported several times [2, 3, 4, 5]. The number of included patients increased from year to year. Up to the end of 1985 it amounted 1069 CF-patients. Of these patients, 266 were deceased and 803 (75.1%) were still alive and under special outpatient care in one of the 26 CF centres of the GDR [4]. 10.6% of these patients were 18 years of age or older. The eldest CF patients at that time were 45 and 47 years old. The diagnosis of CF was established in 6.9% because the family's history gave a suspicion for CF, 17.2% of patients presented with gastrointestinal symptoms, a further 37.5% with both gastrointestinal and pulmonary symptoms, 13.7% of them only with pulmonary symptoms and 9.1% had a meconium ileus. 15.6% of all CF patients were detected by the later described centralized neonatal meconium screening test.

In comparison to the first comprehensive report [3] of the CF register the following positive results could be stated:

- increase of the number of surviving CF patients from 621 to 803 (182 more living CF patients),
- rise of the number of deceased CF patients only by 90 (from 176 to 266),
- further shift of the age distribution to the higher age groups: increase of the median age from 6.9 to 9 years,
- rise of the number of adult CF patients (18 years of age or older) from 19 to 85,

– increase of the median age at death from 4.8 to 6 years and
– increase of the mean life expectancy of CF patients to 25 years of age
  [4] (see Figure 2).

The work at the CF register was steadily continued, even after the German reunification. In October 1991 it included data from 932 living and 391 deceased patients. Up to the 11th October 1993 many changes occurred. Some patients were lost from the outpatient treatment or regular consultations, or went to other doctors. From October 1992 to October 1993 we received reports about 20 new cases of CF. The data from Western Berlin (clinic Heckeshorn) have now been included (with a further 9 new cases from the last year). The register for eastern Germany (now called the "new German States") now lists 1482 persons, among them 1060 (= 71.5%) living CF patients [5]. 873 CF patients (52.8% males) are under regular control. Their mean age is now ¦3.12 ± 7.61 years for males and 14.06 ± 7.8 years for females. Only ¦6.5% are under the age of 7 years and 25% adults (older than 18 years). Figure 1 shows the actual age distribution of all living patients. The important reduction of the birth rate in eastern Germany in the last four years and the possibilities of prenatal diagnosis also resulted in a strong decrease of the number of new CF cases. In the 10 years from 1971 to 1980 in the former GDR altogether 2 107 725 children were born, among them 534 cases of cystic fibrosis. So a mean incidence of 0.0253% or 1:3947 could be calculated [4].

Wachtel made a retrospective analysis of the causes of death among the patients in the CF register [6]. For 198 of 264 patients who had died

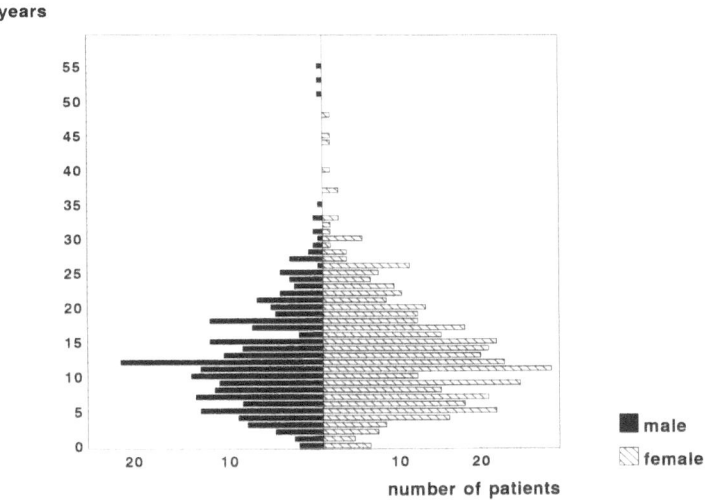

Figure 1. Age distribution of 873 CF-patients. Cystic Fibrosis Register. Dresden 1993.

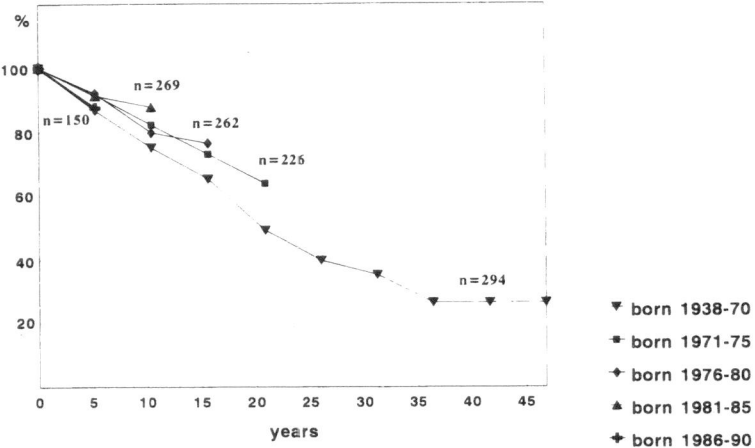

Figure 2. Cumulative survival rates of different cohorts (patients without meconium ileus). Cystic Fibrosis Register. Dresden.

by the end of 1985 detailed records were available. They showed 83.5% of deaths were caused by lung destruction and respiratory insufficiency. There were two cases of pneumothorax and one case of severe haemoptysis. 11.2% of deaths were attributed to a meconium ileus and 5.3% to a liver cirrhosis with bleeding from oesophageal varices, or hepatic coma.

Microbiological Findings

In the last 10 years more and more bacteriological data were reported. In the period from 1985 to 1987 for 55.3%, from 1988 to 1990 for 32.9% and for 1991 to 1993 only in 16.7% no microbiological findings were available per year. For the patients from Heckeshorn only 11% were without bacteriological data.

With greater age of the patients, an increase in *P. aeruginosa* carriers was found. *P. aeruginosa*-positive findings rose from 6.7% (for 1979 to 1981) to at least 27.4% (1991 to 1993) for all patients and 51.3% in patients from Heckeshorn.

In relation to only those patients in whom bacteriological data were reported the portion of *P. aeruginosa* increased even more:

1979 to 1981	18.7%
1982 to 1984	30.6%
1985 to 1987	28.2%
1988 to 1990	23.9%
1991 to 1993	32.9%

From these figures we calculated a cumulative non-pseudomonal infection rate which takes into account the patients' age with Cox-regression (Figure 3). 50% of the *Pseudomonas*-positive register patients received their infection up to the age of 12.55 years. There are no sex-dependent differences [5].

Figure 4 shows the influence of the infection with *P. aeruginosa* upon the life expectancy of older than five years old CF-patients. It can be seen that over the age of 13 years patients with *P. aeruginosa* infection have a decreased life expectancy.

In another retrospective study [7] the course of chronic lung infection in CF was investigated with the aid of the patients' register. For the

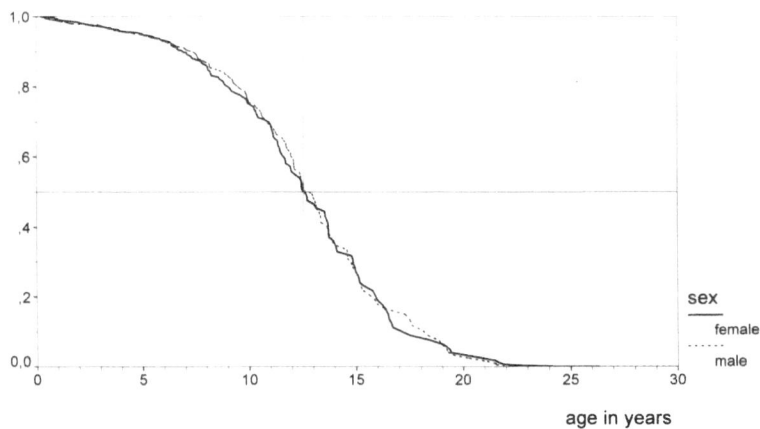

Figure 3. Cumulative non-infection rate with *P. aeruginosa*. Cystic Fibrosis Register. Dresden 1993.

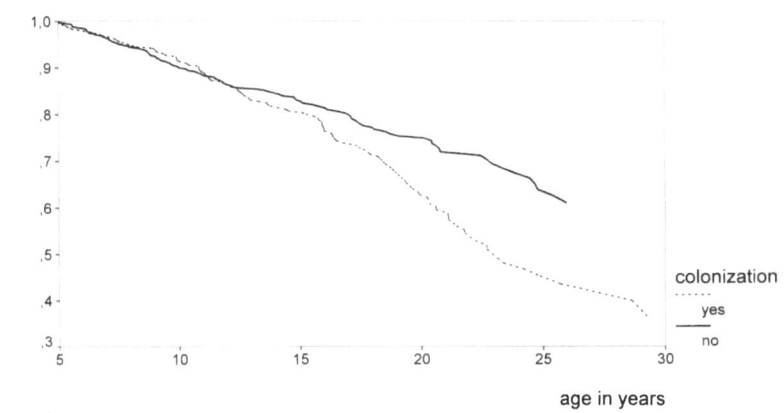

Figure 4. Survival function and *P. aeruginosa* (> = 5 years old, n = 1147). Cystic Fibrosis Register. Dresden 1993.

Table 1. Comparison of CF-patients with permanent lung infection – for longer than 4 years
– by either *Staphyloccocus aureus* or *Pseudomonas aeruginosa* [7]

	S. aureus		*P. aeruginosa*
Number of patients	27		19
Sex (male/female)	16/11		5/14
Mean duration of antibiotic treatment (days per year)	89	(p < 0.05)	199.7
Mean duration of inpatient treatment (days per year)	13.9	(n.s.)	17.3
Body height (HOLT score)	−0.46 ± 1.12	(n.s.)	−0.21 ± 1.10
Body weight (HOLT score)	−1.49 ± 1.44	(n.s.)	−2.07 ± 1.39
Mean X-ray score (SHWACHMAN/KULCZYCKI)	3.5		4.5

period from 1981 to 1985 microbiological data from sputum and/or
bronchial secretions of altogether 1062 patients were available. They
showed an infection rate of 58.7% by *S. aureus* and of 27.8% by *P.
aeruginosa*. The rate of mixed infections amounted to 7.0%. During the
above mentioned five-period the mortality rate in the group of patients
with *Pseudomonas* colonisation was doubled in comparison to the group
with staphyloccal colonisation (32/295 versus 33/623). The mean age of
the deceased patients was 11.2 years in the *Pseudomonas* group and 8.9
years in the *Staphyloccocus* group. Only in 27 patients the chronic
infection with *S. aureus* lasted for four or more years and in 19 patients
a permanent infection of the same duration with *P. aeruginosa* was
found. Table 1 shows the comparative data of these patients. Only the

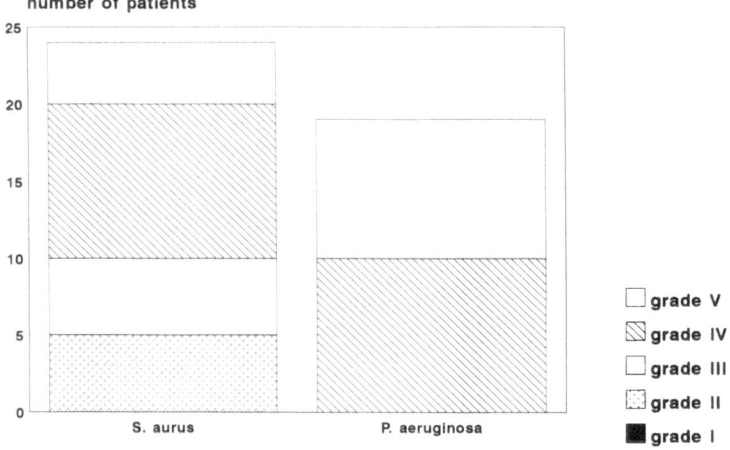

Figure 5. Cystic fibrosis patients with long lasting chronic pulmonary infections. Shwachman-
Kulczycki score (lung X-ray part).

mean duration of antibiotic treatment was significantly higher in the *Pseudomonas* group. The Shwachman–Kulczycki score of the pulmonary x-ray showed more severe changes (Figure 5).

Retrospective Study of a Group of Patients from Leipzig

There are now 300 CF-patients in Saxony, among them 72 (24.0%) older than 18 years. Our clinic is responsible for a third of them [8]. Kunze [9] made a retrospective study of 148 CF-patients who were born between the years 1961 and 1989 and treated at the Children's University Hospital of Leipzig from 1967 to 1991. 51 of these patients remained up to now in the outpatient treatment, 37 moved to other places and 14 to a CF outpatient department. 46 CF-patients (31.1%) have died in the meantime. They were at death between 2 days and 26 years old, their mean age being 5.17 years.

For the evaluation of the microbiological data the patients were divided into two groups, those born before and after the year 1977. From CF-patients born before 1977 *S. aureus* was cultured in 57%, *P. aeruginosa* in 8% and both in 12%. During outpatient treatment in 10 of 51 patients neither of these was found. In at least 41% a chronic pseudomonal infection occurred. In the CF-patients born between the years 1977 and 1985 staphylococci first occurred in 45%, *P. aeruginosa* in 23% and both in 12%. Only in 9 of 74 patients neither of these two could be detected. The proportion of chronic infection with *P. aeruginosa* was 46%.

Pseudomonas infection occurred in the first group of patients at a mean age of 6.5 years (from 6 months to 15 years) and in the second group – with younger patients – much earlier (mean age less than 3 years from 1 month to 8.5 years). In the first group of patients fewer antibiotics were given than in the second. Antibiotic long-term treatment was not performed. Only in acute exacerbations or in cases of chronic deterioration were antibiotics used. In the first group penicillinase-resistant penicillins (49%) dominated against chloramphenicol or cephalosporins (13% for each drug). In the second group of patients the spectrum of antibiotics enlarged. With the increasing problems of *Pseudomonas* infections the application of cephalexin and gentamicin became the therapy of choice. Azlocillin was also used. Other patients – with staphylococcal infections – received erythromycin, cephalexin, oxacillin plus ampicillin or trimethoprim-sulphonamide combinations.

Antibiotic Inhalation Therapy with Azlocillin

The treatment of chronic lung infection with *P. aeruginosa* is a central problem of the whole CF therapy. Many different attempts have been made to achieve better results. Inhalations with antibiotics may be one way to this goal. We have used azlocillin (Securopen from Bayer AG, Leverkusen) as a rapid intravenous infusion alone or in a combination of intravenous and inhalation therapy (unpublished observations).

A cooperative clinical study was performed in the children's university hospital of Leipzig and in our clinic. Between January 1985 and May 1987 we treated 34 patients a total of 60 times with azlocillin. In Leipzig 19 patients were treated a total of 33 times and in Dresden 15 patients a total of 27 times on an in-patient basis. 36 times treatment became necessary because of acute exacerbation and 24 times because of gradual deterioration.

In an open randomized study 30 of the cases were given 100 mg azlocillin/kg three times daily intravenously. A further 30 cases received this treatment plus twice-daily inhalations of 50 mg azlocillin/kg administered as ultrasound aerosol.

This so called sandwich technique was chosen to obtain the maximum possible effective concentrations of the antibiotic in the bronchial wall and the intraluminal secretions. The course of the therapy lasted between 10 and 14 days.

There were no differences between the two groups of patients treated. The majority of patients improved within a few days, fever subsided, auscultation findings and the colour and quality of the sputum improved. According to the clinical criteria the degree of therapeutic success was very good in 15 cases, good in 20 cases and moderate in 17; overall a positive effect was demonstrable in 52 of the 60 cases.

Bacteriological examination of the sputum revealed elimination of *P. aeruginosa* for over two weeks in 20 cases and only short elimination for a shorter period in further 10 cases. Combination (intravenous and inhalation) therapy was more efficacious. It led to elimination of the germs in twice as many (13 compared to 7) cases and also produced a very good clinical outcome in twice as many cases, 10 versus 5. These differences were – due to the small number of patients – not significant. Side-effects occurred in 9 cases: 5 instances of raised temperature, 4 of exanthem, and 2 each of circulatory centralization, dizziness, headache and shortness of breath. The full-blown manifestation of a typical penicillin allergy was observed twice. In 4 patients side-effects necessitated the discontinuation of azlocillin therapy, although the symptoms were definitely or very probably caused by this medication alone only in two of them. Two patients died from the underlying disease before the study was completed. Otherwise azlocillin was tolerated well; monitoring of transaminases, gamma-GT, alkaline phosphatase, bilirubin, creatinine, sodium, potassium, chlorine, haemoglobin, platelets, 5-nucleotidase and urine before and after therapy showed no significant changes. Initial leucocytosis normalized during therapy, stab neutrophils decreased and lymphocytes increased again, thus indicating the regression of an acute inflammation.

Thus azlocillin therapy can be recommended as an alternative to other intravenous therapy in chronic lung infection with *P. aeruginosa*. Often repeated courses should be avoided because the possibility of sensitization and, as with all penicillins, the risk of an allergic reaction. Additional inhalation therapy should be given for all advanced chronic inflammatory processes. The decision in favour of this form of therapy may be facilitated if increased levels of antibodies to specific *P. aeruginosa* exoproteins (exotoxin A, elastase, phospholipase C, alkaline protease) are determined. Unfortunately we had no opportunity to study this.

Inhalation with antibiotics alone (without intravenous therapy) can be continued for several months. It should only be used for recent invasion of the bronchial tree with *P. aeruginosa* and colonization of the bronchial mucosa in the absence of invasion of the deeper layers of the bronchial wall and absent humoral immune response. In this situation total eradication of the pathogen germs may be expected [10].

Neonatal Screening

In the early 1970s investigations in neonatal screening were begun in our clinic. Gottschalk [11] introduced an immunologic test for measuring the albumin content in dried up first passed meconium. Thus he adapted the strip test [12] for the purpose of a centralized procedure. Starting in 1976, the Laboratory of Human Genetics of the Greifswald University (Pomerania) served as a national central screening laboratory. Determination of beta-galactosidase in meconium was used as a further test to improve the discriminating capacity of the screening [13]. Filter paper sheets with dried up meconium probes were sent from all over the GDR to Greifswald. From 1976 until 1985 nearly 1.8 million investigations were made, covering more than 95% of all newborn children during this period. In all patients with a positive meconium test subsequent pilocarpine iontophoresis was performed. Thus 198 children were detected by screening as CF-patients. But as many as 144 CF-patients, who were found out in the same time due to clinical symptoms, had a false negative meconium test (42%). From a further 66 CF-children no meconium probes had been available [14]. These disappointing results led to the decision to stop the test at the end of the year 1985.

Even more marked were the negative results in the CF outpatients department of the children's university hospital at Leipzig [9]. Of 63 CF-children, born between the years 1978 and 1985, only 20 (32%) were diagnosed due to a positive screening test. In 12 patients of this group no screening test was performed and 31 (49%) had a false-negative neonatal meconium screening test. Before the introduction of the neonatal screening in Leipzig the diagnosis was established in 65% in the first year of life, but between 1978 and 1985 in 80%. After the 4th year of life CF was diagnosed in the first group of patients in 15%, in the second only in 9%. The earlier diagnosis was due more to the increased attention of the doctors and less to the screening test itself. According to clinical criteria in Leipzig no benefit could be seen from the neonatal screening. In the meantime 3 of 20 patients detected by the screening test have died.

Follow-Up Study after Neonatal Screening

A follow-up study was performed by Dietzsch and Paul [15, 16] to test the potential benefit of the mass screening. They compared 105 CF-patients (born between 1974 and 1983) diagnosed by screening to the same number of patients found out by clinical symptoms. Neither group of patients included cases of meconium ileus. The results are summarized in the tables 2 to 4. The diagnosis CF was confirmed earlier in the screening group. But as 66 per cent of these patients had already developed clinical symptoms in the first 3 months of life, this is not so important. The study showed no statistical significant advantages in the follow-up for 3 to 12 years.

Table 2. Results of a follow-up-study on the benefit of neonatal mass screening (Dietzsch and Paul [16])

| | CF-patients diagnosed by | |
	screening	clinical symptoms
Number of patients	105	105
Number of boys	53	55
Mean age at follow-up	5.9 years	5.7 years
	(3–12 y)	(3–12 y)
Mean age when diagnosed	85.4 days	361.4 days
Number of deaths	5	2
Number of patients treated as inpatients	19	26
Mean duration of stationary treatment	36 days	48 days
Number of patients with clubbing	31	28
Body height (HOLT-score)	-0.11 ± 1.16	-0.19 ± 1.28 n.s.
Body weight (HOLT-score)	-1.44 ± 0.86	-0.92 ± 0.79 n.s.
Mean x-ray score (Shwachman)	2.63	2.52

Table 3. Comparison of lung functions tests in CF-patients diagnosed either by screening or due to clinical symptoms (Dietzsch and Paul [16])

	CF-patients diagnosed by		
	screening		clinical symptoms
VC	83.7 ± 19.2% (n = 32)	(n.s.)	85.2 ± 17.9% (n = 30)
FEV_1/VC	86.7 ± 15.3% (n = 29)	(n.s.)	81.6 ± 12.8% (n = 29)
paO_2	10.7 ± 4.3 kPa (n = 90)	(n.s.)	9.8 ± 1.5 kPa (n = 92)

Table 4. Bacteriological findings in the sputum or bronchial secretions of CF-patients diagnosed either by screening or due to clinical symptoms (Dietzsch and Paul [16])

	CF-patients diagnosed by	
	screening (n = 44)	clinical symptoms (n = 54)
sterile	6	7
S. aureus	22 (= 50%)	20 (= 37%)
P. aeruginosa	10 (= 23%)	13 (= 24%)
Klebsiella pneumoniae	2	4
Haemophilus influenzae	2	3
E. coli	2	3
Streptococcus pneumoniae	—	3
Proteus vulgaris	—	1

Genetic Analysis

Diagnosis of CF has reached a higher level by the use of polymerase chain reaction and mutation analysis of the CF transmembrane conductance regulator (CFTR). Up to now more than 250 CFTR mutations have been found. In central Europe ΔF508 is the most common mutation and occurs in nearly 75% of all CF chromosomes.

In a recent study our CF patients were analyzed by this method to add information to the open discussion of the genotype/phenotype association [18]. Using probes for only 3 CFTR mutations in 101 CF patients:

ΔF508 homozygotes were found in 46 patients = 45.5%,
ΔF508 compound heterozygotes in 44 patients = 43.6% and
other mutations in 11 patients = 10.9%.

Thus the frequency of the ΔF508 chromosome was 67.3%, the frequency of G551D 3.5% (in 7 patients) and the frequency of R553X 1.5% (in 3 patients).

In 90 patients with at least one ΔF508 mutation a pancreatic insufficiency was found in 76 (84.4%). In 11 patients with non-ΔF508 mutations only 6 (54.5%) showed a pancreatic insufficiency. These findings are in good accordance to the results of the Hannover group [18].

Conclusion

Summarizing some results of CF research from East Germany, it is clear that a computerized patient data register is a valuable tool. The reported data stress the importance of chronic lung infection with *P. aeruginosa* for the prognosis of CF. It remains unexplained why the frequency of this infection is up to now lower in the former GDR than in most other European countries. By no means should it be overlooked that many CF patients die who never became infected by *P. aeruginosa* but had a chronic lung infection with *Staphyloccocus aureus*.

References

1. Dietzsch H-J. Die Entwicklung der Mukoviszidose-Betreuung in der DDR. Z Erkr Atm-Org 1988; 170: 8–16.
2. Gottschalk B. Die Mukoviszidose in der Deutschen Demokratischen Republik. Dtsch Gesundh-wes 1972; 27: 2292–2296.
3. Mittenzwey KW. Bericht über das Mukoviszidose-Register der DDR. Dresden 1982.
4. Paul K-D, Wunderlich P. Bericht des Mukoviszidose-Registers 1986. Dresden 1986.
5. Wiedemann B, Paul K-D. Aktueller Stand der Mukoviszidose-Betreuung in den neuen Bundesländern. 14.CF-Ambulanzärzte-Tagung (22./23.10.1993) Titisee/Germany Tagungsbericht.
6. Wachtel K. Analyse der Todesfälle bei Mukoviszidose in der DDR. Med. Diplomarbeit, Dresden 1988.
7. Dietzsch H-J, Kossatz A, Lerche M. Zur Häufigkeit der Lungeninfektionen bei Patienten mit Mukoviscidose und zum Krankheitsverlauf bei unterschiedlichem Erregerspektrum. Kinderärztl Prax 1989; 57: 81–87.
8. Wunderlich P, Paul K-D, Wiedemann, B. Mukoviszidose in Sachsen. Ärztebl Sachsen 1993; 3: 120–122.
9. Kunze K. Retrospektive Analyse des Krankheitsverlaufs von 148 Mukoviszidosepatienten der Geburtsjahrgänge 1961–1989 im Behandlungszeitraum von 1967 bis 1991. Med Thesis, Leipzig 1994.
10. Wunderlich P, Paul K-D, Wehner J. Value of inhaled antibiotics in cystic fibrosis patients. Acta Univ Carol med (Prague) 1990; 36: 34–36.
11. Gottschalk B. Entwicklung und Optimierung eines Massencreening-Programmes für das Krankheitsbild der Mukoviszidose. Dissertation B, Dresden 1980.
12. Stephan U, Busch E-W, Kollberg H, Hellsing K. Cystic fibrosis detection by means of an teststrip. Pediatrics 55 (1975) 35–38.
13. Machill G, Petruschka L. Früherfassung genetischer Stoffwechselstörungen in der DDR. 2. Mitt.: Mukoviszidose Z klin Med 1986; 41: 255–258.
14. Hein J, Dietzsch H-J, Machill G, Henker J. Aktuelles zum Mukoviszidose-Screening in der DDR. Kinderärztl Prax 1986; 54: 547–551.
15. Dietzsch H-J, Burkhardt J, Paul KD. Hat die Frühdiagnose der Mukoviszidose mittels Screening der Neugeborenen Einfluß auf den Krankheitsverlauf? Z klin Med 1986; 41: 1923–1925.
16. Dietzsch H-J, Paul K-D. Zur Langzeitprognose von Kindern mit Zystischer Fibrose, die durch neonatales Screening diagnostiziert wurden. pp 71–80. In D. Kaiser u, G. Döring: CF-Symposium Wildbad 1987. Hannover 1987.
17. Winkler A, Gerisch S, Wiedemann B, Henker J, Ulbrich K, Paul K-D. Genotype/phenotype association in cystic fibrosis: analysis of the DF508, R553X and G551D mutations in 101 cystic fibrosis patients. Paper for the 4th Int CF Symposium Hannover (1994).
18. Kubesch P, Dörk T, Wulbrand U, Kalin N, Neumann T, Wulf B et al. Genetic determinants of airways colonisation with *Pseudomonas aeruginosa* in cystic fibrosis. Lancet 1993; 341: 189–193.

Cystic Fibrosis Pulmonary Infections
Lessons from Around the World
ed. by A. Bauernfeind, M. I. Marks and B. Strandvik
© 1996 Birkhäuser Verlag Basel/Switzerland

CHAPTER 21
Pulmonary Infection and its Management in Cystic Fibrosis Patients in the Czech Republic

Věra Vávrová[1], Zdenka Jedličková, Otto Lochmann[1], Dana Zemková[1], Hana Krásničanová[1], Milan Macek[1], Milan Macek Jr[10], Alois Zapletal[1], Jiří Biolek[2], Alena Holčiková[3], Helena Honomichlová[4], Antonín Kolek[5], Jaromír Musil[1], Ivana Sekyrová[6], Miroslava Šuláková[7], Lenka Ťoukálková[8], Hubert Vaníček[9]

[1]*2nd Medical Faculty, Charles University Prague, University Hospital Prague-Motol, 15018 Prague, Czech Republic;* [2]*Department of Pediatrics, Hospital Most, 43464 Most, Czech Republic;* [3]*University Children's Hospital, Brno, 66263 Brno, Czech Republic;* [4]*Department of Pediatrics, University Hospital Plzeň, 30599 Plzeň, Czech Republic;* [5]*Department of Pediatrics, University Hospital Olomouc, 77520 Olomouc, Czech Republic;* [6]*Department of Pediatrics IPVZ, České Budějovice, 37087 České Budějovice, Czech Republic;* [7]*1st Department of Pediatrics, University Hospital Brno, 65691 Brno, Czech Republic;* [8]*Department of Pediatrics, Batta's Hospital, Zlin, 76001 Zlin, Czech Republic;* [9]*Department of Pediatrics, University Hospital Hradec Králové, 50036 Hradec Králové, Czech Republic,* [10]*Johns Hopkins University, Baltimore, USA*

Summary. Since 1985, a total of 384 CF patients have been treated in the Czech Republic. Seventy five percent of patients have been treated in Prague, where a research center is also located, and 25% have been managed in other university and large regional hospitals. The mean age of 295 living patients is 12.3 ± 7.4 years. Eighty nine patients died at the mean age 13.2 ± 8.35 years. Fifty percent of our patients survive 21.7 years.

The management of pulmonary infection is based on the bacterial sensitivity to antibiotics. *Staphylococcus aureus* was present in 75% and *Pseudomonas aeruginosa* in 49.5% of the patients respectively (in 43.7% of living and 69.7% of deceased patients). The mean age of the first positive *Pseudomonas* culture was 9.6 ± 6.5 y. *Burkholderia cepacia* was found in 4.4% of our CF patients.

During the first year of life, all CF infants have been given continuous prophylactic antistaphylococcal antibiotics. If clinical or laboratory signs of infection are present at a later age, antibiotics in full dosage are administered for at least three weeks depending on the bacterial sensitivity. Patients chronically infected with *Pseudomonas aeruginosa* have been given i.v. treatment 3–4 times a year for a period of 14 days. The dosage of aminoglycosides is adjusted to the monitored plasma levels. Between the periods of i.v. therapy courses, quinolones *per os* and/or colomycin inhalations are given frequently. During 1993 i.v. home therapy was started. Antimycotic drugs are provided when indicated.

Introduction

In the Czech Republic with a population of 10 million inhabitants, approximately 120 thousand children are born every year and the incidence of CF newborns is 1:2 500. The first child with cystic fibrosis

Correspondence address: Věra Vávrová, Associate Professor of Pediatrics, 2nd Department of Pediatrics, V úvalu 84, 150 18 Prague 5-Motol, Czech Republic.

(CF) in the Czech Republic territory was diagnosed in the 2nd Department of Pediatrics in Prague in 1946 [1]. During the following years, a total of 432 children have been treated in this institution [2] and the system of diagnosis and treatment of patients with CF has been established.

Since no official CF center for the whole republic exists, the majority of CF patients have been treated in the Pediatric Clinics of the university hospitals. The clinical course, biochemical, bacteriological, anthropometrical data and chest X-rays are regularly followed-up by the team of specialists in special laboratories. In the CF patients older than 6 years, pulmonary function tests have been regularly performed (Spiroscope Ganshorn in Prague and similar instruments in other centers). Seventy five percent of the patients have been treated in Prague, where the CF research center is also located, and 25% have been managed in other university and large regional hospitals (Hradec Králové, Plzeň, České Budějovice, Brno, Olomouc, Most and Zlín).

Pediatricians handling CF patients in these centers are members of the CF Committee of the Czech Pediatric Society belonging to the Medical Society of J. E. Purkyně. Therefore, the system of care virtually unifies the whole country.

In some cases, the patient is followed-up regularly by a regional paediatrician who is given recommendations and a program of therapy from the CF specialist after a detailed assessment of the patient carried out in a particular CF center once a year.

The purpose of this paper is to show the system of health care in CF patients under the conditions which differed in the past from the conditions in more developed countries of the world.

The Czech Cystic Fibrosis Population

Since 1985, 384 CF patients have fulfilled the diagnostic criteria stated by the CF committee of the Czech Pediatric Society. The group of patients consists of 201 boys and 183 girls, 295 of them (155 boys and 140 girls) are alive at the end of 1994. The mean age of living patients is 12.3 ± 7.4 years (range: 0.55 to 63.3 years). The mean age at death of 89 deceased CF patients was 13.2 ± 8.3 years (range: 0.1 to 37.5 years). The difference in age at death between the boys (14.1 ± 8.4) and girls (12.4 ± 8.1) was not significant. Fifty percent of our patients survived 21.7 years (Quick-stat method). The diagnosis of the disease was established in all patients on the basis of personal and/or family history of CF, and was confirmed in all of them by the pilocarpine iontophoresis-induced sweat test [3]. The mean sweat chloride concentration was 93.4 ± 4.8 mmol/l (range: 42 to 142). The mean age at diagnosis was 2.4 ± 4.9 years (range: 0.1 to 60.9 years).

Table 1. Basic anthropometric characteristics of Czech CF patients

Parameter	n	Mean	SD	Min.	Max.
age (years)	332	11.93	7.07	0.08	60.9
height (SDS)	330	−1.12	1.22	−4.84	2.1
weight (SDS)	332	−1.42	1.12	−4.90	1.7

SDS = $x − \bar{x}/SD$, where x is the measured value, $\bar{x}$ and SD are mean and standard deviation value of the population specific reference sample [9, 10].

Since 1990, routine genotype analysis has been performed in our 256 patients with CF. DeltaF508 mutation was present in 70% of the chromosomes and 12 other mutations were also identified. The genotype–phenotype correlation has been studied in collaboration with the institutes of genetics in Berlin and Baltimore [4].

The growth and nutritional data of the patients (Table 1) document a great variation in the course of the disease. Longitudinal studies of the patients [5] have shown a significant deterioration of the nutritional status during puberty accompanied by worsening of the pulmonary function. It is not possible to explain the variability of the patients phenotype by means of the present methods of the molecular genetics. The greatest influence on the nutrition and pulmonary function of the patient is *Pseudomonas aeruginosa* infection.

Therefore, our attention has been focused on this special topic. Sputum specimens and/or deep throat swabs have been obtained for bacterial culture at every visit of the patient to the clinic. However, the exact analysis of the frequency of the different microbiological and mycotic agents in our patients will be possible in the future when the data base is established.

Pulmonary Infection

The present results of microbiological analysis revealed in the majority of our studied CF children *Staphylococcus aureus* as a dominant pathogen in the respiratory tract, i.e. present in approximately 75% of the patients. The latter pathogen was found either as the only one present or in combination with other bacteria, most frequently with Gram-negative pathogens. Sometimes *Staphylococcus aureus* was revealed with *Pseudomonas aeruginosa*, especially in its mucoid form. Serologically, the most frequent type of *Pseudomonas aeruginosa* was 010, but further serotypes 06 and 03 were isolated [6]. *Candida* was often identified in more severe course of the disease; different types of *Aspergillus* were rare.

In order to differentiate *Pseudomonas aeruginosa* from other *Pseudomonas species*, classical biochemical analyses were carried out in the majority of the microbiological laboratories. In our Prague CF center,

Table 2. Predicted values of the lung function tests (percentage) and the nutritional state in *Pseudomonas* infected and non-infected CF patients

	Pseudomonas +	*Pseudomonas* −	Total number
n	78:134 resp.*	48:70 resp.*	126:204 resp.*
mean age* (yrs)	14.0 ± 4.0	13.1 ± 4.6	13.7 ± 4.2
FVC*	64.3 ± 21.4	79.1 ± 20.1	77.2 ± 26.4
FEV$_1$*	54.8 ± 24.6	77.2 ± 26.4	62.5 ± 25.3
PEF	69.1 ± 21.4	76.4 ± 25.3	71.8 ± 23.0
MEF 75% VC	57.1 ± 27.3	72.5 ± 31.7	63.0 ± 29.0
MEF 50% VC	45.7 ± 29.2	67.4 ± 34.8	53.9 ± 31.5
MEF 25% VC	33.0 ± 23.8	57.2 ± 35.1	42.2 ± 28.6
weight (SDS)*	− 1.7 ± 1.1	− 1.0 ± 1.0	− 1.5 ± 1.0

*Mean age. FVC. FEV$_1$ and weight were calculated in 134 Ps. aer. infected and 70 non infected patients.
Mean values ± SD are presented.

during the second half of 1994 we had the opportunity to use the Crystal system (Beckton-Dickinson) with computer analysis, which enabled us to perform an exact bacteriological diagnosis and specification of *Pseudomonas*.

Pseudomonas aeruginosa was found in 190 patients (49.5%) of the total group of 384 patients. It was isolated in 43.7% of living and in 69.7% of deceased patients. The mean age of the first positive *Pseudomonas* culture was 9.6 ± 6.5 years and was not statistically different in living and deceased patients.

The differences in the lung function tests and the nutritional state in *Pseudomonas*-infected and non-infected patients older than 6 years are shown in Table 2. Longitudinal study of 69 pairs matched for sex and age [7] proved that the patients colonized by *Pseudomonas aeruginosa* were already in a worse nutritional and pulmonary function status at the time of the first positive culture. In the following 3 years further deterioration occurred.

Burkholderia cepacia has been found sporadically in 18 patients before 1988. Its occurrence was not constant and its bacterial resistance very low. In the period between the years of 1988 to 1993 "*Pseudomonas* sp." was identified. In 1994, with better diagnostic methods *Pseudomonas cepacia* was found in 4.4% of our CF patients. The evaluation of its influence on the clinical course of the disease is still under investigation.

Treatment of Infection

The good nutritional status of the patients has been considered as an important factor in the prevention of *Pseudomonas* infection. The greatest emphasis is therefore put on the optimalisation of antiinfectious treatment.

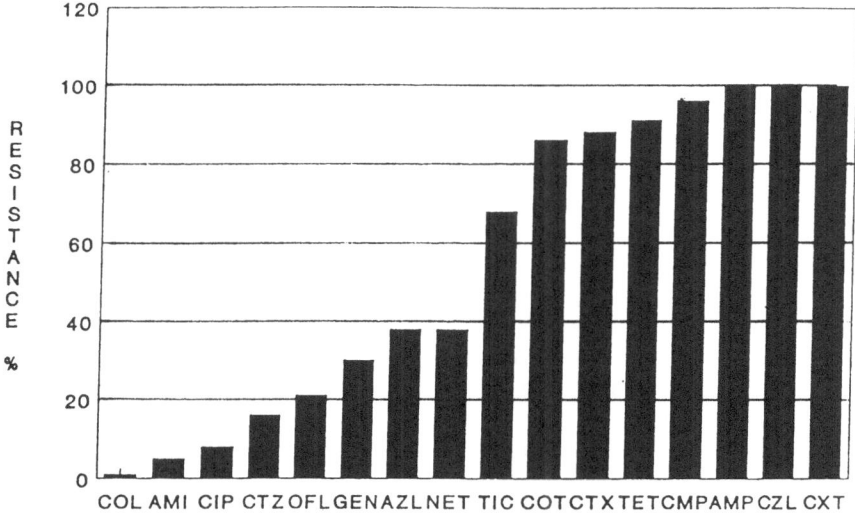

Figure 1. *Pseudomonas aeruginosa* resistance in the University Hospital Prague-Motol.

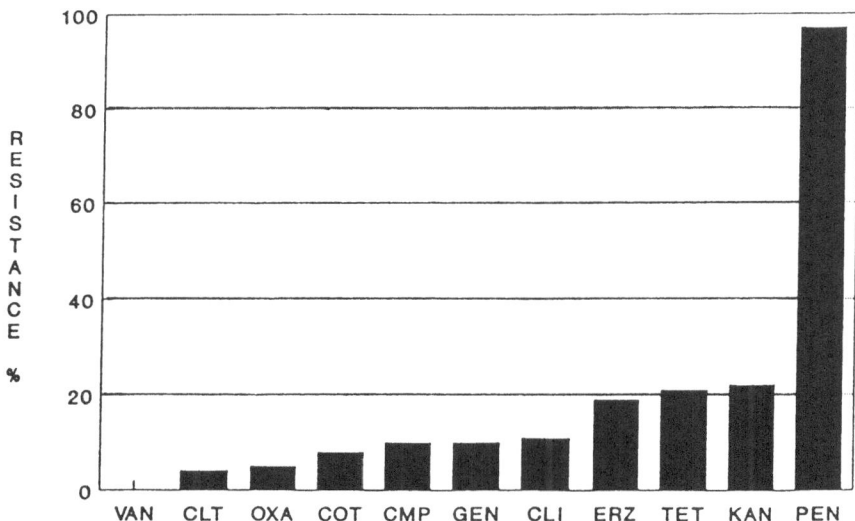

Figure 2. *Staphylococcus aureus* resistance in the University Hospital Prague-Motol. Abbreviations used: AMI = Amikacin, AMP = Ampicillin, AZL = Azlocillin, CIP = Ciprofloxacin, CLI = Clindamycin, CLT = Cefalotin, CMP = Chloramphenicol, COL = Colistin, COT = Cotrimoxazol, CTX = Ceftotaxime, CTZ = Ceftazidime, CXT = Cefoxitin, CZL = Cefazolin, ERY = Erythromycin, GEN = Gentamicin, KAN = Kanamycin, NET = Netilmicin, OFL = Ofloxacin, OXA = Oxacillin, PEN = Penicillin, TET = Tetracyclin, TIC = Ticarcillin, VAN = Vancomycin.

Both bacteriological diagnosis and antibiotic sensitivity have been monitored regularly. Figure 1 shows the results of *Pseudomonas aeruginosa* resistance obtained in our CF center in Prague in 1993. In 1994 the spectrum of antibiotics was enlarged by imipenem/cilastin and piperacillin. The bacteriological resistance to imipenem/cilastin was lower than 5% and to piperacillin 25%. Figure 2 shows the resistance of the second important pathogen in our CF population, i.e. *Staphylococcus aureus*. The resistance is rather stable and the latest tested drugs (fluoroquinolones or imipenem/cilastin) had resistance lower than 10%.

The treatment strategy is similar throughout the whole country. During the first year of life, all CF infants are given continuously antibiotics as prophylaxis. Antistaphylococcal antibiotics have been used and switched according to the bacterial sensitivity or tolerance. If clinical or laboratory signs of infection are present in the later age, antibiotics according to bacterial sensitivity are used in full doses for at least three weeks. When *Pseudomonas aeruginosa* is detected in the following 2–3 bacterial cultures, quinolone treatment *per os* with colomycin inhalation is started. In chronically infected patients, i.v. antibiotic treatment is given for 14 days 3–4 times a year. We nearly always use a combination of aminoglycosides (netilmicin, tobramycin or amikacin) with cephalosporines of the third generation (ceftazidime), carbapenems, imipenem/cilastin, semi-synthetic penicillins or fluoroquinolones. The dosage of aminoglycosides is adjusted to the plasma levels monitored. Between the i.v. therapy courses, quinolones *per os* and/or colomycin inhalations are given frequently. During 1993 i.v. home therapy was started following the careful education of parents in the hospital.

In mycotic infections, antimycotic drugs are given regularly. In severe *Asperigillus fumigatus* infections, amphotericin B has been used.

Conclusion

The analysis of our results from the past showed that the mortality in our patients was higher, the survival rate shorter, and the nutritional status worse than in other Western countries [8]. We believe that the lack of medicaments and new antibiotics, less intensive antibiotic treatment, inefficient pancreatic substitution and the absence of nutritional supplements before November 1989 was the cause of the unfavourable course of the disease in our patients.

It seems that the disease in our country in the past had almost a natural course, not influenced by the advances in the therapy.

However, anybody involved in the health care of CF patients in our country can observe the progress made over the last four years. Therefore, the outlook for our CF patients is the same as for other CF patients in the world.

Acknowledgement

This work was supported by grants form IGA MZ Czech Republic 0728-3 (1990-1993) and 2056 5 (since 1994) to V.V.

References

1. Švejcar J, Benešová D, Houštěk J. Cystická fibrosa pankreatu. Čas lék Čes 1948; 87: 1116 22.
2. Houštěk J, Vávrová V. Cystická fibrosa v minulosti, přitomnosti a budoucnosti. Čs Pediat 1987; 42(11): 645 9.
3. Gibson LE, Cooke RE. A test for concentration of electrolytes in sweat in cystic fibrosis of the pancreas utilizing pilocarpine by iontophoresis. Pediatrics 1959; 23: 545 9.
4. Macek M, Jr, Vávrová V, Böhm I, Stuhrmann M, Reis A, Duspivová R, et al.: Frequency of the Δ F508 mutation and flanking marker haplotypes at the cystic fibrosis locus from 167 Czech families. Hum Genet 1990; 85(4): 417 8.
5. Vávrová V, Zemková D, Krásničanová H, Zapletal A, Macek M, Jr, Macek M. Factors influencing the course of cystic fibrosis in Czech patients: experience of the Prague clinic. Paediatr Paedol 1995; 30: 19 24.
6. Jedličková Z, Vávrová V. Infekce *Pseudomonas aeruginosa* u děti s mukoviscidosou. Prakt lékař 1972; 52(11): 423 7.
7. Zemková D, Krásničanová H, Macek M, Jr, Zapletal A, Vávrová V. Relation between *Pseudomonas* infection, nutritional state and lung function. Proceedings of the 19th European Cystic Fibrosis Conference, 1994 May 29 June 3, Paris, 1994: abstr. P61.
8. Corey M, McLaughlin FJ, Williams M, Levison H. A comparison of survival, growth, and pulmonary function in patients with cystic fibrosis in Boston and Toronto. J Clin Epidemiol 1988; 41: 583 91.
9. Bláha P, Šedivý V, Čechovský K, Kosová A, Havel K, Trzynecki P et al.: Anthropometric studies of the Czechoslovak population from 6 to 55 years. 1986 UNZ VS Praha.
10. Bláha P, Bošková R, Krásničanová H, Riedlová J, Sup R, Zemková D et al. Anthropometric studies of the Czech pre-school children from 3 to 7 years. Institute of Sports Medicine Publ., Prague 1990.

Cystic Fibrosis Pulmonary Infections:
Lessons from Around the World
ed. by A. Bauernfeind, M. I. Marks and B. Strandvik
© 1996 Birkhäuser Verlag Basel/Switzerland

CHAPTER 22
The General Approach to Cystic Fibrosis Pulmonary Infection in Hungary

Kálmán Gyurkovits

Hospital for Chest Diseases of County Somogy, 7257 Mosdós, Hungary

Summary. Hungary has ten million multi-ethnic inhabitants, among whom the frequency of CF is 1:4000 live births. There are more than 300 patients under the care of 12 centres; and nearly 30 CF homozygote newborns are expected per year.

Up to 7–8% of our CF patients reach adulthood, and to date two of them have become the mothers of healthy children.

The complex management of CF respiratory complications has therefore to be directed to the underlying pathophysiological changes.

The principle of the policy relating to the use of antibiotics in Hungary does not differ from the international consensus, but their aggressive use is rare (only in two to three centres), and home intravenous treatment with antimicrobial regimens has not yet started.

Introduction

As elsewhere, cystic fibrosis (CF) is the most common life-threatening recessively inherited genetic disease in Hungary. This country has ten million multi-ethnic inhabitants, among whom the frequency of CF is 1:4000 live births. There are more than 300 patients under the care of 12 centres; and nearly 30 CF homozygote newborns are expected per year.

The CF population had been investigated for the main mutation of the CF chromosome, and the specific three base pair deletion (delta F 508) has been found in 65% of cases [1].

The median survival age has increased from 3 to 13 years during the last two decades, and the median life expectancy of a child with CF born today in Hungary, is likely to be 20 years. There are no significant differences between the two sexes as regards the incidence and the severity of the disease, however, the two eldest patients are males (aged 43 and 32 years respectively). Up to 7–8% of our CF patients reach adulthood.

Some Historical Data – Landmarks in the Fight Against Cystic Fibrosis in Hungary

The recognition and treatment of CF was started in Hungary 25 years ago. Before then it was widely believed that CF was a rarity in this country, as in Finland and many Asiatic countries. On the basis of meconium ileus occurrence, active screening was started and more than 100 new CF cases were detected in one centre (Szeged) during 10 years (1968-77).

In 1977 a Medical Working Group for CF was organized with the participation of 12 Departments of Paediatrics. The main goals of these CF centres were: i) to formulate a harmonized approach to diagnosis and therapy; ii) to collect data on CF incidence, together with complications; and iii) to join in with the international activities in the fight against CF. A project for the screening of newborn infants was introduced on a regional basis between 1975 and 1985. More than 200 000 tests have revealed a frequency of CF in Hungary closely corresponding to that found in other European countries. Although it has not been analysed by population screening, the incidence of the most common CF mutation among gipsy families seems to be far lower than among the others. The main advantage of the introduction of screening was that it helped to attract the attention of the general medical profession in Hungary to the problems of CF [2].

The European Working Group for CF held its 14th Annual Meeting to coincide with the 3rd Conference of IACFA in Budapest in 1986. Prenatal diagnosis based upon abnormal microvillar enzymes in the amniotic fluid was changed for the genetic method used in the first trimester of chorionic villus sampling since 1987; a CF Parents' Association was established in 1981, and was expanded to a nationwide organization since then; regular CF summer camps, two weeks twice a year, have been organized with medical and physiotherapists' assistance for 30-40 CF families at Dömös for 6 years; in addition the first book in Hungarian on CF was published in 1991 [3].

The activity on CF has become wider than ever during the last three years. We were able to set up the Hungarian CF Foundation for supporting CF care and therapy; in 1991 the Hungarian CF Adults Association was established. The National Working Group for CF acts as a medical advisory committee, and the recently established Hungarian CF Association (1993) took over the task of coordinating all the work of the different branches, making it possible for others to join as well, e.g. allied health personnel, laymen, and sponsors [4].

Thanks to the improving health care, and also to the increase in health-education, life-expectancy is increasing gradually, and CF patients' general state of health and quality of life are now far better than they previously were.

The Changing Face of the General Approach to Cystic Fibrosis Pulmonary Care in Hungary

Trends in the therapeutic policy of pulmonary care in CF patients are summarized in the Table 1. The sequence follows the three chronologi-

Table 1. Pulmonary care of CF patients in Hungary (management of pulmonary infection)

Years	Pathomechanism	Aetiology	Symptomatology
	Preventive	Curative	Palliative
1968–93			
1968–77	Postural drainage	Penicillin Ampicillin	OXYGEN
	CHEST PERCUSSION	Cephalosporin II. gen	DIGITALIS
	REGULAR EXERCISE*	Cotrimoxazole	FUROSEMIDE
	Mucosolvin 5% aerosol	Oleandomycin	mech.ventilation
	mist tent	Kanamycin	hospitalization
	PANCREATIC ENZYMES*	GENTAMICIN	SALT ORAL*
1977–86	AUTOGENIC DRAINAGE*	AUGMENTIN	Ca CHANNEL BLOCKERS
	HUFFING (FET)	CEPHALOSPORIN III. GEN	ANTI-ALDOSTERONE
	N-ACETYLCYSTEINE*	TOBRAMYCIN	BRONCHODILATORS
	ORAL and aerosol	VANCOMYCIN	bronchial lavage
	Zaditen (ketotifen)	DOXYCYCLIN	lobectomy (3 cases)
	unsaturated oils	Clindamycin	NASAL POLYPECTOMY
	Zn, VIT. A,D,E,K	MACROLIDES	PSYCHOTHERAPY
1986 95	FLUTTER VRP₁*	NETILMYCIN	OXYGENATOR
	Clini-Jet. PEEP*	QUINOLONES	ANTI-INFLAMMATORY AGENTS
	SALT AEROSOL	IMIPENEM	(antiprotease)
	HIGH FAT DIET	(immunotherapy	(Gelsolin)
	ANTIOXIDANTS	amiloride	NON-SEDATIVE TRANQUILLANTS
	MULTIVITAMINS*	triphosphate	PULMOZYME
	ACTIVE IMMUNIZATION	nucleotides	(lung artery embolization)
	PATIENT EDUCATION	CFTR gene transfer)	(heart lung transplant)

Small letters (lowercase) indicate earlier system, CAPITAL LETTERS indicate currently applied methods, standard ones with asterisk (*), and the future therapy is indicated with brackets ().

cal phases mentioned earlier, separating the preventive, causative and palliative approaches. By prevention, we mean the efforts to improve mucociliary clearance, i.e. prevention of bronchial obstruction; causative or aetiological treatment is limited only to antimicrobial chemotherapy; and palliative methods are directed towards the symptomatological care of the patients. The drugs and methods listed in Table 1 do not cover the whole spectrum of CF clinical management; these are its cornerstones, which have remained substantially unaltered: i.e. *optimized nutrition, antibiotics* and *chest physiotherapy.*

Recent Strategies in the Care of Pulmonary Infections in Cystic Fibrosis

First of all, it is essential to mention that adequate management of respiratory tract infection in CF not only consists of anti-microbial therapy, but also includes intensive chest physiotherapy, inhalation therapy, mucolytics, pancreatic enzymes and high-calorie nutrition, treatment of respiratory, cardiac and metabolic complications, and psychosocial support. The influence of these latter measures on lung infection is indirect. It is well accepted that long-term maintenance of normal weight and lung function clearly contributes to prevent both lung colonization and infectious exacerbations.

As regards the choice of treatment with pharmaceuticals, the special features of chronic endobronchial infection in CF must be taken into consideration: The lower airways in CF homozygotes are initially colonized usually by *Haemophilus influenzae,* later by *Staphylococcus auereus,* and finally with *Pseudomonas aeruginosa,* and, in some cases, *Burkholderia cepacia.* The inflammation remains mainly localized: septicaemia rarely occurs: There is a huge number of granulocytes in the endobronchial secretion. Biochemically, the metabolic excitability of leukocytes produces a high amount of oxygen-derived free radicals, the disproportion between the activity of neutrophilic proteases and the total anti-neutrophilic elastase capacity increases, and also an increase in the tumour necrosing factor (TNF = cachectin) occurs, among others, damaging the lung tissues.

The complex management of CF respiratory complications has therefore to be directed to the underlying pathophysiological changes. The method of choice depends mainly on the

– age of the patient,
– physical condition, general state,
– laboratory data, X-ray and lung function results, and
– earlier and recent microbiological examinations.

The principle of the policy relating to the use of antibiotics in Hungary does not differ from the international consensus [5–8], but the aggressive use of these is rare (only in two to three centres), and a home intravenous treatment with antimicrobial regimens has not started yet. All medications for CF patients are financed by the government; however there is a need for improving health care and welfare support regarding e.g. home oxygen therapy, home i.v. antibiotics, etc.

There are three levels of approaches to CF diagnosis and management in Hungary, as follows:

Basic level – conducted by district paediatricians, first hospitalization at the Paediatric Departments of Municipal or County Hospitals (there are close to 60 such places in Hungary). The main goals are: to provide CF diagnosis by sweat test; to estimate the type and severity of organ manifestations; to introduce general substitution and mucolytic therapy.

Medium level – available usually in one of the 12 CF centres, this facility offers among others verification of diagnosis, classification of the disease using score systems, and screening for special complications, with recommendation of antimicrobial therapy.

High level – in very well equipped institutions, suitable for specialized tasks, e.g. genetic techniques, nuclear magnetic resonance imaging, thoracic surgery. Only two or three such places are ready to deal with novel therapeutic techniques in the country. There are two rehabilitation centres for CF adults (Korányi Institute for Pulmonology in Budapest and Hospital for Chest Diseases of County Somogy at Mosdós; the latter is the only one for both children and adults) in Hungary.

A rapid survey of the hospitalized CF patients at two centres (Paed. Dept. Univ. Med. School of Szeged and Mosdós) in the last two years has shown the following microbiological results: Nearly half of the 111 sputum examinations have revealed *Staphylococcus aureus*, 17% *Pseudomonas aeruginosa* and 11% *Haemophilus influenzae*. The total number of patients was 28 (10 boys and 18 girls, aged between 1 and 24 years), one to five microbiological tests were carried out per patient during a two year period. The spectrum of bacteria is listed in Table 2. The most frequently used antibiotics were cephalosporins and aminoglycosides.

In spite of rapid development in various kinds of therapeutic methods and their use uniformly, the pulmonary progression remains individually different; it seems to be genetically determinated.

As regards the use of bronchodilators in CF patients, there is much controversy. For detecting bronchial hyperresponsiveness, both a specific provocation tests and trials for pharmacological broncholysis are suggested. The pharmacocapnographic method was developed first in Hungary. This lung function test proves to be a suitable screening method for the detection of ventilation-perfusion disequilibrium. The main advantages are its simplicity – there is no need for the active cooperation of the child, it is sensitive enough for the detection of even a subclinical bronchospasm, and we can use it in patients from the age of 2 years. In spite of proven reversible bronchial obstruction only the

Table 2. Microbiologically positive results of 28 CF patients in 1992–93

Findings		N =
Staphylococcus aureus	47%	52
Pseudomonas aeruginosa	17%	19
Haemophilus influenzae	11%	12
Escherichia coli		6
Candida albicans		4
Klebsiella pneumoniae		4
Burkholderia cepacia		3
Streptococcus pneumoniae		3
Branhamella catarrhalis		2
Proteus mirabilis		2
Streptococcus viridans		2
Enterobacter aerogenes		1
Neisseria pharyngis		1
Total number of examinations:		111

temporary use of bronchodilators is recommended. It may be supposed that reversible bronchospasms play a role in removing purulent secretions from the lungs.

Nearly 50% of CF patients show a hyperresponsiveness to various kinds of aspecific bronchoprovocation, but the clinical condition (based for example on the Shwachman score) has proved to be better in the hyperreactive group.

Our investigations have also confirmed that both the generation of free radicals in baseline condition in the granulocytes and the reduced glutathione level in the erythrocytes are elevated in CF patients and the metabolic excitability of the granulocytes is highest in CF cases with a severe clinical condition, suggesting a continuous oxidative stress [9].

The measured glutathione instability (determined after *in vitro* acetylphenylhydrazine) and the increase in oxidative derivatives of haemoglobin (methaemoglobin and haemichrome) prove a higher sensitivity and a decreased capacity of the red blood cells of CF patients to overcome oxidant attack. The whole blood selenium concentrations were significantly lower in the patient group in comparison with controls. A more potent antioxidant therapy, including selenium administration, zinc, and high doses of vitamins A and E seems to be indicated, especially in CF with progressive symptoms.

Anti-inflammatory agents (i.e. corticosteroids such as prednisolone) are used only in chronically colonized patients with severe clinical condition.

Only CF cases with potentially reversible respiratory insufficiency may be given mechanical ventilatory support (about one case in a year); otherwise the end-stage patients receive the usual palliative therapy.

Management of such pulmonary complications as pneumothorax, haemoptysis or respiratory failure always needs hospitalization.

References

1. Endreffy, Emöke, Burg K, Gyurkovits K, László, Aranka, Raskó I. Allele frequencies of cystic fibrosis – linked markers and F_{508} deletion in affected Hungarian families. Acta Paediatrica Hungarica 1992; 32: 101 113.
2. Fejes Á, Andrásofszky B, Havass Z, Gyurkovits, K. Cystic fibrosis frequency in Hungary: results of neonatal screening experiments during 10 years. 14th annual meeting of the European working group for cystic fibrosis (Abstracts) Budapest, Hungary, 1986; Sept. 1 2.
3. Gyurkovits K. Cystic Fibrosis (Mucoviscidosis). Medicina, Budapest, 1991.
4. Reports to the ICF(M)A on the CF activity in Hungary. Dublin, 1992.
5. Cystic Fibrosis Foundation: Pulmonary infection in cystic fibrosis "GAP" Conference Report. Sandpiper Bay, Florida, 1993; March 2 4.
6. Fiel SB. Clinical management of pulmonary disease in cystic fibrosis. Lancet i, 1993; 1070 1074.
7. MacLusky B, Levison H. Recent advances in cystic fibrosis. Current opinion in pediatrics 1992; 4: 392 400.
8. Schidlow DW, Taussig, Knowles MR. Cystic fibrosis foundation consensus conference report on pulmonary complications of cystic fibrosis. Pediatric Pulmonology 1993; 15: 187 198.
9. Gyurkovits K, Németh I. Neutrophil superoxide anion production and the red blood cell glutathione redox system in the whole blood of CF children. (Abstract) EWGCF Congress, Copenhagen, 1991.

Cystic Fibrosis Pulmonary Infections:
Lessons from Around the World
ed. by A. Bauernfeind, M. I. Marks and B. Strandvik
© 1996 Birkhäuser Verlag Basel/Switzerland

CHAPTER 23
The General Approach to Cystic Fibrosis Pulmonary Infection in Denmark

Svend Stenvang Pedersen, Niels Høiby and Christian Koch

The Cystic Fibrosis Center, Rigshospitalet, DK-2100 Copenhagen, Denmark

Introduction

The first Danish case of cystic fibrosis (CF) was diagnosed in 1944 [1] and since then approximately 10–15 new cases have been added yearly. The clinical problems presented by these patients have largely dictated the approach to treating them. Because recurrent bacterial pulmonary infections are so prominent a feature, the evolution of CF pulmonary care parallels closely the history of antibiotic development (and is of similarly brief duration).

Present day therapy and the general approach to pulmonary care at the Copenhagen CF centre is based on a tradition of clinical studies and basic research in the pathogenesis of lung infection [2, 3, 4].

CF care has to be individualized and measured out with due respect to the age, pulmonary status, exocrine pancreatic sufficiency, patient acceptability and many other factors. However, the basic concept of the pathogenetic puzzle is the same as simplified in Figure 1.

The approach to pulmonary treatment must be aimed at many points in order to break the vicious cycle of events and comprises both pharmacological and non-pharmacological modalities. The main elements of the pulmonary care are prevention, detection, treatment and evaluation.

The Vicious Cycle of Events in the Cystic Fibrosis Lung

Patients with CF are born with histologically normal lungs, normal cilia and may have a virtually normal lung function [5, 6, 7]. However, the genetic defect renders respiratory secretions more dehydrated, thus impairing the mucociliary clearance [8]. It is not yet known whether the

Correspondence address: Svend Stenvang Pedersen, Department of Infectious Diseases, Rigshospitalet, Blegdamsvej 9, DK-2100 Copenhagen, Denmark.

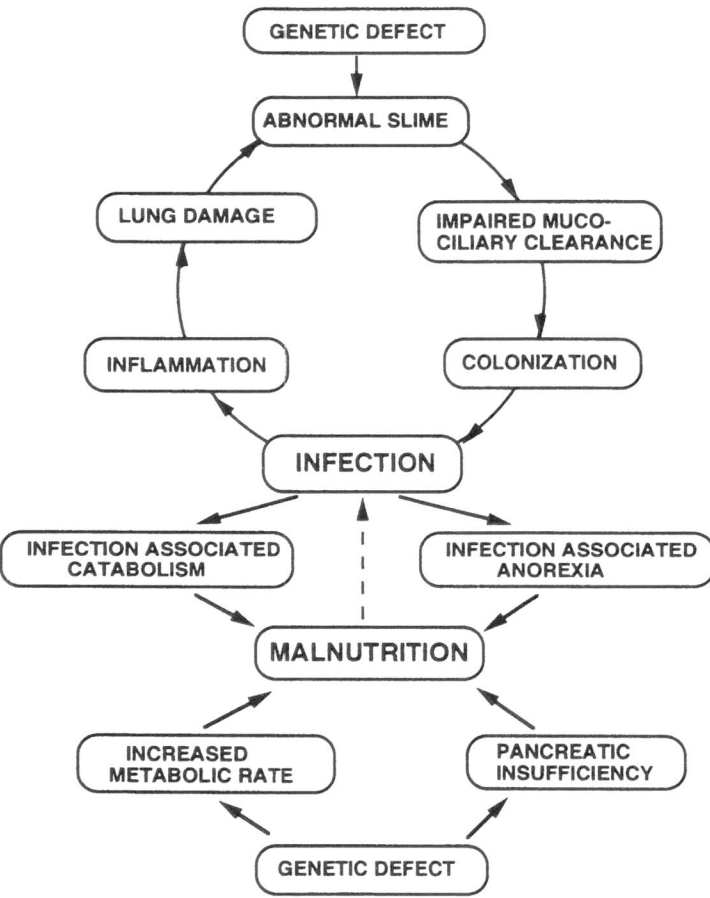

Figure 1. A simplified approach to the pathogenesis and treatment of CF lung disease. For explanation and possibilities for intervention see text.

impaired airway clearance and retention of secretions *per se* is the direct cause of subsequent colonization of the airways with bacteria or if the genetic defect leads to changes of the airways epithelial cells leading to increased bacterial adherence. No matter what the mechanism involved, CF patients are, already from infancy, highly susceptible to infection with *Staphylococcus aureus*, *Haemophilus influenzae* and *Streptococcus pneumoniae* (Figure 2) [9, 10].

Infection of the lungs may be associated with an increased respiratory workload and with infection-associated-anorexia due to cytokine release. This catabolic state – being recurrent – places an increased

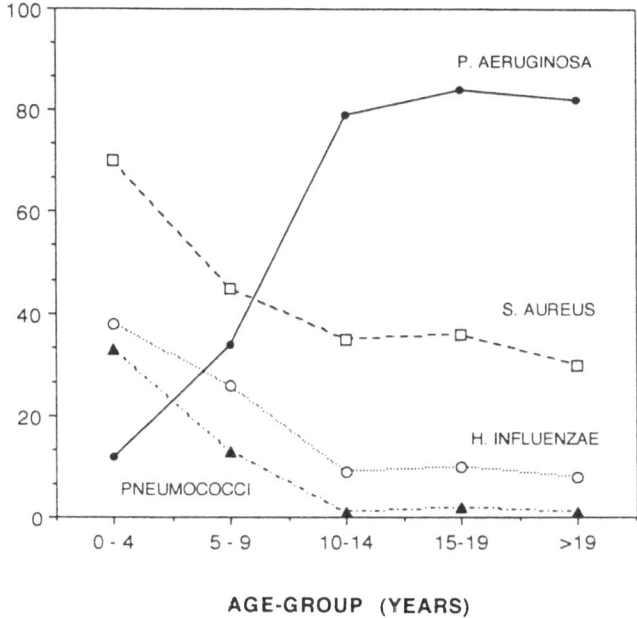

AGE-GROUP (YEARS)

Figure 2. The age-related point prevalence of the 4 major pulmonary pathogens in CF. Reprinted from [4] with permission.

burden on the caloric intake on top of the increased resting metabolic rate of CF patients [11]. Furthermore, the extrinsic pancreatic insuffiency so common in most CF patients impairs even further the ability to maintain energy balance, and hence growth and development, resulting in a vicious cycle where recurrent pulmonary infections aggravates the difficulty to thrive. A vigorous treatment of pulmonary infection is therefore likely to pay dividends in terms of improved nutritional status of the patient. On the other hand, it has never been convincingly demonstrated that moderate malnutrition increases susceptibility to infection, either in CF or in other conditions.

When bacterial colonization results in infection and inflammation of the lung parenchyma tissue degrading enzymes are released in the form of bacterial toxins and enzymes and oxygen radicals from host inflammatory cells [4, 12, 13]. Damage to pulmonary surface lining cells and connective tissue ensues. Some bacterial toxins even possess cilioinhibitory or ciliotoxic properties [14], which further reduces the already compromised mucociliary clearance. The dehydrated airway secretions now become mixed with an abundance of leukocyte debris forming purulent secretion, mainly due to leukocyte DNA [15]. Thus, in CF, a vicious cycle is set up where infection may increase the likelihood of subsequent infection. It has been shown that in the years immediately preceding onset of chronic infection with *Pseudomonas aeruginosa* these patients have a signficantly lower lung function than age-matched controls, indicating that significant damage to the lungs occurred prior to *P. aeruginosa* infection [16].

Although it is the most significant pathogen in terms of morbidity, mortality and cost of CF care, *P. aeruginosa* is therefore not regarded as an initial pathogen in CF lung disease, but rather an opportunistic pathogen which emerges to settle in patients with advanced lung disease [4].

When *P. aeruginosa* becomes chronic, the infection cannot be eradicated by antibiotics, and an immune-complex reaction in the lungs develops, which perpetuates the inflammatory cycle [17, 18].

This simplified outline of the pathophysiology of CF pulmonary infection provides a convenient platform from which to deal with possibilities for prevention, surveillance, early case detection, treatment and evaluation of therapy.

Prevention

Until causal gene therapy of airway cells become a reality only few preventive measures for avoiding pulmonary colonization exists. Lung physiotherapy is aimed at improving airway clearance and a multitude of methods have been presented. Based on clinical studies with documented efficacy Danish CF patients are offered PEP-mask physiotherapy (positive expiratory pressure) in combination with the forced expiratory technique (19). Clapping, postural drainage etc. is no longer recommended.

Liquification of the airway mucus was originally attempted with mist tent use, but this is now considered obsolete. Mucolytics such as N-acetylcysteine have not had a convincing effect and are not generally recommended. Instead some patient with hyperreactive airways benefit from inhalations with saline and beta-agonists.

Several studies have shown an association of onset of *P. aeruginosa* infection to a preceding viral respiratory infection [20, 21]. In order to reduce the latter, preschool children are therefore encouraged to attend small day-care homes having only a few other children instead of larger kindergartens, where the attending children have a much higher incidence of viral respiratory infections.

In addition to the usual child immunization programme CF patients are offered annual vaccinations against influenza virus. *S. aureus*, *H. influenzae* and pneumococci are commonly found in the normal oropharyngeal flora and no proper measures to avoid exposure exist. Infection with *H. influenzae* is usually caused by non-encapsulated strains [9] and the commercially available vaccine against *H. influenzae* (capsulated, type b) is unlikely to be of particular value in this setting.

Contamination of the inanimate surroundings in a CF clinic by *P. aeruginosa* and cross-infection from infected to uninfected patients has convincingly been demonstrated as a significant extrinsic source of infection. Hygienic principles aimed at stopping this transmission have therefore a very high priority at the Danish CF centre. Strict segregation policies are enforced such that infected and non-infected patients are seen on separate days in the out-patient clinic and, when hospitalization is necessary, these groups are admitted to different wards [4, 22]. Currently the following four groups are separted from each other: CF patients without *P. aeruginosa*, CF patients with antibiotic-sensitive, mucoid, *P. aeruginosa*, CF patients with multiply resistant, non-mucoid *P. aeruginosa* and finally patients infected or colonized with *Burkholderia cepacia*.

Vaccination against *P. aeruginosa* has been attempted, initially without beneficial effect [23]. Lately however, new vaccines and immunization strategies have been developed with encouraging results [24]. This approach is still of experimental nature.

Surveillance and Early Case Detection

As outlined above only a few interventions are in practical use for prevention. The main emphasis is therefore placed upon frequent clinical visits for early case detection and hence treatment.

Most patients are seen at monthly intervals and are assessed clinically in terms of lung function, nutritional and metabolic status and, when necessary, appropriate action is taken to optimize the condition of the patient and to prevent deterioration. Furthermore, at each visit samples of airway secretions are examined by microscopy and cultured for presence of pathogenic microorganisms [9]. The microscopy has to verify the origin of the secretions from the lower airways and the culture must be in accordance with the microscopy before therapeutic action (usually antibiotic prescription) is taken. The microbiological data are primarily used for treatment of the individual, but are also compiled to demonstrate changes in the bacterial flora and antibiotic susceptibility. The specific humoral immune response to *P. aeruginosa* is examined at least yearly [2]. This serves several purposes: Firstly, a certain level of antibodies to *P. aeruginosa*. (≥ 2 precipitins) is required to fulfill criteria for chronic infection with *P. aeruginosa*. Secondly, development of antibodies leads to intensified control in order to detect, as early as possible, the transition to chronic infection as this implies initiation of a separate treatment schedule. Thirdly, the rate of increase and the actual level of antibodies is correlated to prognosis and to an aggressive course of infection [2, 4]. Rapid increase in antibodies leads to an intensification of treatment.

Early Treatment

The principle behind this is that the patients should experience as few symptoms as possible before treatment is commenced. It is therefore an act of balance to differentiate between no infection and infection with no or only minor symptoms. The crucial tool for this is the microbiological examination. This approach is based on the assumption that the less inflammation, the less damage to lung parenchyma and better thriving, thus arresting or delaying the vicious cycle of events as outlined above. Patients with overt clinical symptoms like fever, respiratory distress, cyanosis and leukocytosis have a severe inflammation with a systemic reaction to the pathogen with inflammatory mediators spilling over from the lungs. Furthermore, early antibiotic treatment has a greater chance of achieving bacteriological success [25, 26]. The treatment approach can therefore be regarded as secondary prophylaxis. This prophylaxis is only intermittent and relies always on microbiological diagnosis. If a patient is found, by microbiological criteria, to have *S. aureus*, *H. influenzae* and pneumococci in the lungs, treatment is initiated and given for two weeks although infection *sensu strictu* is not necessarily present (Table 1). Rarely, if ever, is it necessary to admit patients with these pathogens for hospital based intravenous treatment.

A similar approach to early *P. aeruginosa* colonization was not possible until the orally absorbed fluoroquinolones became available, which made home-based treatment possible. As soon as *P. aeruginosa* is grown, even in the absence of antibody reaction and other criteria for

Table 1. Recommended antibiotic treatment of pulmonary infection in cystic fibrosis

Pneumoccocci	Phenoxymethylpenicillin (25 000–50 000 IU/kg/day)
S. aureus	*Penicillin sensitive*:
	Phenoxymethylpenicillin (25 000–50 000 IU/kg/day)
	in combination with
	Fusidic acid (50 mg/kg/day)
	Penicillin resistant:
	Dicloxacillin (25 mg/kg/day)
	in combination with
	Fusidic acid (50 mg/kg/day)

Duration of treatment: 14 days
Alternatives: Rifampicin (15 mg/kg/day) or clindamycin (20–40 mg/kg/day)

H. influenzae:	
	Ampicillin sensitive:
	Amoxycillin (25–50 mg/kg/day)
	Ampicillin resistant:
	Amoxycillin + clavulanic acid (25–50 mg/kg/day + 12.5 mg/kg/day)
	Alternatives: Rifampicin (15 mg/kg/day) in combination with Erythromycin
	(30–50 mg/kg/day)

Duration of treatment: 14 days
Probenecid (10–15 mg/kg/day) is added to all courses of beta-lactams eliminated by renal tubular secretion.

Table 2. Antibiotics recommended for treatment of *P. aeruginosa* infection

1: Intermittent colonization:

	Colistin aerosol	Ciprofloxacin orally	Duration weeks
1st isolation	1 MIU b.d	25–50 mg/kg/day	3
2nd isolation	2 MIU t.i.d	25–50 mg/kg/day	3
>3 isolation in 6 months	2 MIU t.i.d.	25–50 mg/kg/day	12

2: Chronic infection:

A. Regular intravenous courses for 2 weeks every 3 months during hospital admission:
       tobramycin (10–20 mg/kg/day)*

        in combination with
            piperacillin 300 mg/kg/day
    or   ceftazidime 150–200 mg/day
    or   imipenem 50–75 mg/kg/day
    or   aztreonam 150–200 mg/kg/day
    or   cefsulodin 150–200 mg/kg/day

B. To all   Aerosolized colistin 2–4 MIU/day is given continuously

C. Patients in unstable condition is given:
    Oral ciprofloxacin (20–40 mg/kg/day) during and between courses.
    Interval between i.v. courses may be shortened and courses prolonged to 3
    weeks until clinical condition becomes stable.

*Adjusted to trough concentrations of 1–2 mg tobramycin/l serum.

chronic infection, patients are started on oral fluoroquinolones and inhalation with colistin (Table 2). By doing this it is possible to significantly delay or perhaps even prevent the infection from becoming chronic [27].

Thus, the principles for early treatment are all the same irrespective of the offending pathogen, namely to prevent the infection from becoming chronic.

Chronic Lung Infection

Most of the effort in the daily CF care is focused on treatment of chronic *P. aeruginosa* infection. The criteria for this condition are positive cultures with *P. aeruginosa* for 6 months and the development of specific antibodies. It typically occurs in the early teens and is associated with a decline in clinical status.

The infection is characteristic because most, if not all, CF patients acquire it; it is the most common cause of death and disability in CF and it cannot be cured with antibiotics [4]. The bacteria grow in a peculiar microcolony mode of growth, where antibiotics do not affect the sessile, slow growing cells, which act as a reservoir for recurrence of growth of daughter cells. Poor prognosis is associated with a high antibody level and the pathogenetic mechanism of lung damage is thought to be due to immune-complex reaction in the lungs. The mainstay of antipseudomonal treatment is regular intravenous 2-week courses given during admission at the center [26]. The courses are repeated every 3 months for an indefinite time, usually for the rest of the patients' lives. In some cases and at certain periods the individual patient may even require more frequent treatment. If the patient is clinically unstable home inhalation of colistin may be added in between intravenous antibiotic courses [28]. The choice of antibiotics is preferably a combination of tobramycin, chosen for its greater antipseudomonal acitivity, and a beta-lactam antibiotic as shown in Table 2. Quinolones have been found to be less effective than the conventional intravenous combination chemotherapy [29]. Quinolones are used mainly in unstable patients between i.v. courses. The aim of the treatment is not to eradicate the bacteria, but to restore and maintain lung function. Thus this treatment principle has been termed 'maintenance' antibiotic chemotherapy. The repetitive antibiotic courses act as chronic suppressive treatment with the purpose of reducing the level of antigens. It is usual to see that the number of organisms in the lungs are reduced by a factor of log 3–5 during treatment. As in early treatment, the principle governing the approach to chronic infection is to prevent overt clinical symptoms associated with inflammation and subsequent parenchymal damage.

Evaluation of Therapy and Monitoring of Side-Effects

By using phage typing for *S. aureus* and biotyping for *H. influenzae* it is possible to differentiate between repeatedly positive cultures due to chronic persistence of the same strain, or reinfection with an unrelated strain [9]. If the same strain persists the treatment period is expanded and generally less than 10% have chronic infection with either *S. aureus* or *H. influenzae* [25]. These two pathogens do not possess the same ability to become chronic as *P. aeruginosa*.

The annual incidence of chronic *P. aeruginosa* infection has fallen to 1–2% [22] and the age at acquisition is increasing [4]. It is possible, on an average, to maintain lung function for at least 10 years in the chronic *P. aeruginosa*-infected patients [16]. The intensive maintenance chemotherapy is associated with a diminished increase in antibody responses and a significantly increased likelihood of survival [30, 31].

The antibiotic selection pressure is considerable and a gradual decrease in antibiotic susceptibility of *P. aeruginosa* has been noted, especially during courses of chemotherapy. The repeated nature of antibiotic treatment gives rise to concern of side-effects and regular surveillance for renal and hepatic toxicity is mandatory. The major problem seems to be hypersensitivity reactions to beta-lactam antibiotics. 62% of the patients with chronic *P. aeruginosa* have had one or more reactions. It can usually be managed by shifting to other drugs [32].

The use of quinolones for intermittent *P. aeruginosa* is usually for children that are still growing. However, no irreversible damage to the joints has yet been seen, although arthralgia is occasionally seen but disappears on cessation of therapy.

Tobramycin is the aminoglycoside of choice and has been used in excessive cumulative doses. Some damage to high frequency hearing has been noted, whereas chronic renal damage is not yet observed. The doses used of aminoglycoside are tailored by bi-weekly determination of serum concentration [33].

Other Treatment Options

Correction of the genetic defect by gene therapy is the ultimate goal. However, there are still a number of symptomatic treatment options that are being explored, which may interfere in the cycle of events.

Amiloride may be used to rehydrate the airway secretions and it has been shown to improve airway clearance [34, 35]. A reduced frequency of lower respiratory colonization has not been shown. Several attempts have been made to intervene much later in the pathogenetic process, mainly at the level of inflammation. Recombinant human DNase is advocated to reduce viscosity of airway secretion by breaking up leukocyte DNA [36, 37]. Alpha-1-antitrypsin given as an aerosol may protect against the proteolytic activity released from leukocytes [38]. At these points of intervention infection and inflammation is already established and use of nonsteroid and steroid antiinflammatory drugs to diminish inflammation seems more rational. Ongoing studies are currently determining the efficacy and side-effects of these therapies.

Despite aggressive and intensive treatment some patients still deteriorate and for those patients lung transplantation has become an established treatment option.

In the future it is conceivable that the approach to CF pulmonary care will include several of the treatment options listed above. Until their efficacy of interrupting the vicious cycle of events has been clearly established antibiotics will still form the basis for treatment of the pulmonary problems in CF.

References

1. Flensborg EW. Om den såkaldte congenitte cystiske pancreasfibrose. – Meddelelse af 5 tilfælde. Nord Med 1948; 39: 1574.

2. Høiby N. *Pseudomonas aeruginosa* infection in cystic fibrosis. Diagnostic and prognostic significance of *Pseudomonas aeruginosa* precipitins determined by means of crossed immunoelectrophoresis. A survey. Acta Pathol Microbiol Scand Sect C 1977; suppl 262: 1–96.

3. Schiøtz PO. Local humoral immunity and immune reactions in the lungs of patients with cystic fibrosis. Acta Pathol Microbiol Scand C 1981; suppl 276: 1–26.

4. Pedersen SS. Lung infection with alginate-producing, mucoid *Pseudomonas aeruginosa* in cystic fibrosis. APMIS; 100 suppl 28: 1–79.

5. Sturgess JM. Mucus secretion and clearance in the pathogenesis of cystic fibrosis. Monogr Pediatr 1981; 14: 60–74.

6. Katz SM, Holsclaw DS. Ultrastructural features of respiratory cilia in cystic fibrosis. Am J Pathol 1980; 106: 303–311.

7. Beardsmore CS, Bar-Yoshay E, Maayan C, Yahav Y, Katznelson D, Godfrey S. Lung function in infants with cystic fibrosis. Thorax 1988; 43: 545–551.

8. Wine JJ. Basic aspects of cystic fibrosis. Clin Rev Allergy 1991; 9: 1–28.

9. Høiby N. Microbiology of lung infections in cystic fibrosis patients. Acta Paediatr Scand 1982; suppl 301: 33–54.

10. Pedersen SS, Jensen T, Pressler T, Høiby N, Rosendal K. Does centralized treatment of cystic fibrosis increase the risk of *Pseudomonas aeruginosa* infection? Acta Paediatr Scand 1986; 75: 840–845.

11. Dodge JA, O'Rawe A. Metabolism and hyperalimentation in cystic fibrosis: an overview. In: N Høiby, SS Pedersen, editors: Cystic fibrosis, basic and clinical research. Amsterdam: Elsevier Science Publishers, 1992; 59–68.

12. Høiby N, Döring G, Schiøtz PO. Pathogenic mechanisms of chronic *Pseudomonas aeruginosa* infections in cystic fibrosis patients. Antibiot Chemother 1987; 39: 60–76.

13. Suter S. Lung inflammation and anti-inflammatory treatment. In: N Høiby, SS Pedersen, editors: Cystic fibrosis, basic and clinical research. Amsterdam: Elsevier Science Publishers, 1992: 177–182.

14. Wilson R, Roberts D, Cole P. Effect of bacterial products on human ciliary function in vitro. Thorax 1985; 40: 124–131.

15. Lethem MI, James SL, Marriott C, Burke JF. The origin of DNA associated with mucoid glycoproteins in cystic fibrosis sputum. Eur Respir J 1990; 3: 19–23.

16. Pedersen SS, Høiby N, Espersen F, Koch C. Role of alginate in infection with mucoid *Pseudomonas aeruginosa* in cystic fibrosis. Thorax 1992; 47: 6–13.

17. Høiby N, Döring G, Schiøtz PO. The role of immune complexes in the pathogenesis of bacterial infections. Ann Rev Microbiol 1986; 40: 29–53.

18. Döring G, Goldstein W, Botzenhart K, Kharazmi A, Schiøtz PO, Høiby N, Dasgupta M. Elastase from polymorphonuclear leukocytes: a regulatory enzyme in immune complex disease. Clin Exp Immunol 1986; 64: 597–605.

19. Falk M, Kelstrup M, Andersen JB, Støvring S, Falk P, Gøthgen IH. Improving the ketchup bottle method with positive expiratory pressure, PEP, in cystic fibrosis. Eur J Respir Dis 1984; 65: 423–432.

20. Petersen NT, Høiby N, Mordhorst CH, Lind K, Flensborg EW, Bruun B. Respiratory infections in cystic fibrosis patients caused by virus, chlamydia and mycoplasma – possible synergism with *Pseudomonas aeruginosa*. Acta Paediatr Scand 1981; 70: 623–628.

21. Johansen HK, Høiby N. Seasonal onset of initial colonisation and chronic infection with *Pseudomonas aeruginosa* in patients with cystic fibrosis in Denmark. Thorax 1992; 47: 109–111.

22. Høiby N, Pedersen SS. Estimated risk of cross-infection with *Pseudomonas aeruginosa* in Danish cystic fibrosis patients. Acta Paediatr Scand 1989; 78: 395–404.

23. Langford DT, Hiller J. Prospective, controlled study of a polyvalent pseudomonas vaccine in cystic fibrosis – three year results. Arch Dis Child 1984; 59: 1131–1134.

24. Bruderer U, Cryz S Jr, Schaad UB, Deusinger M, Que JU, Lang AB. Affinity constants of naturally acquired and vaccine-induced anti-*pseudomonas* antibodies in healthy adults and cystic fibrosis patients. J Infect Dis 1992; 166: 344–349.

25. Høiby N, Friis B, Jensen K, Koch C, Møller NE, Støvring S, Szaff M. Antimicrobial chemotherapy in cystic fibrosis patients. Acta Paediatr Scand 1982; suppl 301: 75–100.

26. Høiby N. Antibiotic therapy for chronic infection of pseudomonas in the lung. Ann Rev Med 1993; 44: 1–10.

27. Valerius NH, Koch C, Høiby N. Prevention of chronic *Pseudomonas aeruginosa* colonisation in cystic fibrosis by early treatment. Lancet 338; 8769: 725–726.

28. Jensen T, Pedersen SS, Garne S, Heilman C, Høiby N, Koch C. Colistin inhalation therapy in cystic fibrosis patients with chronic *Pseudomonas aeruginosa* lung infection. J Antimicrob Chemother 1987; 19: 831–838.

29. Jensen T, Pedersen SS, Høiby N, Koch C. Efficacy of oral fluoroquinolones versus conventional chemotherapy in treatment of cystic fibrosis. Eur J Clin Microbiol 1988; 6: 618–622.

30. Szaff M, Høiby N, Flensborg EW. Frequent antibiotic therapy improves survival of cystic fibrosis patients with chronic *Pseudomonas aeruginosa* infection. Acta Paediatr Scand 1983; 72: 651–657.

31. Pedersen SS, Jensen T, Høiby N, Koch C, Flensborg EW. Management of *Pseudomonas aeruginosa* lung infection in Danish cystic fibrosis patients. Acta Paediatr Scand 1987; 76: 955–961.

32. Koch C, Hjelt K, Pedersen SS, Jensen ET, Jensen T, Lang S et al. Retrospective clinical study of hypersensitivity reactions to aztreonam and six other betalactam antibiotics in cystic fibrosis patients receiving multiple treatment courses. Rev Infect Dis 1991; 13 suppl 7: S608–S611.

33. Pedersen SS, Jensen T, Osterhammel D, Osterhammel P. Cumulative and acute toxicity of repeated high-dose tobramycin treatment in cystic fibrosis. Antimicrob Agents Chemother 1987; 31: 594–599.

34. App EM, King M, Helfesrieder R, Köhler D, Matthys H. Acute and long-term amiloride inhalation in cystic fibrosis lung disease. Am Rev Respir Dis 1990; 141: 605–612.

35. Knowles MR, Church NL, Waltner WE, Yankaskas JR, Gilligan P, King M et al. A pilot study of aerosolized amiloride for the treatment of lung disease in cystic fibrosis. N Eng J Med 1990; 322: 1189–1194.

36. Ranasinha C, Assoufi B, Shak S, Christiansen D, Fuchs H, Empey D et al. Efficacy and safety of short-term administation of aerosolised recombinant human DNase 1 in adults with stable stage cystic fibrosis. Lancet 1993; 342: 199–202.

37. Hubbard RC, McElvaney NG, Birrer P, Shak S, Robinson WW, Jolley C et al. A preliminary study of aerosolized recombinant human deoxyribonuclease 1 in the treatment of cystic fibrosis. N Eng J Med 1992; 326: 812–815.

38. McElvaney NG, Hubbard RC, Birrer P, Chernick MS, Caplan DB, Frank MM et al. Aerosol alfa-1-antitrypsin treatment for cystic fibrosis. Lancet 1991; 337: 392–394.

Cystic Fibrosis Pulmonary Infections:
Lessons from Around the World
ed. by A. Bauernfeind, M. I. Marks and B. Strandvik
© 1996 Birkhäuser Verlag Basel/Switzerland

CHAPTER 24
The General Approach to Cystic Fibrosis Pulmonary Infection in The Netherlands

Lieke V. Möller[1], Jeannette E. Dankert-Roelse[2], J. Margriet Collée[3], Loek van Alphen[1] and Jacob Dankert[1]

From [1]the Department of Medical Microbiology, University of Amsterdam, Academic Medical Centre, 1105 AZ Amsterdam;
[2]Department of Pediatrics, Pediatric Pulmonology, Free University, 1081 HV Amsterdam;
[3]Department of Human Genetics, Free University, 1081 HV Amsterdam, The Netherlands

Summary. In the Netherlands, a national registry provides patient data on the demography of cystic fibrosis (CF). The survival rate of patients with CF has increased considerably over the last decade. The improved survival rate is in part attributable to management and care of these patients by multidisciplinary treatment in CF centres. Early diagnosis of CF, preferably made at the neonatal stage, will lead to improved patient treatment in order to delay deterioration in lung function. Treatment involves a comprehensive approach based on intensive antiobiotic therapy and physiotherapy in addition to nutritional and psychosocial support. Improvement of selective culture media has resulted in enhanced recovery of bacterial pathogens in CF, resulting in better basis for a rational choice of the antibiotic regimen. The complex pathogenic bacterial flora usually requires a combined therapeutic antibiotic treatment, especially for *Pseudomonoas aeruginosa* infections. The cornerstone of pulmonary care in CF is prevention of pulmonary deterioration through physiotherapy in combination with prophylactic antimicrobial therapy, an optimal nutritional state and possibly vaccination.

Demography of Cystic Fibrosis

In the Netherlands, cystic fibrosis (CF) affects approximately 1 in 3600 live births [1]. Currently, it is estimated that about 1000 patients have CF out of a total population of more than 15 million people. The heterozygous carrier frequency has been estimated to be approximately 1:30. Both sexes are equally distributed among CF patients. The disease sporadically occurs in non-whites.

A national CF registry was started in 1983 (Prof. Dr. L. P. ten Kate, Department of Human Genetics, Free University, Amsterdam). Dutch pediatricians and pulmonologists have been requested to report demographic data considering CF patients periodically. The latest report of

Correspondence address: Lieke V. Möller, University Hospital Groningen, Department of Medical Microbiology, Oostersingel 59, P.O. Box 30.001, 9700 RB Groningen, The Netherlands.

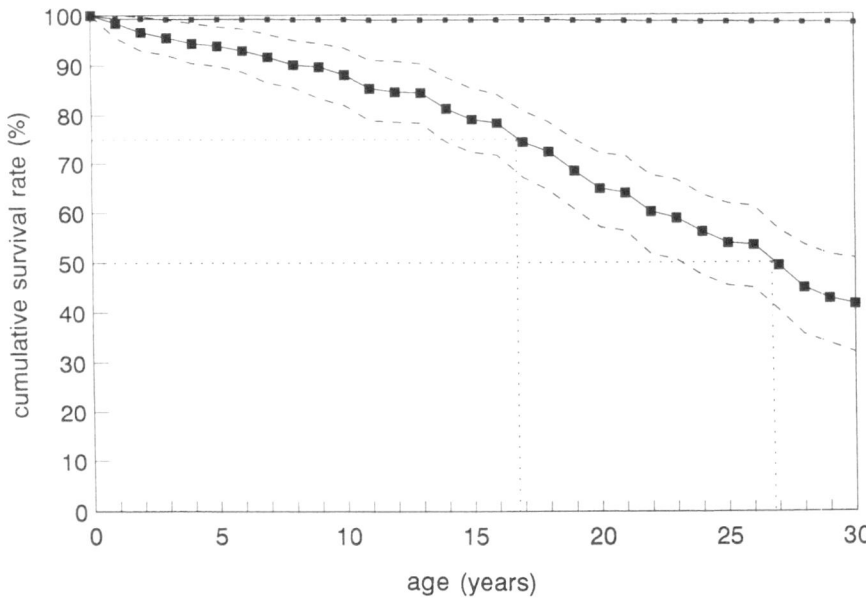

Figure 1. Cumulative survival rate (percent) of newborn CF-patients (■ – ■ – ■) with 95 percent confidence interval based on 3302 observed patient years compared to the Dutch population in general (■ – ■ – ■). Results are based on data collected in 1985–1990. Source: Dutch Cystic Fibrosis Foundation Patient Registry, 1993 (with permission) and the CBS (Central Bureau for Statistics).

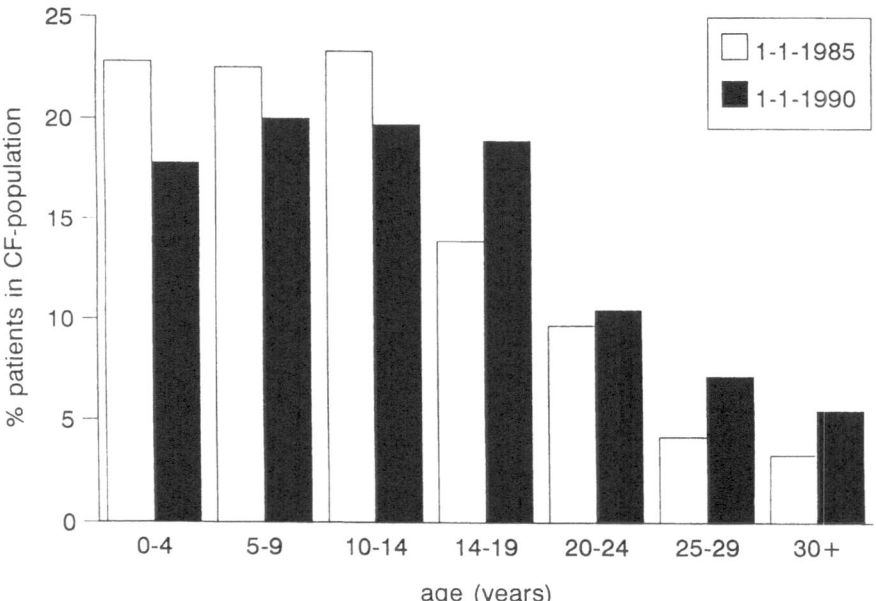

Figure 2. Percentage of the CF-patient population present in different age-groups in 1985 and 1990. Source: Dutch Cystic Fibrosis Foundation Patient Registry, 1993 (with permission).

this registry showed that about 75% of CF patients are diagnosed before the age of 2 years, increasing to 90% at the age of 15. This implies that 10% of CF is diagnosed at a rather advanced age. The survival rate of patients with CF in the Netherlands has increased considerably over the last decades. Estimates on cumulative survival based on data collected in 1985–1990 showed that 75% of newborns will reach the age of 17 and 50% of them the age of 27 years (Figure 1) [2]. In 1975 only 50% of newborns with CF reached the age of 10 years [1]. At present, the median survival age is 27, with an increasing number of patients surviving over 30 years of age [2]. The improvement of survival is also reflected in the age distribution as shown in Figure 2. The proportion of patients of 15 years or older was about 31% in 1985, while in 1990 this proportion was 42%. The proportion of patients of 20 years or older increased from 17% to 23%, respectively.

Care of Cystic Fibrosis Patients

In the Netherlands, most CF patients are treated in CF centres or in close collaboration with these centres. However, the CF centres are not officially registered. Management of the majority of CF patients is provided by most university hospitals in the division of pediatric pulmonology of the departments of pediatrics. Due to improvement of long-term survival and an increasing number of adult CF patients, CF centres for adult patients are required in order to guarantee continuous care for such patients. At present, the largest number of Dutch adult CF patients are treated in the adult CF centre in the Hague, although pulmonologists in various university hospitals are also involved in the care of adult CF patients. A CF centre providing multidisciplinary treatment in close collaboration with local practitioners is desirable in the Dutch situation. A prerequisite for this approach in hospitals caring for CF patients, is the availability of a CF team which gives advice and recommendations. Essential members of a CF team are a pulmonologist, gastro-enterologist, dietitian, physiotherapist, psychologist, social worker and a specialized nurse and preferably also a medical microbiologist, E.N.T. specialist, surgeon and medical geneticist. For the transition of adolescent to adult CF patient care, it is recommended that both pediatricians as well as internal medicine physicians are members of the team. This ensures the continuity of care and better insight into the problems occurring at the different stages of life. An important task of the CF team is to determine the goals of treatment, to develop treatment protocols, to introduce new methods of treatment for each discipline involved and to design the appropriate management for the individual patient together with the family or partner. Current treatment programmes ensure at least a stable condition of the patient for a long time, but require intensive attention and close cooperation between patients, parents and practitioners.

In our opinion, management and care for CF patients should start immediately after diagnosis, preferably made at the neonatal stage. This view is supported by the results of a 10–16 year clinical follow-up study after an experimental neonatal screening programme for CF. It was demonstrated that patients diagnosed at neonatal age maintain a nearly normal lung function and a practically normal weight and height for age during the whole period of follow-up [3]. The success of this approach is based on the following main principles:

1) *Intensive antibiotic treatment.* This should start soon after the first symptoms of the onset of an exacerbation of a respiratory tract infection appear. Due to the often insidious deterioration of the CF patient, early recognition of a (bacterial) infection of the lower airways is important in order to start the antibiotic treatment before the infection leads to a clinically manifest exacerbation. Easy accessibility to the CF team and broad experience of the team members with the first symptoms of lower airway infections are mandatory for effective management of CF patients. In addition, appropriate guidelines for antibiotic treatment and prophylaxis should be available.

2) *Intensive physiotherapy.* Physiotherapy should be performed at least once daily to facilitate sputum clearance, preceded by nebulisation of mucolytic agents, starting from the moment of CF diagnosis. In case of increased cough, the frequency of physiotherapy needs to be intensified to 2 to 4 times daily. Participation in sports with peers is encouraged, as well as going by bicycle to school. When the severity of the lung disease restricts a normal participation in sports, special training programmes should be organised to improve the physical condition.

3) *Intensive nutritional support.* Most CF patients can grow and develop somatically within the expected percentiles when they consume a high-calorie diet supplemented with pancreatic enzymes and fat-soluble vitamins. In the case of growth retardation more intensive nutritional supplementation is required, varying from extra snacks between meals to tube feeding overnight.

4) *Psychosocial support.* Despite the intensive treatment, most children with CF can live a life like other children do and participate in school activities and sports. However, many children and their parents need encouragement and support to continue and to perform the daily intensive treatment programmes. Due to the consequences of the disease and the requirements of its treatment it is not easy for patients to choose the best suitable education programme and profession. Often help and advice is provided in this field by CF team members.

Etiology of Cystic Fibrosis Pulmonary Infection

Although a variety of microorganisms are involved in infections of the lower respiratory tract of CF patients, the major pathogens are *Staphylococcus aureus*, nonencapsulated *Haemophilus influenzae*, and mucoid *Pseudomonas aeruginosa*. *S. aureus* is commonly the first microorganism recovered from CF patients and a main cause of permanent lung damage [4, 5]. In a 1986 survey of CF centres in the United States, *S. aureus* was found in 27% of the respiratory tract cultures and this was confirmed by a recent study performed in the Netherlands [6, 7]. *H. influenzae* is predominantly found in the early years and is responsible for 14% of the acute respiratory exacerbations [4, 8]. In a 1990 study of 2 CF centres in the Netherlands, *H. influenzae* was isolated from 23% of the sputum samples. This high recovery rate of *H. influenzae* can primarily be ascribed to the use of selective culture techniques, but using an immunochemical staining this bacterium was detected in 37% of the sputum samples [7, 9]. Although the clinical significance of *H. influenzae* in the respiratory tract of CF patients has yet to be elucidated, it is suggested that initial lung injury caused by *S. aureus* and *H. influenzae* predisposes to infection with *P. aeruginosa* [4]. *P. aeruginosa* usually appears in early adolescence with the highest incidence in the late twenties [4, 6]. Once infection with *P. aeruginosa* is established, this microorganism is hardly, if ever, eradicated. In some centres in the Netherlands the prevalence of *P. aeruginosa* is 70–80% [7, 10]. *Burkholderia cepacia*, an important pathogen in CF patients, especially in asymptomatic adults, may cause rapidly fatal deterioration after mild infection [11]. The prevalence of *B. cepacia* is centre-restricted and varies between geographic areas [6]. In the Netherlands, the prevalance of *B. cepacia* is not known, but *B. cepacia* seems to be uncommon.

Strategies for Routine Culturing of Respiratory Tract Specimens from Cystic Fibrosis Patients

To determine the etiologic agent of acute exacerbations, washed sputum specimens or throat swabs obtained after forced coughing are cultured on standard media as well as on various selective media in the Netherlands. Standard media included are horse blood agar, enriched chocolate agar, and MacConkey agar or cystine-lactose-electrolyte-deficient (CLED) medium for isolation of *P. aeruginosa* and other glucose fermenters and nonfermenters. Selective media are used to isolate specific microorganisms associated with pulmonary disease in CF [6, 9]. For the recovery of *S. aureus* a mannitol–salt agar is mainly used. This selective medium also supports the growth of thymidine-dependent *S. aureus*. Additionally, this medium enhances the recovery of *S. aureus* in the presence of mucoid *P. aeruginosa* [9]. For the recovery of *H. influenzae* the use of selective media is strongly advocated [6, 9]. N-acetyl-D-glucosamine agar is superior to chocolate agar plus bacitracin for the isolation of *H. influenzae* [12]. Both media suppress overgrowth by *P. aeruginosa* (which obscures the growth of *H. influenzae*). A selective medium containing ticarcillin and polymyxin B (PC agar) or alternatively a medium containing polymyxin B and bacitracin (OF-PBL agar) is used for the recovery of *B. cepacia* [6, 9]. For isolation of *Aspergillus* spp. and *Candida* spp. culturing of sputum on Sabouraud agar is recommended [6].

The use of an immunochemical staining technique with a monoclonal antibody against *H. influenzae* is a valuable addition in the laboratory diagnosis of this microorganism since its isolation from sputum is often hampered by the presence of antimicrobial agents in these samples and the growth of *P. aeruginosa*, despite the use of various selective culture media [12].

Indications for Starting Antimicrobial Therapy

Antimicrobial therapy in CF patients is indicated in case of an acute respiratoray tract infectious exacerbation [13]. Since the onset of an exacerbation is insidious, its presence is not always easy to determine. In addition, uniform criteria to define the onset of an exacerbation are not available. Therefore the diagnosis is usually made on the basis of clinical symptoms including increased cough, increased sputum production coinciding with a change in volume and appearance of the sputum, weight loss and decreased exercise tolerance. In contrast to the erythrocyte sedimentaion rate which generally becomes elevated in CF patients, C-reactive protein is a reliable indicator for an exacerbation. This diagnostic marker generally returns to normal as the acute episode of infection resolves [14]. There is a general tendency to start antibiotic treatment in CF patients as soon as the first signs suspected for the onset of an exacerbation appear. The occurrence of fever and leucocytosis associated with alterations of chest roentgenograms, are an absolute indication to start antimicrobial therapy [15, 16]. A decrease in spirometric indices, in particular of FEV_1, is also often considered to be indicative for treatment of an exacerbation [16].

Strategies for Antimicrobial Therapy

CF patients have a large volume of distribution and an increased total body clearance for certain antibiotics compared to other patients. Therefore, dose and/or frequency of administration are increased in CF patients to achieve antimicrobial efficacy. Some centres in the Netherlands use antimicrobial serum levels to determine dosing requirements in order to achieve a better clinical outcome than is observed with conventional dosing schedules [10].

Antimicrobial therapy is usually based on identification and sensitivity patterns of the isolated bacterial pathogens. Guidelines for antibiotic treatment of pulmonary exacerbations caused by the most common bacterial pathogens in CF patients are shown in Table 1 and 2. Patients with mild to moderate exacerbations caused by *S. aureus* and/or *H. influenzae* are usally treated with oral antibiotics. Patients with severe exacerbations are sometimes hospitalized for treatment with intravenous antimicrobial agents. *H. influenzae* may be treated with amoxicillin, however β-lactamase producing strains occur quite frequently (5–15%) [17]. In mixed infections with *S. aureus*, amoxicillin with clavulanic acid (Augmentin[R]) is used for oral treatment [16]. Parenteral therapy with amoxicillin and flucloxacillin or Augmentin[R] has proven to be effective for treatment of mixed infections with *H. influenzae* and *S. aureus* [18]. *S. aureus* infections are treated with flucloxacillin, if necessary combined with fusidic acid [6, 18]. When patients exhibit penicillin allergy, macrolides can be given as mono- or combination therapy. In the future, the new macrolides clarithromycin or azithromycin will probably replace erythromycin. Relatively infrequent dosing is possible which is beneficial for gastro-intestinal side effects [19]. *P. aeruginosa* infections are usually treated intravenously with a two-drug regimen of an aminoglycoside and a third-generation cephalosporin or semisynthetic penicillin [16]. Beta-lactams and aminoglycosides show a synergistic effect while the inducement of resistance is minimized. Ceftazidime is active against *P. aeruginosa* and preferably should be combined with tobramycin [16]. The use of ciprofloxacin for mono- or combination therapy to treat infections with *P. aeruginosa* is limited by the rapid emergence of bacterial resistance, especially of *P. aeruginosa* [20]. In some centres, patients with incipient or mild infections caused by *P. aeruginosa* receive oral treatment with a fluoroquinolone [16].

The duration of antibiotic treatment following an exacerbation is usually 2–3 weeks and is determined by the improvement of spirometric indices to previous levels or to a plateau level. The FEV_1 is a reliable index for the effect of treatment [10]. It has to be determined whether early onset of antibiotic therapy, before clinical manifestation of the exacerbation, may shorten the duration of therapy.

Intravenous Antibiotic Therapy in the Home Situation

Home intravenous antibiotic treatment of patients with cystic fibrosis was started in 1990 in the Netherlands. Nowadays, continuous intra-

Table 1. Guidelines for antibiotic treatment of pulmonary exacerbations caused by the most common bacterial pathogens in cystic fibrosis

Pathogen(s)	Antibiotic	Route of administration
unknown	amoxicillin/clavulanic acid[a] + ciprofloxacin	oral
	flucloxacillin + ciprofloxacin	oral
	flucloxacillin + cefazidime	iv
	penicillin allergy:	
	erythromycin + ciprofloxacin	oral
	erythromycin + ceftazidime	iv
H. influenzae		
β-lactamase negative	amoxicillin	oral/iv
β-lactamase positive	amoxicillin/clavulanic acid[a]	oral/iv
	penicillin allergy:	
	co-trimoxazole[b]	oral/iv
	ciprofloxacin	oral
	cefotaxime	iv
S. aureus	flucloxacillin + fusidic acid	oral/iv
	penicillin allergy:	
	erythromycin + fusidic acid	oral/iv
	rifampicin + fusidic acid	oral/iv
	vancomycin	iv

H. influenzae + *S. aureus*	amoxicillin/clavulanic acid[a]	oral/iv
	amoxicillin + flucloxacillin	iv
	penicillin allergy:	
	co-trimoxazole[b] + fusidic acid	oral
	ciprofloxacin + fusidic acid	oral
	cefotaxime + fusidic acid	iv
	co-trimoxazole[b] + fusidic acid	iv
P. aeruginosa + (*H. influenzae*)	ciprofloxacin	oral/iv
	ceftazidime + tobramycin	iv
	ticarcillin + tobramycin	iv
	penicillin allergy:	
	aztreonam + tobramycin	iv
P. aeruginosa + *S. aureus*	flucloxacillin + fusidic acid + ciprofloxacin	oral
	flucloxacillin + ceftazidime + tobramycin	iv
	flucloxacillin + ticarcillin + tobramycin	iv
	penicillin allergy:	
	ciprofloxacin + rifampicin + fusidic acid	oral
	aztreonam + rifampicin + fusidic acid	iv

[a] Augmentin.
[b] Sulfamethoxazole + trimethoprim.

Table 2. Dosage of antimicrobial agents for treatment of pulmonary infections in cystic fibrosis

Antibiotic	Route of administration	Dose (mg/kg/day)	No. of doses per day	Maximum daily dose (g)
amoxicillin	oral	50	3–4	4
	iv	100–150	6	12
amoxicillin/clavulanic acid[a]	oral	50 + 12.5	3–4	4 + 1
	iv	150 + 15	6	12 + 1.2
flucloxacillin	oral	75–100	3–4	4
	iv	100–150	6	12
ticarcillin	iv	500–750	4–6	30
cefotaxime	iv	100–150	4	12
ceftazidime	iv	150–200	4	12
	iv	100	continuous[b]	12
aztreonam	iv	150–200	3–4	8
tobramycin	iv	10–20	2–3	*
fusidic acid	oral/iv	50	3–4	1.5
erythromycin	oral	50	4	2
	iv	50	4	4
rifampicin	oral/iv	20	2	1.2
vancomycin	iv	40	4	2
sulfamethoxazole-trimethoprim	oral/iv	40 + 8	2–3	2.4 + 0.48
ciprofloxacin	oral	30	2	1.5
	iv	10	2	0.6

*Dosage based on plasma levels: peak 8–12 mg/l, trough 1–2mg/l.
[a]Augmentin".
[b]Initial dose of 100 mg/kg followed by continuous infusion.

venous antibiotic therapy in the home situation is feasible for most of the CF patients. A recently performed multicentre study in the Netherlands showed that home intravenous treatment of pulmonary infections in CF was as effective as treatment in the hospital [21]. Patients prefer home treatment because it enhances the quality of life by avoidance of frequent hospitalization and by improvement of their physical condition. An additional advantage is the earlier start of treatment of exacerbations. Home intravenous antibiotic treatment is cost-saving but requires a well-organized team operating outside the hospital, while remaining in touch with the hospital CF team.

Prevention of Infections

Acute as well as chronic infection of the respiratory tract in CF patients risks lung damage. Appropriate measures for the prevention of infection postpone the period after which pulmonary damage will develop. Generally, the following approaches are recommended:

1) *Physiotherapy*. Chest physiotherapy together with inhalation of mucolytics and/or bronchodilatators are still considered as effective, supportive measures to degrade thickened mucus and to remove retained airway secretions from CF patients [22]. It is important that the inhaled particle size generated by the nebuliser is small enough to reach the lower airways. Guidelines to decontaminate the nebulizers are provided by the National Cystic Fibrosis Society.

2) *Prophylactic antimicrobial therapy*. Continuous administration of oral antimicrobial therapy is intended to reduce the frequency and severity of exacerbations, but its benefit in the management of CF pulmonary disease has not been clearly proved. In the Netherlands, long-term prophylaxis with co-trimoxazole or flucloxacillin is empirically used when the respiratory tract of the patient is known to harbour *H. influenzae* or *S. aureus*. An improvement in spirometric indices and a reduction of the number of hospital admissions for treatment of exacerbations are obtained by nebulizing antimicrobial agents as maintenance therapy in patients colonized with *P. aeruginosa* [23]. This observation has led to the frequent use of nebulized colistin in CF patients with *P. aeruginosa*. Inhaled tobramycin is also efficacious for the prevention and treatment of chronic *P. aeruginosa* infection in CF patients. Chronic pulmonary colonisation with *P. aeruginosa* is further suppressed by use of oral ciprofloxacin therapy in conjunction with aerosol inhalations of colistin [24].

3) *Optimal nutritional status*. The maintenance of an optimal nutritional status by a well balanced diet started early during childhood, has shown to improve the condition of CF patients [25, 26].

4) *Vaccination*. In the Netherlands, the regular childhood vaccination programme includes vaccination against diphtheria, pertussis, tetanus, poliomyelitis, measles, rubella, mumps, and *H. influenzae* type b. Additionally, the influenza vaccine is used for the prevention of pulmonary influenza infections in CF patients. Influenza vaccination should be repeated yearly. In the Netherlands, vaccination against *P. aeruginosa* has not regularly been performed.

Conclusion

Comprehensive management of pulmonary infections in CF patients by intensive use of antiobiotic therapy in addition to chest physiotherapy and improved nutritional state, has been largely responsible for the increased life span of CF patients during the past decade in the Netherlands. A rational approach to antimicrobial therapy in and outside the hospital may postpone chronic infection, and may delay the pulmonary damage caused by ongoing recurrent infections. In the near future, development of new strategies for prevention and therapy of chronic lung infection is expected to further improve the quality of life and lifetime of CF patients.

References

1. Ten Kate LP. Cystic fibrosis in the Netherlands. Int J Epidem 1977; 6: 23–34.
2. Collée JM, Cobben JM, ten Kate LP. Survival of cystic fibrosis patients in the Netherlands. 11th international cystic fibrosis congress, Dublin, Ireland, August 24–27 1992; TP 104 (abstr.)
3. Dankert-Roelse JE, te Meerman GJ. Long term prognosis of patients with cystic fibrosis in relation to early detection by neonatal screening and treatment in a cystic fibrosis centre. Thorax 1995; 50: 712–8.
4. Hoiby N. Microbiology of lung infections in cystic fibrosis patients. Acta Paediatr Scand 1982; 301: suppl: 33–54.
5. Abman SH, Ogle JW, Harbeck RJ, Butler-Simon N, Hammond KB, Accurso FJ. Early bacteriologic, immunologic anc clinical courses of young infants with cystic fibrosis identified by neonatal screening. J. Pediatr 1991; 119: 211–17.
6. Gilligan PH. Microbiology of airway disease in patients with cystic fibrosis. Clin Microbiol Rev 1991; 4: 35–51.
7. Möller LVM, Ruys GJ, Heijerman HGM, Dankert J, van Alphen L. *Haemophilus influenzae* is frequently detected with monoclonal antibody 8BD9 in sputum samples from patients with cystic fibrosis. J Clin Microbiol 1992; 30: 2495–97.
8. Rayner RJ, Hiller EJ, Ispahani P, Baker M. *Haemophilus* infection in cystic fibrosis. Arch Dis Child 1990; 65: 255–58.
9. van Doern G, Brogden-Torres B. Optimum use of selective plated medium in primary processing of respiratory tract specimens from patients with cystic fibrosis. J Clin Microbiol 1992; 30: 2740–42.
10. Mouton JW. Pharmacokinetic and pharmacodynamic studies of beta-lactam antibiotics in volunteers and patients with cystic fibrosis [dissertation]. Rotterdam, The Netherlands: Univ. of Rotterdam, 1993.
11. *Pseudomonas cepacia* – more than a harmless commensal [editoral]. Lancet 1992; 339: 1385–86.

12. Möller LVM, van Alphen L, Grasselier H, Dankert J. N-acetyl-D-glucosamine medium improves recovery of *Haemophilus influenzae* from sputum of patient with cystic fibrosis. J Clin Microbiol 1993; 31: 1952 54.
13. Fiel SB. Clinical management of pulmonary disease in cystic fibrosis. Lancet 1993; 341: 1070 74.
14. Glass S, Hayward C. Serum C-reactive protein in assessment of pulmonary exacerbations and antimicrobial therapy in cystic fibrosis. J Pediatr 1988; 113(1): 76 79.
15. Greene KE, Takasugi JE, Godwin JD, Richardson ML, Burke W, Aitken ML. Radiographic changes in acute exacerbations of cystic fibrosis in adults: a pilot study. Am J Roentgenol 1994; 163(3): 557 62.
16. Mouton JW, Kerrebijn KF. Antibacterial therapy in cystic fibrosis. Med Clin North Am 1990; 74: 837 55.
17. Hoiby N. *Haemophilus influenzae, Staphylococcus aureus, Pseudomonas cepacia,* and *Pseudomonas aeruginosa* in patients with cystic fibrosis. Chest 1988; 94: 97S 102S.
18. Michel BC. Antibacterial therapy in cystic fibrosis. A review of the literature published between 1980 and February 1987. Chest 1988; 94: 129S 139S.
19. Aldons PM. A comparison of clarithromycin with ampicillin in the treatment of outpatients with acute bacterial exacerbation of chronic bronchitis. J Antimicrob Chemother 1991; 27: A: 101 108.
20. Bosso JA. Advances in the pharmacotherpy of cystic fibrosis. J Clin Pharm Ther 1992; 17: 263 70.
21. Bakker W, Vinks AATMM, Mouton JW, de Jonge P, Verzijl JG, Heijerman HGM. Continue intraveneuze thuisbehandeling van luchtweginfecties met ceftazidim via een draagbare pomp bij patiënten met cystische fibrose, een multicentrisch onderzoek. Ned Tijdschr Geneeskd 1993; 137: 2486 91.
22. Oberwaldner B, Theissl B, Rucker A, Zach MS. Chest physiotherapy in hospitalized patients with cystic fibrosis: A study of lung function effects and sputum production. Eur Respir J 1991; 4: 152 58.
23. MacLusky IB, Gold R, Corey M, Levison H. Long-term effects of inhaled tobramycin in patients with cystic fibrosis colonized with *Pseudomonas aeruginosa*. Pediatr Pulmonol 1989; 7: 42 48.
24. Valerius NG, Koch C, Hoiby N. Prevention of chronic *Pseudomonas aeruginosa* colonisation in cystic fibrosis by early antibiotic treatment. Lancet 1991; 338: 725 26.
25. Corey M. McLaughlin FJ, Williams M, Levison HA. Comparison of survival, growth and pulmonary function in patients with cystic fibrosis in Boston and Toronto. J Clin Epidemiol 1988; 41: 583 91.
26. Heijerman HGM. Studies in the clinical management of cystic fibrosis [dissertation]. Leiden, The Netherlands: Univ. of Leiden, 1991.

CHAPTER 25
Cystic Fibrosis Pulmonary Infection: The Swedish Experience

Birgitta Strandvik[1], Lena Hjelte[2] and Anna-Stina Malmborg[3]

Department of Pediatrics[1], Faculty of Medicine, Göteborg University, Göteborg, and Departments of Pediatrics[2] and Clinical Microbiology[3], Karolinska Institutet, Huddinge Hospital, Stockholm, Sweden

Introduction

Since the late 1960s, centres for cystic fibrosis (CF) patients have slowly been able to grow and now care for most of the patients with the disease in Sweden. At present there are close to 400 patients with CF out of a population of about 8 million inhabitants. About 340 of these are known to the three centres at the university clinics in Lund, Göteborg and Stockholm. Local screening programmes and genetic studies have indicated that the incidence in Sweden, as well as in the other Nordic countries, is lower than in central Europe and North America, approaching 1:4000 live births [1, 2].

Patient Population

During the 25 years of specialised care in Sweden the median age of patients under care has increased from 7.5 years of age in 1968 to 16 years in 1992 [3, 4]. The figures differ between the different centres and especially between patients regularly controlled at a centre and those not attending any centre. Our oldest patient died at the age of 72 years. The largest centre in Sweden is the one in Stockholm (developed after the first centre, which was established in Uppsala) caring for about 160 patients. It also presents the best results with a median age of patients under care of 20 years, and also a slight, but not significantly higher expected mean survival rate of 30 years [5]. The newest centre is the one in Göteborg, established in 1992, supervising about 100 patients. Each

Correspondence address: Professor B. Strandvik, Dept of Paediatrics, Göteborg University, S-416 85 Göteborg, Sweden.

centre provides a holistic view and works in a team consisting of physicians experienced in CF, nurses, physiotherapists, social worker, psychologist, dietitian and secretary. Their location at university hospitals guarantee the cooperation of clinical physiologists and chemists, microbiologists and other specialists according to international recommendations [6, 7]. The improved survival of the patients offers increasing experience of adults with CF. We have had the privilege to guide patients through several pregnancies without deterioration of their pulmonary function. Recently we have also had successful pregnancies with healthy babies born after *in vitro* fertilisation with sperms from male CF patients [8].

Interestingly, there seems to be a small difference in the genotype distribution between the south of Sweden and the rest of the country [2, 9]. The southern part, which is close to Denmark, has a high prevalence of $\Delta F508$, approaching 77%, in comparison with the middle and upper part, where $\Delta F508$ is found in about 63% of the chromosomes.

Altogether 14 patients have undergone lung or heart–lung transplantation; two were heart–lung transplanted at Harefield, UK before the procedure was possible in Sweden. Now three patients have been transplanted in Lund and 9 in Göteborg. Most of them have had double-lung transplantation. Twelve patients are alive and well with a good quality of life.

Most patients are studying or working full time or 75% of full time [10]. They are encouraged to use the 25% saved time for physical activities, for inhalation and when necessary for physiotherapy. According to our experience those working full time have either to restrict their social life (if they are not happy to be in a family physically very active) or neglect part of the important treatment. In order to have spare time for special activities similar to a healthy person we therefore recommend a reduction of working hours.

Strategies of Treatment

The strategies of treatment of the pulmonary infections are similar for the three centres and identical for the Stockholm and Göteborg centres. As soon as the diagnosis is suspected the patients and the parents are invited to the centre for confirmation of the diagnosis, information about the disease and education about treatment.

The patients living close to the centre (within 100 km) are preferably and most often seen monthly (or otherwise by their local doctor at the same intervals with telephone contact with the centre when necessary). All patients should be seen at a centre yearly. Newly diagnosed or severely ill patients might be seen twice to four times a year at the centre. At the monthly visit height, weight, clinical investigation and sputum – if possible – culture or nasopharyngeal swab culture are checked and children above 6–7 years of age have lung function tests (Vitalograph[R] or corresponding measurement). More extensive tests, including biochemistry, immunology, liver and renal function, lung and cardiac function and roentogenological investigations are usually confined to the yearly assessment when the individual treatment strategy for each patient is reconsidered.

In order to prevent mucus plugging in the airways, bromhexin therapy is instituted orally 0.5 mg/kg · day^{-1} divided in 3 doses at diagnosis. If there are absolutely no clinical, physiological or roentgenological indications of pulmonary engagement other mucus-dissolving measures are postponed to infectious exacerbations. The most important of these are inhalation with saline mixed with β-agonists (most used inhalator, Aiolos[R]) or use of mist tent nightly with sterile water nebulised in disposable tents with an ultrasonic nebulisator. Patients with very tenacious mucus might prefer N-acetylcysteine or occasionally mercaptoethanosulphate (Mesna, Mistabron). At acute exacerbations of pulmonary infections in heavy mucus producers, bromhexin or N-acetylcysteine are sometimes given intravenously for a few days.

The shortness of time in the morning for schoolchildren makes it difficult for them to both inhale and do physical activity or physiotherapy. This is the main reason why we still recommend mist tent nightly, which means that the patients do not need to inhale to dissolve the mucus. Similarly it is often difficult for infants and small children to understand and cooperate to obtain an efficient inhalation technique. The mist tent helps the parents by sparing inhalation in the morning.

In the strategy of prevention we vaccinate the patients for whooping-cough and tuberculosis and yearly for influenza. Other vaccinations, such as those against polio, rubella, measles, diphtheria, haemophilus (encapsulated) and mumps are included in the general health care programme for all Swedish children.

The policy to treat bacterial colonisation of the airways is based on prevention more than waiting for biochemical abnormalities or clinical disease to present [11]. About half of the patients are chronically colonised with *Staphyloccoccus aureus*, i.e. the bacteria are regularly isolated from the patient in sputum or from nasopharyngeal swabs for more than 6 months. Usually the youngest patients harbour *S. aureus* but sometimes adults persist being chronically colonised solely with *S. aureus* into the 4th decade of life. In patients free from pulmonary symptoms we prescribe flucloxacillin at minor viral infections, also when no sputum can be produced. Serum IgG antibodies against the staphylococcal toxins α-toxin and teichoic acid are regularly checked [12, 13], and if pathological titres are found the patients are treated with flucloxacillin (100 mg/kg body weight · day^{-1}, divided in 3 doses orally) for long periods of time, even years if necessary, for normalisation of titres. We have never seen any resistance against this penicillinase-resistant penicillin although frequently used for decades. Many younger patients – and occasionally older ones as well – are in addition repeatedly colonised with *Haemophilus influenzae*, which we always try to eradicate. In a few patients *Escherichia coli*, even mucoid strains, are isolated and *Proteus mirabilis* was a chronic coloniser for years in one patient.

Pseudomonas aeruginosa is regularly found in about 60% of the patients. It usually appears at about 10 years of age, but it sometimes present already during the first year of life, especially if the patient has developed pulmonary damage before diagnosis. According to our experience there is very often a co-colonisation of *S. aureus* and *P. aeruginosa* over years. During this time the patient presents with higher antibody titres both against staphylococcal toxins and against pseudomonal toxins [12–16]. We therefore believe that this period of time needs extra attention to prevent deterioration of pulmonary function, and sometimes long term treatment with flucloxacillin is recommended, superimposed by antipseudomonal treatment with high dosages of antibiotics at signs of mild infection [17].

The development of new β-lactams has probably been one of the major factors in the improved survival of patients with CF. As soon as pseudomonas is isolated – even if the patient has no actual symptoms and no deterioration of lung function, intravenous antibiotic treatment is instituted for about 10 days, with an aminoglycoside, nearly always tobramycin, and a β-lactam. The doses are high due to the fact that the patients with CF have both an increased renal and non-renal clearance [18–20]. Frequently there is a period of intermittent colonisation for months and even years before the pseudomonas strains constitute a chronic colonisation. During the time of intermittent colonisation the antibody titres against specific pseudomonas antigens are negative [14, 15]. We do not consider *pseudomonas* to be as life-threatening as before the time when efficient β-lactams became available. Most of our patients manage to keep their lung function stable for decades after the chronic colonisation [17, 21]. It is not clear if this is due to different genotypes of patients in Sweden [2, 9] or to our strategy to treat patients with very mild symptoms [17]. The strategy implies that some patients need intravenous antipseudomonal therapy monthly and some only once or twice a year. This individualised treatment makes the monthly clinical visits very important since a gradual deterioration, which is very common in CF, is hardly noticed by the patient until more pronounced symptoms present.

During recent years there have been an emerging problem of colonisation with *Stenotrophomonas maltophilia* in about 8% of our patients

[22]. *S. maltophilia* may be present together with *P. aeruginosa* but sometimes alone or together with *S. aureus*. At first presentation the strains are often sensitive to cotrimoxazole but very often develop multiresistance. *Burkholderia cepacia* has not hitherto been a problem since it has only been seen in a few isolated patients, who seldom visit the centres and in those cases the strains have been sensitive to most antibiotics.

Since 1985 we have preferred to teach the patients, who need intravenous antibiotic treatment, to manage the treatment at home [23]. This policy has been very successful and the patients prefer this kind of treatment to hospitalisation. Most patients continue to go to school or work, and some of the patients not even miss an hour. They are taught to mix the antibiotic with sterile water or saline and to administer it as a short time infusion. The first infusions of the aminoglycoside and the β-lactam at each treatment course are always given in hospital to control any severe allergic reactions but all others are given at home. Some severely ill patients still prefer hospitalisation where they can obtain more regular help of a physiotherapist but even these patients usually do not stay in hospital for the whole course. Also the patients who have a central venous access, usually Port-a-cath[R], are allowed to follow home intravenous treatment and no side effects or serious complications have occurred so far. Besides, many of the patients with essential fatty acid deficiency treat themselves with intravenous fat emulsions during three to four days when having the venous access. The burden on patients and/or parents is heavy but they prefer home treatment to hospitalisation since the ordinary family life is better preserved by staying at home. The home treatment has been facilitated during recent years by an infusion device (Intermate[R], Home pump[R]) which makes it possible to load the antibiotic solution for infusion in the device at the pharmacy. By using this the patients save time because they do not have to mix the antibiotics at home. It is also safe and the only drawback so far is the cost and that it is not usable for all kinds of β-lactams. Similarly good results are obtained as those with conventional home intravenous treatment or hospitalisation [23, 24].

The new quinolones are only used when intravenous therapy can not be given, usually for psychological or social reasons. The efficacy of intravenous treatment with ciprofloxacin has not been superior to the oral route since the drug has an extremely high bioavailability [25, 26]. Since ciprofloxacin is used comparatively infrequently, the *Pseudomonas* strains have remained sensitive. The treatment with ciprofloxacin orally is sometimes combined with inhalation therapy with tobramycin or when less sensitive strains are present, like *S. maltophilia*, with colomycin. We usually try to avoid using the same β-lactam in two consecutive treatment courses, and believe that this rule together with the rules of short time courses and a combination of an aminoglycoside and a

B. Strandvik, L. Hjelte and A.-S. Malmborg

Table 1. Antimicrobial susceptibility (%) of *Pseudomonas aeruginosa* isolated during the first part of 1984 (73 isolates), 1991 (352 isolates) and 1994 (391 isolates)

	Break points mg/l S ≤ /R ≥	S			I			R		
		1984	1991	1994	1984	1991	1994	1984	1991	1994
Piperacillin	16/32	85	80	84	10	8	7	5	12	9
Ceftazidime	4/16	82	77	84	8	14	11	10	9	5
Imipenem	4/16	90	76	81	7	5	4	3	19	15
Aztreonam	4/16	—	61	62	—	26	27	3	13	11
Tobramycin	4/8	90	98	99	6	0	0	4	2	1
Netilmicin	4/8	78	61	87	8	14	0	14	25	13
Trimethoprim-Sulfamethoxazole	32/64	23	0	0	18	0	0	59	100	100
Ciprofloxacin	1/8	—	93	92	—	3	4	—	4	4

S = Sensitive; I = Intermediate; R = Resistant.

Table 2. Antimicrobial susceptibility (%) of *Stenotrophomonas maltophilia* isolated during the first part of 1991 (38 isolates) and 1994 (70 isolates)

	Break points mg/l S≤/R≥	S		I		R	
		1991	1994	1991	1994	1991	1994
Piperacillin	16/32	5	13	13	41	82	46
Ceftazidime	4/16	19	56	26	18	55	26
Imipenem	4/16	0	0	0	0	100	100
Aztreonam	4/16	0	6	8	17	92	77
Tobramycin	4/8	26	27	0	0	74	73
Netilmicin	4/8	32	34	3	0	66	66
Trimethoprim-Sulfamethoxazole	32/64	82	73	5	4	13	23
Ciprofloxacin	1/8	63	70	8	10	29	20

S = Sensitive; I = Intermediate; R = Resistant.

β-lactam have been the factors behind the very low development of resistant strains of *P. aeruginosa* despite a very aggressive antibiotic treatment policy [17].

Antimicrobial Susceptibility

The low frequency of resistant strains of *P. aeruginosa* and *S. maltophilia* can be shown by a comparison of sensitivity pattern over time (Tables 1 and 2). The antimicrobial susceptibility has been determined by ICS method [27] using paper discs (Biodisk, Sweden). Sensitivity was defined as sensitive (S), intermediate (I) or resistant (R) [28]. Marked development of resistance to trimethoprim-sulpha-methoxazole was seen from 1984 to 1991. Imipenem was a rather new drug in 1984, and a low development of resistance can now be noted. The discrepancy between the sensitivity to netilmicin between years may be due to methodological changes. Aztreonam and ciprofloxacin were not on the market in 1984. *S. maltophilia* has only been isolated from our CF patients during recent years [22], and the number of isolates is low. It is therefore difficult to draw any conclusions from the sensitivity pattern between 1991 and 1994. It seems however that the sensitivity pattern has been stable.

Other Factors of Importance for Treatment

In some patients with an unexpected and inexplicable deterioration we have found atypical mycobacteria and in one patient even tuberculosis as causative factors [29]. All patients lived in good socio-economic situations, and no special risk factor for those patients could be found. After appropriate treatment all patients recovered. It is thus important to investigate for this possibility even in patients vaccinated against tuberculosis.

Parallel to all antibiotic treatment, the physiotherapy has to be intensified to obtain optimal result of the treatment at clinical as well as subclinical exacerbations. Some patients can proceed with their usual activities such as jogging, horse-riding etc., but some need more rest and thus more help from more conventional physiotherapy. The forced expiratory technique is the most often used therapy but different kinds of physiotherapy are used depending on the preference of the patients. In severely ill patients both PEEP-mask and autogenic drainage seem to be of value, and even clapping may sometimes be valuable together with the forced expiratory technique [30]. In patients who desaturate at night, oxygen is prescribed nightly and if possible also during the physiotherapy sessions.

We also consider the nutritional status of the patients very important and do not accept a divergence from the growth chart [31]. When that occurs – the tendency is very often seen in prepuberty – we check for pulmonary infection, food intake, adequacy and/or compliance of pancreatic supplementation and essential fatty acid deficiency and treat accordingly. In the severely ill patient anorexia may develop and tube-feeding nightly via gastrostomy or jejunostomy might then be necessary to improve the nutrition. In that way normal growth can be maintained in practically all patients and lung function can more easily be preserved.

Gene therapy is under development but we still do not know when it will be clinically possible to treat patients. Until that time we have to rely on the development of different mucus-dissolving agents (like rhDNas, amiloride together with UTP) and new antibiotics to keep the lungs as clear as possible. Lung transplantation should only be considered as the last resort when we have failed to help the patients keep their lungs in a good function. The most important parts in this strategy are probably early diagnosis, centralised care with treatment of very mild pulmonary symptoms, and optimal nutrition.

References

1. Kollberg H, Hellsing K. Screening for cystic fibrosis by analysis of albumin in meconium. Acta Paediatr Scand 1975; 64: 477–482.
2. Dahl N, Grandell U, Martinsson T, Allen M, Johansson L, Stolpe L, et al. Frequency of four cystic fibrosis mutations in a Swedish population. Acta Paediatr 1993; 82: 609.
3. Kollberg H. Incidence and survival curves of cystic fibrosis in Sweden. Acta Paediatr Scand 1982; 71: 197–202.
4. Lannerfors L. Cystic fibrosis in Sweden – a report of the care situation in different parts of the country. Swedish Cystic Fibrosis Association, 1992–94, Uppsala, Sweden.

5. Kollberg H. Increasing survival of Swedish patients with CF. Acta Univ Carol Med 1990; 36: 213–214.
6. The Cystic Fibrosis Foundation Center Committee and Guidelines Subcommittee. Cystic fibrosis foundation guidelines for patient services, evaluation, and monitoring in cystic fibrosis centers. Amer J Dis Child 1990; 144: 1311–1312.
7. Neilson OH, Thomsen BL, Green A, Andersen PK, Hauge M, Schiotz PO. Cystic fibrosis in Denmark 1945–1985. An analysis of incidence, mortality and influence of centralised treatment on survival. Acta Paediatr Scand 1988; 77: 836–841.
8. Fogdestam I, Hamberger L, Hjelte L, Strandvik B. Successful pregnancies after *in vitro* fertilisation with sperm from patients with cystic fibrosis. 18th Cystic Fibrosis Congress Paris, France, 29th May–2nd June, 1994.
9. Kornfält R, Andreasson B, Holmberg L. Cystic fibrosis mutations in southern Sweden: relationship to clinical severity. Acta Paediatr 1992; 81: 262–263.
10. Carlsson M. A psychosocial study of adolescents and adults with cystic fibrosis in Sweden. 10th Intern Cystic Fibrosis Congress, Sydney, Australia, 5–10 March, 1988, p. 130–131.
11. Hollsing AE, Lantz B, Bergström K, Malmborg AS, Strandvik B. Granulocyte elastase – alpha 1 – antiproteinase complex in cystic fibrosis: sensitive plasma assay for monitoring pulmonary infections. J Pediatr 1987; 111: 206–211.
12. Ericsson A, Granström M, Möllby R, Strandvik B. Antibodies to staphylococcal teichoic acid and alpha toxin in patients with cystic fibrosis. Acta Paediatr Scand 1986; 75: 139–144.
13. Ericsson-Hollsing A, Granström M, Strandvik B. Prospective study of serum staphylococcal antibodies in cystic fibrosis. Arch Dis Child 1987; 62: 905–911.
14. Granström M, Ericsson A, Strandvik B, Wretlind B, Pavlovskis OR, Berka R, Vasil ML. Relation between antibody response to *Pseudomonas aeruginosa* exoproteins and colonization/infection in patients with cystic fibrosis. Acta Paediatr Scand 1984; 73: 772–777.
15. Ericsson-Hollsing A, Granström M, Vasil M, Wretlind B, Strandvik B. Prospective study of serum antibodies to *Pseudomonas aeruginosa* exoproteins in cystic fibrosis. J Clin Microbiol 1987; 25: 1868–1874.
16. Strandvik B, Hollsing A, Möllby R, Granström M. Antistaphylococcal antibodies in cystic fibrosis. Infection 1990; 18: 170–172.
17. Strandvik B. Antibiotic therapy of pulmonary infections in cystic fibrosis. Dosage and dose schedules. Chest 1988; 94: 146–149.
18. de Groot R, Smith AL. Antibiotic pharmacokinetics in cystic fibrosis. Differences and clinical significance. Clin Pharmacokinet 1987; 13: 228–253.
19. Spino M. Pharmacokinetics of drugs in cystic fibrosis. In: Clin Rev Allergy. Cystic fibrosis. E Gershwin, editor. Humana Press Inc 1991; 9: 169–210.
20. Taburet A-M, Tollier C, Richard C. The effect of respiratory disorders on clinical pharmacokinetic variables. Clin Pharmacokinet 1990; 19: 462–490.
21. Ericsson A, Strandvik B, Troell S, Freyschuss U. Relation between clinical and roentgenological scores and measures of lung function in cystic fibrosis with special reference to pulmonary Xenon[133] elimination. Clin Physiol 1987; 7: 275–283.
22. Karpati F, Malmborg A-S, Alfredsson H, Hjelte L, Strandvik B. Bacterial colonization with Xanthomonas maltophilia – a retrospective study in a cystic fibrosis patient population. Infection 1994; 22: 258–263.
23. Strandvik B, Hjelte L, Malmborg A-S, Widén B. Home intravenous antibiotic treatment of patients with cystic fibrosis. Acta Paediatr Scand 1992; 81: 340–344.
24. Widén B, Ljung M, Hjelte L, Strandvik B. Home intravenous antibiotic treatment in cystic fibrosis with Intermate[R]. XIth Int Cystic Fibrosis Congress, Dublin 1992 (abstract TP26, p. 150).
25. Strandvik B, Hjelte L, Lindblad A, Ljungberg B, Malmborg A-S, Nilsson-Ehle I. Comparison of efficiency and tolerance of intravenously and orally adminstrated ciprofloxacin in cystic fibrosis patients with acute exacerbations of lung infection. Scand J Inf Dis 1989; suppl 60: 84–88.
26. Christensson BA, Nilsson-Ehle I, Ljungberg B, Lindblad A, Malmborg A-S, Hjelte L, Strandvik B. Increased oral bioavailability of ciprofloxacin in cystic fibrosis patients. Antimicrob Agents Chemother 1992; 36: 2512–2517.

27. Ericsson HM, Sherris JC. Antibiotic sensitivity testing. Report of an international collaborative study. Acta Pathol Microbiol Scand 1971; 217 (suppl): 1–90.
28. The Swedish Reference Group for Antibiotics. Antimicrobial susceptibility testing of bacteria. National Bacteriological Laboratory, Stockholm 1990.
29. Hjelte L, Källenius G, Petrini B, Strandvik B. Prospective study of mycobacterial infections in patients with cystic fibrosis. Thorax 1990; 45: 397–400.
30. Blomquist M, Freyschuss U, Wiman LG, Strandvik B. Physical activity and self treatment in cystic fibrosis. Arch Dis Child 1986; 461: 362–367.
31. Strandvik B. Nutritional management in cystic fibrosis. In: Cystic Fibrosis. Ann Nestlé 1991; 49: 38–46.

Cystic Fibrosis Pulmonary Infections:
Lessons from Around the World
ed. by A. Bauernfeind, M. I. Marks and B. Strandvik

CHAPTER 26
Cystic Fibrosis Pulmonary Infections: The UK Experience

Stuart Elborn[1], John Dodge[2] and James Littlewood[3]

[1]*Adult Cystic Fibrosis Unit, Belfast City Hospital, Belfast, UK*
[2]*Department of Child Health, Queens University, Belfast, UK*
[3]*Regional Paediatric Cystic Fibrosis Unit, St. James' University Hospital, Leeds S9 7TF, UK*

Introduction

There were over 6000 patients with cystic fibrosis resident in the United Kingdom in 1991 [1, 2]. Of these patients, 41% are over the age of 15 years, with 12% 25 years and over. The population of patients in the UK is growing at a rate of about 120 patients per year and by the end of the millennium will be over 7000 [1, 2]. By this time about 50% of patients will be over the age of 15 [2].

Median survival for patients with cystic fibrosis in the United Kingdom is currently of the order of 26–28 years though this is increasing annually [1, 2]. After the first year of life age specific mortality is lower in males than in females and this is particularly evident during the late teenage years [1]. Predictions for children born in England and Wales in 1990 have suggested that median survival, if it continues to increase at the current rate, during the next 30 years will extend towards about 40 years, assuming no further advances in treatment, such as gene therapy [2].

The age of diagnosis for patients with cystic fibrosis varies in the United Kingdom depending on whether neonatal screening for immunoreactive trypsin (IRT) is undertaken [3]. A number of regions currently routinely screen all newborn babies using the IRT method and this leads to earlier diagnosis, but where neonatal screening does not take place the age of diagnosis is higher [4]. It is not yet clear if early diagnosis by such methods results in improved survival [3].

Correspondence address: Stuart Elborn, Adult Cystic Fibrosis Unit, Belfast City Hospital, Belfast BT9 7AB, UK.

Organisation of Care for Patients With Cystic Fibrosis in the UK

The organisation of clinical care for patients with cystic fibrosis varies according to the Regional Health Authority (RHA) [5]. The majority of regions have a specialist centre for the care of patients with cystic fibrosis, usually in a University or Teaching Hospital. These centres have between 40 and 500 patients attending for clinical care. Most regions have a separate paediatric and adult service with transition from the paediatric unit to adult care occurring between the ages of 15 and 18 years. There are, however, a few centres in which care of adults is undertaken by the paediatric services [6]. The majority of patients with cystic fibrosis attend specialist centres but 25% are not in contact with a regional centre and receive care from local hospitals and a few receive most of their care from their general practitioner.

A number of groups including the British Paediatric Association, British Thoracic Society, The Royal College of Physicians (London) and the Clinical Standards Advisory Working Group on Cystic Fibrosis (set up by the Department of Health) have recommended that all patients should have access to specialist care [5, 7]. Shared care arrangements, with routine care provided at the local general hospital in collaboration with expert advice from a regional centre, exist in some regions. This sometimes involves specialist teams visiting the local hospital, or annual visits by the patient to the regional centre for a comprehensive assessment.

Approach to the Management of Respiratory Infections

Respiratory infection is the main cause of morbidity and mortality in cystic fibrosis. Lung damage can be demonstrated histologically from the early months of life and this is probably a consequence of early infection [8]. Many organisms may cause pulmonary infection in patients with cystic fibrosis (Table 1). Non-pseudomonal bacterial infection predominates in the first decade of life while *Pseudomonas aeruginosa* is the most common infecting organism by the end of the second decade [9]. Other organisms will often cause co-infection with *P. aeruginosa*.

Non-Pseudomonal Bacterial Infection

Most centres in the United Kingdom take an aggressive approach to the management of pulmonary infection. The presence of respiratory symtoms and/or the culture of specific organisms, such as *Staphylococcus*

Table 1. Pathogens infecting the respiratory tract in cystic fibrosis

Bacteria	*Staphylococcus aureus*
	Haemophilus influenzae
	Streptococcus pneumoniae
	Pseudomonas aeruginosa
	Stenotrophomonas maltophilia
	Burkholderia cepacia
	Mycobacterium tuberculosis
	Atypical *mycobacterium*
Viruses	Respiratory Syncytial Virus
	Adenovirus
	Rhinoviruses
Fungi	*Aspergillus fumigatus*

aureus, Haemophilus influenzae or *Streptococcus pneumoniae* from sputum or throat swab culture, as many children produce little or no sputum, is an indication for treatment with antiobiotics. The choice of antibiotic is usually obvious when specific organisms are isolated from sputum culture. Most treatment schedules are for two weeks duration and it is useful to re-culture sputum after 10 days of a course of antibiotics. We advocate that patients are treated until these organisms are eradicated. When no organism is identified then treatment is started on the basis of changing symptoms and lung function tests, if available. Many symptomatic exacerbations, particularly in children, are not associated with positive sputum isolation of bacteria and may be due to viral infection or non-specific airways obstruction. In this situation *H. influenzae* and *S. aureus* should be covered in the antibiotic therapy.

Treatment of non-pseudomonal infection can usually be achieved using oral antibiotics and, therefore, will often take place in the community. Patients are encouraged to increase the frequency of physiotherapy to three times daily. Bronchodilator medication may also need to be increased as organisms may elaborate bronchoconstrictor substances, such as histamine. Pulmonary infection is often associated with anorexia and weight loss and appropriate nutritional supplements may be required to maintain or regain weight.

Staphylococcus aureus

A number of centres in the UK treat children with prophylactic anti-staphylococcal agents, such as flucloxacillin, from the first isolation of *S. aureus* in sputum culture or, in some, from early in life [10]. This approach has recently been validated in children during the first year of life [11]. In this study newborn infants treated continuously with flucloxacillin from diagnosis by immunoreactive trypsin (IRT) assay had fewer admissions to hospital and required fewer courses of extra antibiotics compared to a group treated with placebo. Further studies are required to confirm longer term benefit from the use of prophylactic anti-staphylococcal agents.

If *S. aureus* is isolated while the patient is on long-term flucloxacillin the addition of a second anti-staphylococcal agent is indicated. The combination of oral flucloxacillin and fusidic acid, oral clindamycin or intravenous flucloxacillin combined with gentamicin or tobramycin for two weeks, usually eradicates *S. aureus* from sputum culture (Table 2).

Table 2. Drugs used to treat *S. aureus* infection

Flucloxacillin	80 mg/kg/24 h
Fusidic acid	50 mg/kg/24 h
Erythromycin	50 mg/kg/24 h
Clindamycin	20–40 mg/kg/24 h
Gentamicin	5–8 mg/kg/24 h
Tobramycin	10–15 mg/kg/24 h

Haemophilus influenzae

Haemophilus influenzae is a relatively common pathogen particularly in children with cystic fibrosis. It occurs more frequently than in patients with asthma and probably plays an important pathogenic role [12]. *H. influenzae* is usually sensitive to an aminopenicillin but increasing resistance to penicillin has been observed in the past decade. In the UK most centres report that approximately 10% of isolates are resistant to ampicillin [13]. The antibiotic of choice should be dictated by local sensitivity patterns for organisms resistant to ampicillin *in vitro*. The addition of clavulanic acid to amoxycillin (co-amoxyclav) is likely to be useful, or a cephalosporin, such as cefuroxime axetil or cefaclor may be used (Table 3). The new macrolides, such as clarithromycin and azithromycin, have better *in vitro* activity against *H. influenzae* and may be useful in cystic fibrosis. We would suggest that treatment for *H. influenzae* should be continued for two weeks and if repeat sputum culture at the end of this time still isolates the organism the antibiotic should be changed according to sensitivity patterns and continued until the organism is eradicated.

Table 3. Drugs used to treat *H. influenzae* infection

Amoxycillin	50–100 mg/kg/24 h
Amoxycillin & Clavulanic acid (Amoxiclav)	50 mg + 12.5 mg/kg/24 h
Cefuroxime Axetil	50–75 mg/kg/24 h
Chloramphenicol	50–100 mg/kg/24 h

Other Non-Pseudomonal Infections

Streptococcus pneumoniae, Moraxella catarrhalis, coliforms *Legionella pneumophilia* and *Mycoplasma pneumoniae* may also cause intermittent airways infection in patients with cystic fibrosis [14]. Treatment should be dictated by clinical suspicion and antimicrobial sensitivity in consultation with a microbiologist. Treatment should be continued until eradication of the organism from sputum culture is obtained.

Mycobacterial Infections

The incidence of *Mycobacterium tuberculosis* infection is increased in patients with CF [15]. When isolated from sputum, treatment for this organism should be as for non-cystic fibrosis patients and modified, when necessary, according to anti-microbial sensitivity patterns. Pulmonary infection with environmental mycobacteria (atypical mycobacteria) is also increased in patients with cystic fibrosis (Table 4) [16]. Deciding when to treat such infections is often difficult as isolation may indicate transient colonisation or supra-infection. Repeated isolation of the organism in heavy growth from a patient with compatible clinical and radiological features of infection should be treated with appropriate anti-tuberculosis drugs according to sensitivity patterns [17].

Table 4. Mycobacterial organisms causing pulmonary infection in cystic fibrosis

M. tuberculosis
M. avium-intracellulare complex (MAC)
M. kansasii
M. fortuitum

Pseudomonas aeruginosa

Pseudomonas aeruginosa is the major pathogen affecting patients with cystic fibrosis from the second decade of life [18]. Prevention, or postponement, of infection may be achieved by isolation of patients harbouring *P. aeruginosa* from non-infected patients [19]. This has been achieved in some European centres and is practiced in a few centres in the UK. Vaccination against pseudomonal infection has not been found to be successful [20].

Treatment of first isolation of *P. aeruginosa* has been the subject of some recent research. It has been demonstrated that an inflammatory response occurs at the time of first isolation of this organism from adults with cystic fibrosis and it is likely that this pertains in children

[21]. It has also been demonstrated that aggressive treatment of first isolation of *P. aeruginosa*, with intravenous anti-pseudomonal antibiotics or a combination of oral ciprofloxacin and nebulised colomycin, can result in a medium term eradication of this organism from sputum culture for up to two years [22, 23]. We would recommend that such an aggressive policy be considered at first isolation of this organism, as once established in the airways *P. aeruginosa* plays a major part in the establishment and continuation of a vicious cycle of infection and host inflammation [18].

P. aeruginosa is responsible for initiating a continuous process of infection and inflammation resulting in bronchiectasis, airways damage and eventually interstitial pulmonary damage [18, 24]. It is likely that most of the damage to the airways and the lungs is a result of the host response to infection and treatment of early colonisation may be important in postponing the onset of severe lung injury [21]. Once chronically infected with this organism aggressive treatment of respiratory exacerbations may be helpful in attenuating the inflammatory process. The mainstay of treatment is antibiotic drugs and physiotherapy to aid airways clearance. It is, however, unclear if the effect of antibiotics is only due to killing organisms or whether they have more subtle effects in reducing the production of virulence factors from organisms [25]. Antibiotics may also have some direct effects on host inflammatory response, such as diminution of mucus producton [26].

The antibiotic treatment of respiratory exacerbations in patients who are chronically infected with *P. aeruginosa* usually involves two antibiotics combining an aminoglycoside, such as tobramycin or gentamicin, plus a second antpseudomonal agent (Table 5) [27]. Intravenous antibiotic therapy is usually continued for 14 days though there have been few studies to confirm that this is the appropriate length of time for treatment. In addition some centres have shown that single agent treatment using ceftazidime, without the addition of an aminoglycoside, may be as effective as combined therapy [28, 29]. In patients with

Table 5. Drugs used to treat exacerbations of *P. aeruginosa* and *B. cepacia* infection

Aminoglycosides†		**Quinolones**	
Gentamicin	5–8 mg/kg/24 h	Ciprofloxacin	20–40 mg/kg/24 h
Tobramycin	5–8 mg/kg/24 h		
Amino-penicillins		**Carbapenems**	
Azlocillin	200–300 mg/kg/24 h	Imipenem	50 mg/kg/24 h
Piperacillin	200–300 mg/kg/24 h		
Ticarcillin	250–300 mg/kg/24 h		
Cephalosporins		**Monobactams**	
Ceftazidime	150–250 mg/kg/24 h	Aztreonam	150–250 mg/kg/24 h
Cefpirome	75–100 mg/kg/24 h		

†Plasma concentrations should be measured after 5th dose.

increased systemic markers of inflammation at the beginning of a course of antibiotics, attenuation of their host inflammatory response can be demonstrated by reduction of serum C-reactive protein and neutrophil elastase alpha-1-antiproteinase complex after antibiotic therapy. In addition an improvement in spirometry is usually observed [30]. It has been recently demonstrated that resting energy expenditure (basal metabolic rate) is reduced following a course of intravenous antibiotics in patients chronically colonised with *P. aeruginosa* [31, 32]. This suggests that the inflammatory process within the lung has important systemic effects and can be down-regulated by treatment with antibiotics.

Some centres in the UK advocate regular three monthly intravenous antibiotics regardless of symptoms while others treat on a symptom determined basis. The use of regular antibiotics has primarily been advocated from the Copenhagen CF centre but a controlled trial has never been performed to show the true extent to which this policy may improve morbidity or survival [25]. A study comparing this approach is currently under way in the UK and results will be available in five years. Most centres treat exacerbations in patients chronically infected with *P. aeruginosa* on the basis of increased respiratory and sytemic symptoms, changes in spirometry and, sometimes, evidence of an acute phase response (e.g. raised neutrophil count or C-reactive protein). Some centres also use colony counting but we have not found this to be consistent or reproducible enough to be helpful.

In vitro antimicrobial sensitivity testing is an important aid to the choice of chemotherapy and should be used in deciding antibiotic choice. Some studies now suggest that treatment with an antibiotic to which an isolated organism is apparently resistant *in vitro* can result in clinical improvement [33]. We "rotate" antibiotic courses in an attempt to reduce the incidence of resistant organisms. Many patients with cystic fibrosis develop hypersensitivity reactions to antibiotics and this may limit the choice available [34]. Successful densensitisation to allergy due to intravenous antibiotics has been described [34].

Treatment with oral quinolones is sometimes useful but is limited by the rapid development of *in vitro* resistance and reduction in clinical effect with repeated doses [35]. *In vitro* bacterial sensitivity to ciprofloxacin may return following an interval of three months or more.

New approaches to the treatment of patients chronically colonised by *P. aeruginosa* include the use of recombinant human DNase. In patients treated with DNase the requirement for intravenous antibiotic treatment is reduced and this may be a direct result of improved clearance of infected mucus from the lungs [36, 37]. However, it is possible that the increased clearance attenuates the host inflammatory response by aiding removal of the stimulating antigen and this may account for the reduced need for IV antibiotics. Other novel approaches, such as the use of nebulised anti-elastases (e.g. alpha-1-antitrypsin and secretory leuko-

Table 6. New and potential future treatments for cystic fibrosis related lung disease

Treatment	Problem addressed
Gene Therapy	Gene defect (CFTR)
Amiloride UTP/ATP	Membrane/secretory defect/chloride sodium transport
Antiproteases Anti-inflammatory agents Immunotherapy	Infection/inflammation
DNase	Mucus viscosity

protease inhibitor) may also reduce the host inflammatory response and reduce the need for antibiotics though long term studies using these agents have not yet been reported [38, 39]. (Table 6).

Nebulised Antibiotics

Nebulised antibiotics have an important role in the treatment of chronic *pseudomonas* infection. There is no uniform policy regarding their use in UK clinics. Patients chronically infected with *P. aeruginosa* are candidates for regular therapy if they are having an increased frequency of respiratory exacerbations requiring intravenous antibiotics or a progressive decline in pulmonary function tests. A number of agents (Table 7) have been shown to produce symptomatic improvement [40–42]. Most centres in the UK use tobramycin or colomycin (colistin). Colomycin has the advantage of not being a routine intravenous antibiotic and *P. aeruginosa* rarely becomes resistant to it. Some patients, however, may develop bronchoconstriction though this can usually be overcome by dose reduction or the use of β-agonists prior to antibiotic nebulisation [43]. Care must be taken to use an appropriately powered compressor and nebuliser device with these drugs.

Table 7. Drugs delivered by nebuliser for treatment of *P. aeruginosa*

Tobramycin	80–160 mg twice daily
Colomycin	1–2 mega units twice daily
Gentamicin	80–160 mg twice daily

Burkholderia cepacia

Following reports from Canada, *Burkholderia cepacia* was first recognised in the United Kingdom centres in the 1980s and currently most centres have a proportion of patients chronically infected with *B.*

cepacia [44, 45]. The percentage of patients with this organism regularly isolated from their sputum varies from 5% to 45% [46]. Most cystic fibrosis centres in the UK now have separate outpatient clinics for patients with *B. cepacia* and inpatients are managed in separate wards or in isolation cubicles [45, 47, 48].

The approach to antibiotic treatment of *B. cepacia* is similar to that for *P. aeruginosa* but *B. cepacia*, in general, is more resistant to the usual antipseudomonal antibiotics [47]. However, *in vitro* resistance to antibiotics does not necessarily indicate that the patient will not respond clinically. The combination of ceftazidime and an aminoglycoside, or newer antibiotics such as temocillin and meropenem with an aminoglycoside, are useful combinations in the management of respiratory exacerbations. Preliminary studies suggest that the response to antibiotics of patients infected with *B. cepacia* is qualitatively similar to exacerbations in patients infected with *P. aeruginosa* [49]. No significant differences were observed in the improvement in lung function, increase in body weight or reduction in markers of the host inflammatory response, such as C-reactive protein or neutrophil elastase alpha-1-antiproteinase inhibitor. These effects may, however, be due to treatment of concomitant *P. aeruginosa* or *H. influenzae* infection. It may also be possible that antibiotics have an effect on virulence factors from this organism rather than simple reduction of bacterial numbers. The advent of *B. cepacia* represents, perhaps, the most important and difficult adverse factor in cystic fibrosis to emerge in recent years [50].

Fungal Infections

Invasive fungal infections are rare in patients with cystic fibrosis [51]. Many patients, however, become colonised with *Aspergillus fumigatus* and develop an immunologic response with symptoms of asthma. Allergic broncho-pulmonary aspergillosis (ABPA) is diagnosed according to the criteria for non-CF individuals (Table 8). The symptoms of ABPA are simlar to those of an infective exacerbation due to bacteria or viruses. It is, however, important to differentiate ABPA from other infections for its proper treatment. Symptomatic treatment of asthma symptoms with oral corticosteroids is appropriate and usually effective. Patients with aspergillus species isolated consistently from sputum culture and awaiting heart/lung, or lung transplantation should be treated with antifungal agents (such as itraconazole) to eradicate the organism. Nebulised amphotericin may also have a role in reducing the load of aspergillus in the lung but is unlikely to eradicate the fungus. In patients with fungal infection immunosuppression following transplantation may lead to systemic mycoses.

Table 8. Diagnostic features of allergic broncho-pulmonary aspergillosis

Main Criteria	Asthma
	Pulmonary infiltrates
	Blood eosinophilia
	Positive skin reaction to *A. fumigatus*
	Serum precipitins to *A. fumigatus*
	Elevated IgE
	Central bronchiectasis
Minor Criteria	Brown plugs in sputum
	Culture of *A. fumigatus* from sputum
	Elevated IgE or IgG antibodies to *A. fumigatus* (RAST)

Viral Infections

Viral infection is common in cystic fibrosis patients [52]. Confirmation of viral infection is difficult as it relies primarily on retrospective serological techniques. It has been estimated that some 40% of respiratory exacerbations in children with cystic fibrosis may be due to viral infection. The viruses most commonly associated with infection in CF are respiratory syncytial viruses, influenza virus and adenovirus [52, 53] (Table 1). In adults chronically infected with *P. aeruginosa* viruses may act as co-factors, inducing and amplifying the host inflammatory process [54, 55].

Antiviral therapy is limited, though patients with lung disease and herpes zoster or influenza infection may benefit from specific therapy with acyclovir or amantidine, respectively. The adverse effects of the influenza virus also suggest that older children and adults should receive annual vaccination against influenza [53] and this policy operates in most clinics in the UK [54].

References

1. Dodge JA, Morison S, Lewis PA, Coles EC, Geddes D, Russell G, et al. Cystic fibrosis in the United Kingdom, 1968–1988; incidence, population and survival. Paediatr Perin Epidemiol 1993; 7: 137–166.
2. Elborn JS, Shale DJ, Britton JR, Cystic fibrosis: Current survival and population estimates to the year 2000. Thorax 1991; 46: 881–885.
3. Chatfield S, Owen G, Ryley HC, Williams J, Alfaharn M, Goodchild MC, et al. Neonatal screening for cystic fibrosis in Wales and the West Midlands. Clinical assessment after 5 years of screening. Arch Dis Child 1991; 66: 29–33.
4. Dankert-Roelse JE. Neonatal screening for cystic fibrosis. In: Dodge JA, Brock DJH, Widdecombe JIF, editors: Current Topics. London: John Wiley & Sons, 1993.
5. Clinical Standards Advisory Group (CSAG). Cystic Fibrosis: Access and availability of services. HMSO 1993.
6. Dodge JA, Goodall J, Geddes D, Littlewood JM, Mearns M, Owen JR, Russell G, et al. Cystic fibrosis in the United Kingdom 1977–85; an improving picture. Brit Med J 1988; 297: 1599–1602.

7. The care of adults with cystic fibrosis. Roy Col Phys, London, 1992.
8. Oppenheimer EH, Esterly JR. Pathology of cystic fibrosis. Review of the literature and comparison with 146 autopsied cases. Prospect Pediatr Pathol 1978; 2: 241–278.
9. Boat TF, Welsh MJ, Beaudet AL. Cystic fibrosis. In: Scriver CR, Beaudet AL, Sly WS, Valle D, editors: The metabolic basis of inherited disease. New York: McGraw Hill 1989; 2649–2680.
10. Oades P, Bush A. Modern management of cystic fibrosis. Matern Child Health 1992; 2: 202–207.
11. Weaver LT, Green MR, Nicholson K, Mills J, Heeley ME, Kuzemko JA, et al. Prognosis in cystic fibrosis treated with continuous flucloxacillin from the neonatal period. Arch Dis Child 1994; 70: 84–89.
12. Rayner RJ, Hiller EJ, Ispahani P, Baker M. Haemophilus infection in cystic fibrosis. Arch Dis Child 1990; 65: 255–258.
13. Jankowskie R, Wayoff M, Lion C, Burdin JC, Foliguiet B. Virulence of *Haemophilus influenzae*. In: Rigelmann R, editor. Update of *Haemophilus influenzae*; how virulence, incidence and resistance affect treatment. London: Roy Soc Med Serv (Publ 128), 1988: pp 41–48.
14. Petersen NT, Høiby N, Mordhorst CH, Lind K, Flensborg EW, Brunn B. Respiratory infection in cystic fibrosis patients caused by virus, chlamydia and mycoplasma – possible synergism with *Pseudomonas aeruginosa*. Acta Paediatr Scand 1981; 70: 623–628.
15. Aitken ML. The role of mycobacterial infections in cystic fibrosis pulmonary disease. Ped Pulmonol 1991; suppl 6: 160–161.
16. Olivier KN, Gilligan P, Yarkaskas J, Knowles MR. Pulmonary non-tuberculous mycobacteria in cystic fibrosis. Ped Pulmonol 1992; suppl 8: 116–117.
17. American Thoracic Society. Treatment of tuberculosis and other mycobacterial diseases. Am Rev Respir Dis 1983; 336: 128.
18. Elborn JS, Shale DJ. Lung injury in cystic fibrosis. Thorax 1990; 45: 970–973.
19. Høiby N, Pedersen SS. Estimated risk of cross infection with *Pseudomonas aeruginosa* in Danish cystic fibrosis patients. Acta Paediatr Scand 1989; 78: 395–404.
20. Langford D, Hiller J. Prospective controlled study of polyvalent pseudomonas vaccine in cystic fibrosis – three year results. Arch Dis Child 1984; 59: 1131–1134.
21. Elborn JS, Cordon SM, Shale DJ. Inflammatory responses to first isolation of *Pseudomonas aeruginosa* from sputum in cystic fibrosis. Pediatr Pulmonol 1993; 15: 287–291.
22. Steinkamp G, Tummlar B, Malottke R, Von der Hardt A. Treatment of *Pseudomonas aeruginosa* colonisation in cystic fibrosis. Arch Dis Child 1989; 64: 1022–1028.
23. Valerius N, Koch C, Høiby N. Prevention of chronic *Pseudomonas aeruginosa* colonisation in cystic fibrosis by early treatment. Lancet 1991; 338: 725–726.
24. Berger M. Inflammation in the lung in cystic fibrosis. Clin Rev Allergy 1990; 9: 119–142.
26. Høiby N, Koch C. *Pseudomonas aeruginosa* infection in cystic fibrosis and its management. Thorax 1990; 45: 881–884.
26. Sakala K, Yajima H, Tanaka K. Erythromycin inhibits the producton of elastase by *Pseudomonas aeruginosa* without affecting its proliferation *in vitro*. Am Rev Respir Dis 1993; 148: 1061–1065.
27. Nelson JD. Management of acute pulmonary exacerbations in cystic fibrosis. A critical appraisal. J. Pediatr 1985; 106: 1030–1034.
28. Pederson SS, Jensen T, Høiby N, Koch C, Flensborg EW. Management of *Pseudomonas aeruginosa* lung infection in Danish cystic fibrosis patients. Acta Paediatr Scand 1987; 76: 955–961.
29. Salh B, Bilton O, Dodd M, Abbot J, Webb K. A comparison of aztreonam and ceftazidime in adults with cystic fibrosis. Scand J Infect Dis 1992; 24: 215–218.
30. Norman D, Elborn JS, Cordon SM, Rayner RJ, Wiseman MS, Hiller EJ, et al. Plasma tumour necrosis factor alpha in cystic fibrosis. Thorax 1991; 46: 91–95.
31. Naon H, Hack S, Shelton MT, Gotthoffer RG, Gozal D, et al. Resting energy expenditure. Evolution during antibiotic treatment for pulmonary exacerbations in cystic fibrosis. Chest 1993; 103: 1819–1825.
32. Steinkamp G, Drommer A, Van der Hardt H, et al. Resting energy expenditure before and after treatment for *P. aeruginosa* infection in patients with cystic fibrosis. Am J Clin Nutr 1993; 57: 685–689.

33. Smith A. Antibiotic resistance is not relevant in infections in cystic fibrosis. Ped Pulmonol 1990 (suppl 5): 93.
34. Moss RB. Drug allergy in cystic fibrosis. Clin Rev Allergy 1990; 9: 211–229.
35. Jensen T, Pedersen SS, Høiby N, Koch C. Efficacy of oral fluroquinolones versus conventional intravenous antipseudomonas chemotherapy in treatment of cystic fibrosis. Eur J Clin Microbiol 1988; 6: 618–622.
36. Hubbard RC, McElvaney NC, Birrer P, Shak S, Robinson WW, Jolley C, et al. A preliminary study of aerosolised recombinant human deoxyribonuclease in the sputum of cystic fibrosis. N Engl J Med 1992; 326: 812–815.
37. Ranasinna C, Assouri B, Shak S, Christiansen D, Fuchs R, Empey D, et al. Efficacy and safety of short-term administration of aerosolised recombinant human DNase in adults with stable stage cystic fibrosis. Lancet 1993; 342: 199–202.
38. McElvaney N, Hubbard R, Birrer P, Chernick MS, Conlan DB, Frank MM, et al. Aerosol α_1-antitrypsin treatment for cystic fibrosis. Lancet 1991; 337: 392–394.
39. McElvaney NC, Dougall R, Moan MJ, Burnham MR, Wu MC, Crystal RG. Pharmacokinetics of recombinant secretory leukoprotease inhibitor aerosolised to normals and individuals with cystic fibrosis. Am Rev Respir Dis 1993; 148: 1055–1060.
40. Hodson ME, Penketh ARC, Batten JE. Aerosol carbenicillin and gentamicin treatment of P. aeruginosa infection in patients with cystic fibrosis. Lancet 1981; ii: 1137–1135.
41. Littlewood JM, Miller MG, Ghoneim AT, Ramsden CH. Nebulised colomycin for early P. aeruginosa colonisation in patients with cystic fibrosis. Lancet 1985; i: 865.
42. Ramsey BW, Dorkin HL, Eisenberg JD, Gibson RL, Harwood IR, Kravitz RM, et al. Efficacy of aerosolized tobramycin in patients wtih cystic fibrosis. N Eng J Med 1993; 328: 1740–1746.
43. Maddison J, Dodd M, Webb K. Nebulised colistin causes chest tightness in adults with cystic fibrosis. Respir Med 1994; 88: 145–147.
44. Thomassen MJ, Demko CA, Doershuk CF, Stern RC, Klinger JD. Pseudomonas cepacia: Decrease in colonization in patients with cystic fibrosis. Amer Rev Resp Dis 1986; 134: 669–671.
45. Govan JRW, Brown PH, Maddison J, Doherty CJ, Nelson JW, Dodd M, et al. Evidence for transmission of Pseudomonas cepacia by social contact in cystic fibrosis. Lancet 1993; 342: 15–19.
46. Editorial. Pseudomonas cepacia – more than a harmless commensal. Lancet 1992; 339: 1385–1386.
47. Smith DL, Smith EG, Gumery LB, Stableforth DE. Pseudomonas cepacia infection in cystic fibrosis. Lancet 1992; 339: 252.
48. Gladman G, Connor PJ, Williams RF, David TJ. Controlled study of P. cepacia and P. maltophilia in cystic fibrosis. Arch Dis Child 1992; 67: 192–195.
49. Elborn JS, Maddison J, Nelson J, Dodd M, Shale DJ, Webb KA, et al. Clinical and inflammatory responses in patients with cystic fibrosis infected with Pseudomonas aeruginosa and cepacia. Am Rev Resp Dis (Abstract) (In press).
50. Lewin LO, Byard PO, Davis PB. Effects of Pseudomonas cepacia colonisation on survival and pulmonary function of cystic fibrosis patients. J Clin Epidemiol 1990; 43: 125–131.
51. Knutsen AP, Slavin RG. Allergic bronchopulmonary in patients with cystic fibrosis. Clin Rev Allergy 1991; 9: 103–118.
52. Wang EEL, Prober CG, Manson B, Corey M, Levison H. Association of respiratory viral infections with pulmonary deterioration in patients with cystic fibrosis. N Engl J Med 1984; 311: 1653–1658.
53. Shale DJ. Viral infections: A role in the lung disease of cystic fibrosis? Thorax 1992; 47: 69.
54. Conway SP, Simmonds EJ, Littlewood JM. Acute severe deterioration in cystic fibrosis associated with Influenza A virus infection. Thorax 1992; 47: 112–114.
55. Petersen NT, Høiby N, Mordhorst CH, Lind K, Flensborg EW, Bruun B. Respiratory infections in cystic fibrosis patients caused by virus, chlamydia and mycoplasma – possible synergism with Pseudomonas aeruginosa. Acta Paediatr Scand 1981; 70: 623–628.

Cystic Fibrosis Pulmonary Infections
Lessons from Around the World
ed. by A. Bauernfeind, M. I. Marks and B. Strandvik
© 1996 Birkhauser Verlag Basel/Switzerland

CHAPTER 27
The General Approach to Cystic Fibrosis Pulmonary Infection in Mexico

Jose Luis Lezana-Fernandez and Douglas Maza-Gonzales

Mexican Cystic Fibrosis Association, Altavista 21, CP 01000, Mexico D.F.

Summary. Serious research work on Cystic Fibrosis (CF) in Mexico started back in 1980. CF is still regarded as a rare disease, which accounts for its late diagnosis (4.4 years). CF patients have a life expectancy of only 9 years.

In this chapter we analyse what has been published in our literature on the basic respiratory aspects of the disease, as well as providing an epidemiologic and genetic overview of the situation in Mexico.

The actual incidence of CF is unknown. However, the genetic study of our patients in 4 CF centers showed that the main mutation (ΔF508) appears with a frequency of 39 to 41%.

Pseudomonas aeruginosa prevails as the main pathogen (60 to 68%) with the isolation of some strains of *Burkholderia pseudomallei* and *mallei* (13%).

The annual mean number of out-patient visits to CF Care Centers is 3.1; 27% of patients are hospitalized for IV therapy for a mean of 18 days. Fifteen percent receive IV home therapy, with hypercapnia as the main pulmonary complication (20%).

Ethnic and economic factors hinder the development of more research programs and the establishment of additional Care Centers to provide better treatment to these patients.

Introduction

Cystic fibrosis (CF) is the most common recessive disease among Caucasians, but it has not been possible to establish the actual incidence of the disease in the Mexican population, due to its heterogeneous nature [1, 2].

The first publications on CF in Mexico date back to the 1960s and 1970s and refer to some clinical and radiological data in isolated cases of the disease [3–6]. A prominent work was carried out by Armendares *et al.* in 1974 (Centro Medico Nacional de Mexico), in which CF is mentioned as the most frequent autosomal-recessive disease in 3421 autopsies [7]. In 1990, Lopez-Corella *et al.* (Instituto Nacional de Pediatria, Mexico) documented 32 CF cases in 3260 consecutive autopsies carried out in Mexican children, suggesting an incidence of 0.98% [8].

When the Mexican Cystic Fibrosis Association (AMFQ) started to operate in 1982, the Gibson and Cooke diagnostic method [9] was

Correspondence address: Jose Luis Lezana, Altavista 21, CP 01000, Mexico D.F.

established in Mexico. Up to December 1991 351 CF patients (National CF Registry, Mexico), distributed in 4 Care Centers at the national level, were recorded.

A new and a more hopeful time in CF research began with the discovery, cloning and characterization of the CF gene in 1989, encoding for the cystic fibrosis transmembrane conductance regulator, the CFTR protein. The most common mutation, ΔF508, found in 70% of the chromosomes of CF patients in northern Europe and North America [10, 11], were found in 63% of CF chromosomes in Argentina as revealed in the first study of a Latin American country [10].

In 1992, Rojas-Martinez et al. carried out the first study on molecular genetics of CF in Mexican families, with a frequency of 59% for the ΔF508 mutation [12]. Later in two consecutive works, Orozco et al. reported 1993 an incidence of 39 and 41% for the ΔF508 mutation in Mexican patients [13, 14]. The authors suggested that the frequency of the disease and of the heterozygotes in this population may be similar to that described in 1/2.500 and 1/25 Caucasians, respectively. The low frequency of the ΔF508 mutation in this study may be due to the small size of the sample studied, to the heterogeneous genetic composition, or it may also be due to the fact that a significant number of the cases in Mexico could be homozygotes for the ΔF508 mutation and die undiagnosed at an early age. The purpose of this review is to provide an overview of the status of CF in Mexico, from an epidemiological point of view and from the standpoint of the pulmonary infection.

Epidemiology of Cystic Fibrosis

351 CF patients were recorded at the Mexican Cystic Fibrosis Association (AMFQ) during the period covering January 1982 to December 1991. In all cases, the diagnosis was based on the case history, the determination of chloride levels in sweat by the Gibson and Cooke method [9] and the symptomatology. In each case, the birth date, sex, age at the time of diagnosis and date of death were obtained. A database was made for the descriptive-statistical analysis, using the Kaplan Meier method [15] and the log-rank chi-squared test. Life expectancy at birth, survival after diagnosis and the mean age at the time of diagnosis were analyzed by sex. Cases diagnosed during autopsy and those in which full information was missing were excluded from the study (Table 1). Out of the 244 patients available for this analysis, 55% were males, the mean age being almost 10 years, with no significant difference between sexes. The mean age of the patients at the time of diagnosis was 4.4 years (SD $\pm$ 5.7) with a statistically significant difference in males, 3.8 years versus 5.1 in females ($p < 0.05$). 70 deaths were reported during this period; 36 of them (51%) were male patients. The

Table 1. Survival in Cystic Fibrosis patients, January 1982 to December 1991 (AMFQ, Patient Registry 1991)

	n	%
REGISTERED CASES	351	100.0
EXCLUSION:		
a) Revealed by autopsy	96	27.4
b) Lack information	13*	5.1
STUDIED CASES	242	67.5

*Two cases were included in the analysis by sex, mean age and mean survival after birth.

Table 2. Life table analysis after diagnosis, including both sexes (AMFQ, Patient Registry 1991)

Years	Number of Death	All CF Patients	Cumulative Survival
1	27	242	0.835
2	7	202	0.748
3	8	181	0.616
4	4	149	0.517
5	1	125	0.421
6	2	102	0.331
7	0	80	0.293
8	0	71	0.240
9	1	58	0.211
10	2	51	0.182

Table 3. Life analysis after birth, including both sexes. (AMFQ Patient Registry 1991)

Age (years)	Number of Death	All CF Patients	Cumulative Survival
1	15	244	0.922
2	10	225	0.877
3	5	214	0.840
4	5	205	0.754
5	3	184	0.697
6	1	170	0.664
7	2	162	0.594
8	3	145	0.541
9	0	132	0.492
10	1	120	0.443

simple analysis showed that the mean age at death was 8.3 years (SD $\pm$ 9.9) with a statistically significant difference in females ($p < 0.05$), who died at an older age, 9.0 years compared to the males at 7.5 years.

Estimation of the unspecific cumulative survival in 242 cases showed that only 52% of the CF patients lived four years after diagnosis, with no significant difference between sexes. Life expectancy at birth was similarly analyzed in 244 patients. It was found that 49% reached the age of nine, with no significant difference between sexes (Tables 2 and 3).

Clinical Findings in the Patients

CF is an extremely pleomorphic disease. According to world literature, the symptoms and the age of onset of the disease vary widely from one individual to another [16] and Mexico is no exception in this respect.

Published works regarding CF in Mexico are scarce. In 1989, Perez-Fernandez et al. [17] carried out a retrospective study of 39 cases in which the mean age of onset of symptoms was 14.2 months, with a prevalence of chronic pulmonary suppurative disease secondary to interstitial fibrosis, emphysematous lesions and bronchiectasis. *Pseudomonas aeruginosa* was the causal agent in most cases, followed by *Staphylococcus aureus* and *Hemophilus influenzae*. An important conclusion was that the persistently high frequency of atelectasis of the right middle lobe which was detected, should lead us to suspect the existence of CF, after ruling out conditions which are endemic in our population, such as tuberculosis.

In 1990, Quezada et al. studied 9 CF cases over 15 years of age (Instituto Nacional de Enfermedades Respiratorias, Mexico), highlighting the fact that 100% of these patients experienced a chronic pulmonary suppuration syndrome. The most frequent previous diagnosis was pulmonary tuberculosis in three of the cases, interstitial disease in two, bronchiectasis of unknown etiology and chronic bronchitis, highlighting the fact that in only one case was CF detected at the onset of the symptoms.

The mucoid variety of *P. aeruginosa* was the most frequently isolated germ in this series, followed by *S. aureus* in three cases.

In a preliminary study carried out in 1990, Larracilla-Alegre et al. [19], reported the clinical and laboratory findings of 29 CF patients treated at Centro Medico La Raza in Mexico. Mean age was 7.5 years, with a prevalence of males (59%). Respiratory symptoms were reported initially in 62% of cases, including mainly chronic or recurrent cough, dyspnoea and bronchospasm. The most frequent radiological findings were pulmonary hyperinsufflation, condensation and fibrosis. Bronchial secretion was cultured, and *P. aeruginosa* grew in those from 88% of the patients and *S. aureus* in 50%.

A study carried out at the AMFQ included 50 CF patients (unpublished observation), 21 females with a mean age of 11.7 years (SD ± 4.5) and 29 males with a mean age of 11.5 years (SD ± 4.4). Comparisons were made between the clinical-radiological assessment parameters

(Shwachman-Brasfield) by sex as well as by spirometric variables, and sputum cultures positive for *P. aeruginosa*. $MFEF_{25-75}$ was the most affected spirometric variable, with a mean of 61% of predicted values, and no significant difference between sexes. $FEV_{1.0}$ was the second most affected variable, with a mean of 71% of the predicted values. The mean value obtained with the Shwachman-Brasfield test was 72.4 (69.7 for females and 74.3 for males). *P. aeruginosa* was isolated in 68% of the cases (34 patients). A significant statistical correlation was established between the clinical-radiological assessment and each of the spirometric variables, FVC, $FEV_{1.0}$ and $MFEF_{25-75}$, respectively ($p < 0.001$). No correlation was found to the presence of *P. aeruginosa*.

Microbiology

In 1989, Lezana *et al.* [20] analyzed 32 sputum samples from 32 CF patients with a mean age of 12 years. Pseudomonas species were found in 80% of positive cultures (Table 4). *P. aeruginosa* was the most frequently isolated microorganism in 18 cases (60%), followed by *S. aureus* in 50% and *Candida albicans* in 43% of cases. An outstanding finding of this study was the isolation of *Burkholderia pseudomallei* in 3 of the cases (10%), *B. cepacia* in 2 cases (7%), and *B. mallei* in one patient (3%). The *in vitro* suspectibility to antipseudomonas antibiotics showed the best results for ceftazidime and cefoperazone.

In another study, Coria-Jimenez *et al.* (unpublished observation) collected 92 sputum samples from 63 CF patients, and found that 68.5% of the samples were positive for *P. aeruginosa*. A total of 88 strains of *P. aeruginosa* were isolated, 51 of which correspond to the mucoid phenotype, and the remaining 37 to the rough phenotype. In the *in vitro* assay, ceftazidime showed the lowest presence of bacterial resistance, 5% of mucoid strains and 6.5% of rough strains. However, resistance to gentamicin was found in 36% of the mucoid strains and 23% of the rough strains (MIC at 50% and 90%).

Table 4. Frequency of isolation in sputum of different microorganisms in cystic fibrosis patients (20)

Microorganisms	n	%
Pseudomonas species	24	80.0
P. aeruginosa	18	60.0
Burkholderia cepacia	2	6.7
B. pseudomallei	3	10.0
B. mallei	1	3.3
Staphylococcus aureus	15	50.0
Candida Albicans	13	43.3
Others	4	13.3

Treatment Strategy

There are no comparative studies in Mexico about the clinical and bacteriological response to the various antipseudomonal antibiotic therapy regimens in CF; therefore, our experience is based on what has been published in the international literature, as well as on our own unpublished observations.

The main purpose of respiratory function assessment is to maintain optimal respiratory function in patients, as well as to prevent disease progression and treat pulmonary complications. To this purpose, the following procedure has been established,

1. Complete chest examination at each visit. A minimum of 4 annual visits are proposed.
2. Spirometry every 6 months or on a more frequent basis according to the course and/or stage of the disease. It is used as an indicator of improvement after antibiotic therapy.
3. Pulse oxymetry at each visit and each follow-up visit during antibiotic therapy due to pulmonary exacerbation. Arterial blood gases yearly when $FEV_{1.0}$ is less than 30% of predicted values.
4. Sputum culture once a year, before starting IV antibiotic therapy or as indicated according to clinical findings.
5. Chest X-rays yearly or as indicated according to clinical findings, and Shwachman-Brasfield evaluation.
6. Check of the physiotherapy techniques 4 times a year.
7. Nutritional and psychological assessment and genetic counselling.

During 1992, the CF center at the AMFQ in Mexico City followed up 140 CF patients, and recorded a total of 473 visits with a mean number of outpatient visits of 3.1. Twenty-seven per cent of the patients were admitted one or more times on account of respiratory complications or exacerbations of their pulmonary condition. Mean days per hospitalization was 18.0. During the past 3 years, our center has provided IV home treatment in order to reduce hospitalization costs and to avoid the adverse psychological impact on the patients and their families. Currently, 15% of our patients receive IV treatment at home with a mean of 42 days/patient.

The most frequent complication in the 140 patients monitored during 1992 was the persistent increase of PCO_2 in 20% of the cases, followed by congestive cardiac failure in 10% of the patients. Other complications included atelectasis (4%), hemoptysis (3%), pneumothorax (1.5%) and pleural effusion (0.7%).

Similarities and Dissimilarities to other countries

As this review clearly shows, there are few publications on CF in Mexico and in fact, knowledge about this disease was rather poor before 1980. While it is true that the known incidence of CF in our country is low, more epidemiological studies are required to determine the real incidence of the disease.

The source of the epidemiological data included in our review are recent statistical reports prepared at the AMFQ's Care Center. The remarkably life expectancy of patients (9 years) is the result of late diagnosis in our population, as compared with the results reported by developed countries. As a matter of fact, the mean age at the time of diagnosis was 4.4 years in our study, with a significant difference in males, who were diagnosed earlier. However, this difference was not maintained in survival after diagnosis, which was 4 years in average. As a consequence of this late diagnosis, the patients present with irreversible pulmonary lesions that have an unfavorable influence on mean survival. Other unfavorable factors are the adverse economic conditions that prevail in our country, and the high infant and child morbidity and mortality rates due to the high incidence of pulmonary and gastrointestinal endemic disease, which in certain instances mask the symptomatology of CF.

From the clinical point of view, CF occurs with the same variants as those described in the international medical literature. The causes of hospital admission leading to detection of CF among our patients at the Care Center are mainly chronic multi-treated pulmonary disease, with or without long-standing diarrhoea. Most patients were treated for long periods of time by the clinician without suspicion of CF.

The frequency of sputum cultures positive for *P. aeruginosa* ranged from 60 to 88% in different studies. Coria *et al.* (unpublished observation) reported remarkable findings showing that 59% of the 88 strains of *P. aeruginosa* corresponded to the mucoid phenotype, which had never before been described in our literature. The mucoid strains did not show a higher resistance *in vitro* to the antibiotics most commonly used in the treatment of CF. In the analysis of clinical characteristics observed among the patients colonized with pseudomonas species, the most significant finding was that they had a six times higher risk than patients without such colonization to be classified as moderate or critically ill (according to Shwachman's and Brasfield classification).

The isolation of *B. pseudomallei* in CF patients has already been described by other authors [21]; however, it will be necessary to carry out studies with a larger number of patients to clarify the role of this germ in CF. It is worth notifying that the three cases with *B. pseudomallei* and one more case with the mallei variant reported in our study died at an average of 12 months after proved infection.

In Mexico, with only 4 comprehensive CF Care Centers, patients must sometimes travel long distances, which makes the follow-up of cases more difficult. This fact, together with the poverty affecting a large proportion of our population, further complicates the provision of prophylactic IV treatment, and even treatment during the exacerbation of pulmonary infection.

The antimicrobial treatment of CF is not different from what is reported in the medical literature, based on the results of cultures and dilution antibiograms. It consists of combined antibiotic therapy (cephalosporins or monobactams, plus aminoglycoside) for about 14 days, the extent of therapy determined according to clinical response by pulmonary function test every week. That means that clinical findings and pulmonary function tests are considered as parameters of improvement during IV antibiotic therapy.

Finally, it should be observed that the frequency of the ΔF508 mutation in our population is low, about 40%. This might be due to the limited number of patients studied and/or to the large heterogeneous nature of the Mexican population. Another possible explanation for the low frequency of the ΔF508 mutation may be that the homozygotes for that mutation have a more serious clinical symptomatology with early pulmonary and gastrointestinal manifestations, and die before their fourth year of life without being diagnosed.

References

1. Lisker R, Perez-Briseño R, Granados J. Gene frequences and admixture estimates in a Mexico City population. Am J Phys Anthropol 1986; 71: 203–207.
2. Lisker R, Ramirez E, Perez-Briseño R, Granados J, Babinsky V. Gene frequencies and admixture estimates in four Mexican urban centers. Hum Biol 1990; 62: 791–801.
3. Garcia MP, Velasco CL. Fibrosis Quistica del pancreas en recien nacido. Ginecol Obstet Mex 1965; 20: 811–815.
4. Cuellar A, Rangel L. Aleman P. Mucoviscidosis, Description de un caso con especial atencion al diagnostico y tratamiento. Rev Mex Pediatr 1971; 40: 477–490.
5. Aristizabal DG, Leal QF, Ruiz VE, Franco RG. Actualizacion sobre mucoviscidosis. Presentacion de 2 casos. Bol Med Hosp Infant Mex 1978; 35: 65–77.
6. Gomez MS, Rojas DV. Correlacion clinico-radiologica de 18 casos de mucoviscidosis en niños. Rev Mex Pediatr 1968; 39: 213–218.
7. Armendares S, Cortes R, De la Rosa L. El componente genetico en la mortalidad infantil. Rev Invest Clin 1974; 26: 3–18.
8. Lopez CE, Ridaura SC, Lopez CG. Cystic Fibrosis in Mexican children. A report of 32 cases in 3.260 consecutive autopsies. Pathology 1980; 18: 167–181.
9. Gibson LE, Cooke RE. A test for concentration of electrolytes in sweat in cystic fibrosis of the pancreas utilizing pilocarpine by iontophoresis. Pediatrics 1959; 23: 545–549.
10. Cystic Fibrosis Genetic Analysis Consortium. Worldwide survey of the Δ F508 mutation. Report from the cystic fibrosis genetic consortium. Am J Hum Genet 1990; 47: 354–359.
11. Gasparini P, Nunes V, Savoia A, Dognini M, Morral N, Gaona A, et al. The search for South European cystic fibrosis mutations: identification of two new mutations four variants and intronic sequences. Genomics 1991; 10: 193–200.
12. Rojas-Martinez A, Vazques-Aleman RN, Gustincich S, Cantu JM, Barrera-Saldaña HA. Genetica molecular de la fibrosis quistica: el alelo Δ F508 en familias mexicanas. Bol Med Hosp Infant Mex 1992; 49: 335–341.
13. Orozco L, Salcedo M, Lezana JL, Chavez M, Valdes H, Moreno M. Frequency Δ F508 in a Mexican sample of cystic fibrosis patients. J Med Genet 1993; 30: 501–502.
14. Orozco L, Lezana JL, Chavez M, Valdez H, Moreno M. Carnevale A. Estudio molecular de la mutacion Δ F508 y analisis genetico de una muestra de pacientes con fibrosis quistica. Bol Med Hosp Infant Mex 1993; 50: 457–462.

15. Kaplan EL, Meier P. Nonparametric estimation from incomplete observations. J Am Statist Assoc 1958; 53: 457 481.
16. Maclusky IB, Canny GJ, Levison H. Cystic Fibrosis: an update. Pediatr Rev Commun 1987; 1: 343 389.
17. Perez Fernandez L, Flores-Rojas C, Lopez-Corella E, Parra-Cerdeño W, Lezana-Fernandez J. Cystic Fibrosis in Mexican children. Int Pediatr 1989; 4: 266 270.
18. Quezada ZR, Hernandez FN, Sada DE. Fibrosis quistica en pancreas en mayores de 15 años en poblacion mexicana. Rev Invest Clin 1990; 42: 174–179.
19. Larracilla-Alegre J, Cortez-Martinez M, Flores-Nuñes A, Cruz-Merida A, Aparicio-Frias E. Mucoviscidosis: aspectos clinicos y de laboratorio en 29 casos. Bol Med Hosp Infant Mex 1990; 47: 698 704.
20. Lezana JL, Novoa O, Lezana MA. Epidemiology of Pseudomonas in Mexican CF patients. Pediatr Pulmonol 1989; suppl 4: 138 (abstract).
21. Tullis DE, Corey M, Hyland RH, Levison H. Xanthomonas maltophilia in cystic fibrosis. Pediatr Pulmonol 1992; suppl 8: 294 (abstract).

Cystic Fibrosis Pulmonary Infections:
Lessons from Around the World
ed. by A. Bauernfeind, M. I. Marks and B. Strandvik
© 1996 Birkhäuser Verlag Basel/Switzerland

CHAPTER 28
The General Approach to Cystic Fibrosis Pulmonary Infection in Uruguay

Stella M. Cabeza

Director of the Scientific Medical Advisory Committee, Association of Cystic Fibrosis in Uruguay, Costa Rica 2061 Montevideo, Uruguay

Introduction

Uruguay is a small country in South America located between Brazil and Argentina with a surface area of 186 000 km^2 and a population of three million inhabitants. The infant mortality rate is 21.1 per thousand live births [1] and one of the important contributing factors is genetic diseases. However, general neonatal screening is not performed yet.

Eighty-eight per cent of the population is of Caucasian origin and 12% is negroid or indigenous [2]. Initial immigration mainly came from Spain (it was a Spanish colony until 1915), Italy, Brazil, Western Europe (France, England, Portugal, etc.), Argentina and other countries.

Epidemiology of Cystic Fibrosis

Until the discovery of cystic fibrosis (CF) as a genetic disease, it was thought to be a rarity in our population. However, because the incidence of CF disease in Spain and Italy was higher than expected, (although lower than in Northern Europe), many investigators in Latin America were led to believe that the incidence had to be similar to that in Southern Europe [3]. The first Latin American CF conference was held in May 1986 in Buenos Aires, Argentina. Shortly after that, also during 1986, the Uruguay CF Association ("Asociación de Fibrosis Quística del Uruguay" – "AFQU") was established.

From 1968 to 1986, 68 patients were diagnosed to have CF out of a total of 4000 sweat tests performed in a laboratory in Uruguay. In those

Correspondence address: Dr. Stella M. Cabeza, Costa Rica 2061-11500, Montevideo, Uruguay CP 11500.

days the disease was not studied in a comprehensive way; patients were treated by individual doctors rather than collectively in a centre. The first goal was to create a kind of network to provide comprehensive care of the patients, but, unfortunately, we still do not have a CF centre in Uruguay.

Knowledge of the incidence, prevalence and therapeutic approach to CF is well known in most developed countries but not in Latin America. In a study conducted in Buenos Aires, Argentina, where BM meconium test was performed on 9931 newborn babies, an incidence of 1:4966 was found, somewhat less than the classical 1:2500 described in most European Caucasian countries [4].

If these figures were extrapolated to Uruguay, though there are some differences in the population and BM Meconium test has a percentage of false negatives, there would be 12 new patients yearly and no less than 600 patients would be actual. This figure would be sufficient to ensure the establishment of a CF Centre and special medical personnel devoted to CF. Many factors influence delayed diagnosis [5]:

1) Insufficent professional awareness of the disease among health care staff.
2) Misinformation in primary health care centres.
3) Insufficient economic resources in the health care system (the sweat test is available only in Montevideo and not in other towns in Uruguay).
4) Geographical distance that prevents access to diagnosis in main health care centres.

This situation can be reverted:

– in the long-term through coordinated programs about education, early diagnosis and treatment
– in the short-term, through neonatal screening as a means of early diagnosis.

The latter is an expensive procedure and health authorities have to be aware of the convenience of such a measure. That is the reason why the local CF association, AFQU, promotes a better understanding of CF in every medical conference possible and why it has been decided to create an open office to gather information about CF patients as well as establishing a number of guidelines for better treatment of the disease. AFQU also disseminates knowledge about the disease among doctors who have recently graduated from university and to the public in general.

Present Registration and Care of Patients

AFQU has an open office that sees patients from all over the country. Patients are diagnosed and treated, or simply come to be evaluated and then return to their doctors to be followed-up according to certain guidelines. Since 1986 all the patients have been registered and controls are intended to be carried out on a monthly basis. From July 1986 to August 1993, 19 patients, aged 4 months to 34 years, were controlled at the AFQU office. All the patients were of European Caucasian origin.

There is a complete clinical history for each patient and a follow-up sheet of the disease as well as laboratory findings, chest X-ray, CT scan, blood gases and lung function test when performed. Lung function tests are performed every three months in patients above seven years of age. Since 1993 flow-volume curves are performed in patients under seven years of age, but no comprehensive data is yet available. Because there are no other existing data in our country, comparison between AFQU figures and those obtained from the Latin American Cystic Fibrosis Registry (REGLAFQ) are shown in Table 1 [6, 7, 8]. Other data (not shown) also indicate that the mean number of hospitalization was lower than those shown in REGLAFQ. Three patients died in these seven years. One patient did not return to the office but occasionally made contact by phone.

The medical costs were covered by private health insurances in 64.7% of patients, by Social Security in 12.8% and by Public Health in 23.5% of the patients.

The small number of patients prevents analysis of the figures. A comparison is made more in order to check up the AFQU procedures. The principles established for treatment and follow-up seem to ensure that the rate of survival is as high as in the rest of Latin America as a whole. Nevertheless no conclusions can yet be reached, since there is a higher percentage of patients with pseudomonas strains, three of whom harbour "mucoid" strains. No *Burkholderia cepacia* have been found so far.

Table 1. Comparison between patients known to AFQU and data from Latin American CF Registry (REGLAFQ). For further explanation see text

	AFQU	REGLAFQ
Mean age at diagnosis (yrs)	2.8	4(5.1)
Mean age of patients at follow-up (yrs)	12	10.7
Percentage of patients within the third percentile for weight	12.5	52.1
Percentage of patients without nutritional support	18	71
Percentage of patients on pancreatic enzymes	94	88
Percentage of patients with the main sputum isolate of:		
Pseudomonas aeruginosa	65	50
Burkholderia cepacia	0	2
Staphylococcus aureus	7	29

The low number of hospital admissions can partially be explained by the fact that antibiotic treatments are performed at home and hospitalization is reserved for complicated cases. The goal is to present data to the health authorities to ensure better quality of life and to prolong life expectancy for CF patients, since CF patients are not currently taken into account in any health planning.

Only one brand of pancreatic enzymes is commercially available in Uruguay; the others have to be imported through AFQU. However, this is an improvement because when the Fourth Latin American CF Conference was held in Montevideo in 1991 none were available.

Not all the necessary antibiotics are commercially available in Uruguay. DNase will be introduced in the near future.

No lung transplantation has been performed so far in Uruguay but it is planned to train one surgical team in Argentina.

Our main efforts are directed to establishing a CF Centre in Uruguay, bringing all CF patients together in order to treat them in a more comprehensive way and to achieve the same survival rate as in developed countries. All Latin American countries have a median survival rate 50% less that in developed countries.

Guidelines for Respiratory Management of Cystic Fibrosis

Since 1992 some guidelines for the study and treatment of newly diagnosed CF patients have been practised at the AFQU office. The guidelines have also been proposed to other doctors dealing with CF patients, to ensure that the same procedures are being applied and hence to facilitate comparison of results.

In recent years a paper has been presented with results from the AFQU office and from another office in a Public Health Hospital [9]. Diagnosis was suggested through the usual signs and symptoms described in the main textbooks. Sweat tests were performed using the pilocarpine iontophoresis method described by Gibson and Cook [10]. After diagnosis a complete evaluation was carried out. Shwachman and Brasfield scores were used [11]. References will be made only to measures undertaken to compensate respiratory disease. Complications are dealt within the way usually recommended [12].

Patients without clinical evidence of respiratory disease are assessed using the following procedures: Bacteriological examinations (from sputum or throat swab), chest X-ray, lung function test, CT scan and blood gases.

I. *Treatment of positive bacteriological isolates:*
1. Antibiotics available in the country, no less than three weeks and according to antibiogram.
2. Physical exercises.

3. Physiotherapy: some well-trained professionals teach parents to carry this out at home.
4. Aerosol therapy: no mucolytic drugs are in use, but bronchodilators are commonly used.
5. Environmental protection against smoke, cigarettes, etc.
6. Preventive immunizations against diphtheria, tetanus, pertussis, poliomyelitis, measles, mumps and rubella, and influenza vaccines on an annual basis. *Haemophilus influenzae* vaccine has recently been introduced in the country.
7. Monthly surveillance.

II. *Treatment of negative bacteriological isolates:*
Items 2–7 from the preceding section are applied.
Treatment in patients with pulmonary involvement:
– *without Pseudomonas aeruginosa:*
a. Physiotherapy b.i.d. or t.i.d.
b. Aerosolized antibiotics, i.e. aminoglycosides (colistin is not commercially available).
c. Use of specific antibiotics according to sensitivity, either *per os* or intravenously, for no less than three weeks and at home if possible.

In young infants, anti-staphylococcal therapy is sometimes used on a continuous basis.

– *with colonization by P. aeruginosa:*
a. Initial treatment with: Aerosolized aminoglycosides
(according to sensitivity)
Ciprofloxacin *per os* for three weeks.

Ciprofloxacin is used in patients above five years of age and no problems of joint involvement has been seen. Parents are informed of possible side effects and consent is requested and recorded in the clinical history.

b. If sputum or throat swab remains positive:
Intravenous treatment according to sensitivity; an aminoglycoside plus a third generation cephalosporin is used.

Intravenous treatment is performed on an ambulatory or a semi-ambulatory basis, i.e. the patient is admitted to hospital, one or two days to check on tolerance to treatment and to insert venous device. Sometimes, when complications occur or for economical reasons, patients are admitted for the whole course of treatment.

When *P. aeruginosa* is isolated in every bacteriological culture, treatment is established:

– on a three-monthly basis, especially when bronchiectasis and progressive deterioration of lung function are present.

- according to clinical status and lung function tests, in patients who live "in balance" with the agent.

In patients with bronchiectasis, treatment always includes:

- physiotherapy.
- aerosolized antibiotics.
- *per os* antibiotics twenty days each month.
- intravenous course of antibiotics on a three-monthly basis.

Nutritional support is provided as oral supplements to the diet in all patients with respiratory disease.

These guidelines are "tailored" to each individual case, since there are many circumstances to be considered (economical, social, geographical). The importance of adequate control is emphasized.

References

1. Ministry of Public Health. Epidemiol Bull 1992; 1: 4.
2. Sanz M, Salzano FM, Kacraborty R. Estructura Genética y componentes de la mezcla racial en Uruguay. Resúmenes del XIII Congreso Internacional de Ciencias Antropológicas y Etnológicas, Mexico 1993; 400–401.
3. Pivetta OH. Guiding principles of the formulation of national programs for the prevention and control of cystic fibrosis in developing countries. WHO, 1989.
4. Pivetta OH, Macri CN. Newborn screening meconium BM test for cystic fibrosis. 1st Latin American CF Conference, Buenos Aires. May 1986.
5. Pivetta OH. Cystic fibrosis in Latin America. Screening: a possible solution. Argentinian CF Association (FIPAN), 1992.
6. Macri CN, de Gentile AS. Latin American cystic fibrosis registry: starting life tables. Pediatr Pulmonol 1991; suppl 6: 313 (abstract).
7. Macri CN, Bertero O, Botelli M, Castorina C, D'Astolfo M, Di Yacobo L, et al. Cystic Fibrosis Latin American Multicentric Study. Am Rev Resp Dis 1993; 147(suppl): 579.
8. Macri CN, de Gentile AS. Latin American registry of cystic fibrosis patients 1990. Buenos Aires, Argentina, 1990.
9. Cabeza S, Martínez L, Rivas C, Estevan M, Bazzano M. Perfil Pneumológico de los pacientes con Fibrosis Quística. Resúmenes del VI Encuentro de Pediatras Neumólogos. Mar del Plata, Octubre 1993.
10. Gibson LE, Cooke RE. A test for concentration of electrolytes in sweat in cystic fibrosis of the pancreas utilizing pilocarpine by iontophoresis. Pediatrics 1959; 23: 545–549.
11. Cabeza S. Evaluación de los pacientes con Fibrosis Quística por puntaje de Schwachman y Brasfield. Decimonoveno Congreso Uruguayo de Pediatría, Montevideo, Junio 1993.
12. Goodchild M, Dodge JA. Management of respiratory disease. In: Goodchild M and Dodge JA. Cystic Fibrosis: Manual of diagnosis and management. 2nd ed. Baillière Tindall 1985.

Subject index

Also in this book series:

Airways Smooth Muscle:
Neurotransmitters, Amines, Lipid Mediators and Signal Transduction

Edited by
D. Raeburn, *Rhône-Poulenc Rorer Ltd, Dagenham, UK*
M.A. Giembycz, *Royal Brompton National Heart and Lung Institute, London, UK*

1995. 368 pages. Hardcover • ISBN 3-7643-5141-1

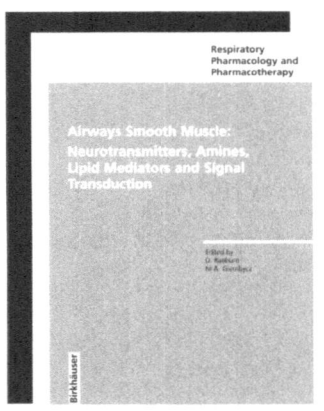

Extending the work of the other titles in the *Airways Smooth Muscle* sub-series, this volume describes in detail current theories concerning the pharmacological control of airways smooth muscle tone. Particular emphasis is placed upon the expression and distribution of receptors that are activated by classical neurotransmitters, lipid mediators and amines. Additionally, special attention is directed to describing the various biochemical signalling pathways that are recruited by these molecules and how they may be manipulated pharmacologically.

Coverage includes chapters on histamine, leukotrienes, GABA and benzodiazepines and 5-hydroxytryptamine. The information presented will serve as an invaluable foundation for understanding both current theories of receptor pharmacology and signal transduction, and provide a basis for drug therapy in treating respiratory disease such as asthma.

Reflecting the latest advances in this important area of respiratory research, this comprehensive and authoritative monograph will prove invaluable to pharmacologists, biochemists and clinicians.

From the Contents:
1. *G.P. Anderson:* Adrenaline and Noradrenaline
2. *A.F. Roffel and J. Zaagsma:* Cholinomimetics
3. *N. Chand and R.D. Sofia:* Histamine
4. *M.G. Belvisi, J.K. Ward and A.J. Fox:*
   5-Hydroxytryptamine
5. *P.J. Gardiner:* Prostanoids

6. *D.W.P. Hay and D. Raeburn:* Leukotrienes
7. *G. Dent:* Platelet Activating Factor
8. *K.J. Broadley:* Purines
9. *P. Devillier, G. Bessard and C. Advenier:*
   GABA and Benzodiazepines
10. *I.M. Richards, J.E. Chin and K.L. Leach:*
    Glucocorticoids

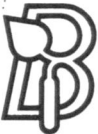

Birkhäuser Verlag • Basel • Boston • Berlin

Pharmacological Sciences:
Perspectives for Research and Therapy in the Late 1990s

Edited by
A.C. Cuello and **B. Collier**
McGill University, Montreal, Quebec, Canada

1995. 544 pages. Hardcover • ISBN 3-7643-5072-5

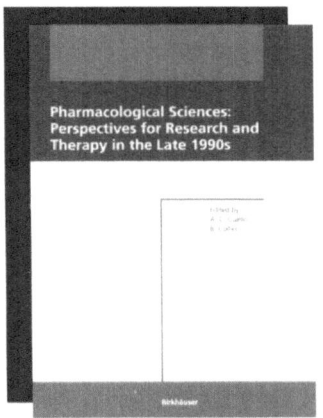

Containing fifty-one outstanding, reviewed chapters, this volume presents a comprehensive picture of the research challenges and novel therapies emerging as we approach the year 2000.

Highly distinguished scientists, all at the very forefront of their fields, were invited to condense into succinct surveys their plenary lectures and symposia from the *XIIth International Congress of Pharmacology*, Montreal, 1994. Highlighting the current developments and future directions in the pharmacological sciences, the chapters span the entire scope from molecular mechanisms to clinical use. They enable the reader to acquire, very rapidly, a panorama of the numerous fields of research. These include drug receptors; signal transduction; ion channels; drug metabolism; neuropharmacology; purines; cardiovascular, endocrine and pulmonary pharmacology; nitric oxide; immunopharmacology; the pharmacology of gene expression; chemotherapy; toxicology; regulatory requirements for drug registration, and pharmacological and instructional methods.

All researchers, teachers, clinicians and graduate students in basic and clinical pharmacology as well as related areas in biochemistry, physiology and pharmacy will find this highly authoritative volume an inspiring and invaluable reference.

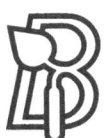

Birkhäuser Verlag • Basel • Boston • Berlin

PHARMACOLOGY • RHEUMATOLOGY • IMMUNOLOGY

This book contains reviewed, edited contibutions which present the latest results from basic inflammation research in the pharmaceutical and biotechnology industries and academia.

Inflammation:
Mechanisms and Therapeutics

Edited by
N.S. Doherty, *Pfizer Central Research, Groton, CT, USA*
B.M. Weichman, *Wyeth-Ayerst Research, Princeton, NJ, USA*
D.W. Morgan, *Abbott Laboratories, Abbott Park, IL, USA*
L.A. Marshall, *SmithKline Beecham Pharmaceuticals, King of Prussia, PA, USA*

1995. 224 pages. Hardcover • ISBN 3-7643-5129-2
Agents and Actions Supplements Volume 47

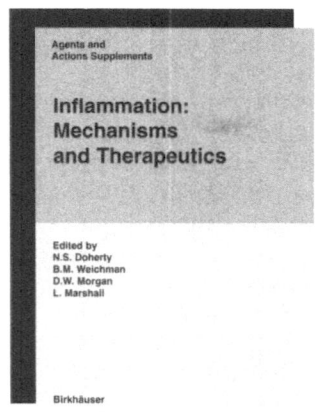

Recent advances in our understanding of the inflammatory process are reviewed in this multi-disciplinary book. It presents the latest results from molecular biology, structural chemistry and fundamental biological and clinical investigations into inflammatory diseases, and discusses their implications for the development of novel therapeutic strategies.

Written by international experts in the field, the chapters include contributions on the role of nitric oxide in inflammation and tissue destruction, cytokine networks in rheumatoid arthritis, antigen specific therapies for the treatment of autoimmune diseases, and gene targeting for inflammatory cell adhesion molecules.

All scientists involved in basic inflammation research in the pharmaceutical and biotechnology industries and academia will find this volume invaluable for their work. The book is primarily intended for pharmacologists, pathologists, immunologists, chemists, and rheumatologists.

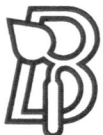

Birkhäuser Verlag • Basel • Boston • Berlin